PHARMACOLOGY for UNDERGRADUATES

Third Edition

PHARMACOLOGY for UNDERGRADUATES

Third Edition

SL Agarwal MD FAMS
Former Professor of Pharmacology
Medical Colleges, Jaipur, Gwalior
Indore, Rewa, Jabalpur and Raipur

Sunil Agarwal MD
Professor of Medicine
University College of Medical Sciences
Delhi

CBSPD

CBS Publishers & Distributors Pvt Ltd
New Delhi • Bengaluru • Chennai • Kochi • Kolkata • Lucknow • Mumbai
Hyderabad • Jharkhand • Nagpur • Patna • Pune • Uttarakhand

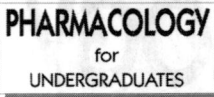

Disclaimer

Science and technology are constantly changing fields. New research and experience broaden the scope of information and knowledge. The authors have tried their best in giving information available to them while preparing the material for this book. Although all efforts have been made to ensure optimum accuracy of the material, yet it is quite possible some errors might have been left uncorrected. The publisher, the printer and the authors will not be held responsible for any inadvertent errors, omissions or inaccuracies.

ISBN: 978-81-239-2390-1

Copyright © Authors and Publisher

Third Edition: 2014
  Reprint: 2016, 2019, **2023, 2024**
First Edition: 2002
Second Edition: 2007
  Reprint: 2007, 2009, 2011

All rights reserved. No part of this book may be reproduced or transmitted in any form or by any means, electronic or mechanical, including photocopying, recording, or any information storage and retrieval system without permission, in writing, from the authors and the publishers.

Published by Satish Kumar Jain and produced by Varun Jain for

CBS Publishers & Distributors Pvt Ltd

4819/XI Prahlad Street, 24 Ansari Road, Daryaganj, New Delhi 110 002, India
Ph: 011-23289259, 011-23266838 Website: www.cbspd.com e-mail: delhi@cbspd.com

Corporate Office: 204 FIE, Industrial Area, Patparganj, Delhi 110 092, India
Ph: 011-4934 4934   Fax: 011-4934 4935   e-mail: publishing@cbspd.com; publicity@cbspd.com

Branches

- **Bengaluru:** Seema House 2975, 17th Cross, K.R. Road, Banasankari 2nd Stage, Bengaluru 560 070, Karnataka, India
  Ph: +91-80-26771678/79   Fax: +91-80-26771680   e-mail: bangalore@cbspd.com
- **Chennai:** 7, Subbaraya Street, Shenoy Nagar, Chennai 600 030, Tamil Nadu, India.
  Ph: +91-44-26680620, 26681266   Fax: +91-44-42032115   e-mail: chennai@cbspd.com
- **Kochi:** 42/1325, 1326, Power House Road, Opposite KSEB, Ernakulam, Kochi-682 018, Kerala, India.
  Ph: +91-484-4059061-67   Fax: +91-484-4059065   e-mail: kochi@cbspd.com
- **Kolkata:** 147, Hind Ceramics Compound, 1st Floor, Nilgunj Road, Belghoria, Kolkata-700 056, West Bengal, India
  Ph: 033-25633055/56   e-mail: kolkata@cbspd.com
- **Lucknow:** Basement, Khushnuma Complex, 7-Meerabai Marg (Behind Jawahar Bhawan), Lucknow-226 001, Uttar Pradesh, India.
  Ph: +0522-4000032   e-mail:tiwari.lucknow@cbspd.com
- **Mumbai:** PWD Shed, Gala No. 25/26, Ramchandra Bhatt Marg, Next to JJ Hospital Gate No. 2, Opp Union Bank of India, Noorbaug, Mumbai-400009, Maharashtra, India
  Ph: +91-22-66661880, 66661889   e-mail: mumbai@cbspd.com

Representatives

• **Hyderabad**	0-9885175004	• **Jharkhand**	0-9811541605	• **Nagpur**	0-8692091830
• **Patna**	0-9334159340	• **Pune**	0-9664372571	• **Uttarakhand**	0-9716462459

Printed at Glorious Printers, Delhi, India

to
my daughter

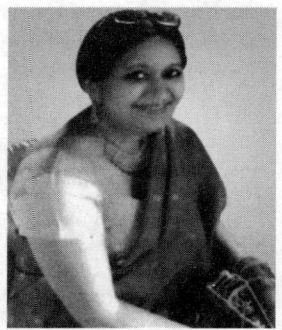

Dr. Madhu Agrawal MS
1951–2011

Recipient of the Pfizer 'Post-Graduate' Medical Award with 'Pfizer Gold Medal in Medicine' in the year 1972

छत्तीसगढ़ आयुष एवं स्वास्थ्य विज्ञान विश्वविद्यालय
रायपुर (छ0ग0)
(छ.ग. अधिनियम क्र. 21/2008 द्वारा स्थापित)
AYUSH AND HEALTH SCIENCES UNIVERSITY OF CHHATTISGARH
RAIPUR (C.G.)

Dr. Arun T. Dabke
M.D., Ph.D.
PADMASHREE
Vice Chancellor

No. Ayush/Gen./
Date: 14.01.2013

Foreword

Pharmacology is one of the most important subjects of medical undergraduate studies. It has shown tremendous changes in the last 50 years. This was mainly because of advances in understanding metabolism of drugs and its interaction with human body as a whole. For keeping oneself updated in medical practice, it is very essential that apart from having knowledge of newer drugs, one also has knowledge of drugs which have lost their importance due to adverse effects or invention of newer better drugs.

Prof SL Agrawal is one of the senior most teachers of pharmacology in India, and has one of the longest undergraduate and postgraduate teaching experience. He was associated with Medical Council of India and was also with National Board of Examination. He was responsible primarily for changing pharmacology subject from animal experiments, chemical structures to practical uses of drugs. Dr Agrawal's one of the greatest qualities is interest of students, for which he had several times fought with the highest authorities in favour of students.

This book reflects the above philosophy of Prof Agrawal. It is very useful for the undergraduate medical students and will help them in understanding pharmacology. This book will also find a place on the table of every practising doctors for quick reference of drugs.

Dr Arun T Dabke

Preface to the Third Edition

The success of *Pharmacology for Undergraduates* continues to exceed my most optimistic expectations. More than six reprints of its previous editions indicate the acceptability of its contents and presentation to the students. In reality, it serves a far greater role, namely, it allows the students to learn in a concise but comprehensive fashion to follow their clinical phase of training more usefully.

The third edition, as the previous two, updates the dynamic discipline of pharmacology. This new edition of book has been extensively revised to reflect the up-to-date treatment of diseases, such as tropical diseases, AIDS, cancer, as well as the latest developments in the treatment of common diseases encountered with changes in lifestyle. Again my hope is that *Pharmacology for Undergraduates* will serve the interests of students judiciously.

SL Agarwal

Preface to the First Edition

Medical Council of India, of recent, have restructured undergraduate curriculum with a reduction in time allotted to basic sciences.

The available textbooks on pharmacology deal with all aspects of pharmacology, which contain many facts and details that a student neither needs nor attempt to learn. The knowledge of the history, source, physical and chemical properties, compounding and biochemical effects of drugs essentially fall in the domain of the industry and serve no useful purpose in learning how and why drugs act.

Thus, students should read selectively and this book is an attempt in that direction. The book deals with the basic concepts of how drugs get into the body, how they produce their effects of their fate, the hazards, their adverse effects, and how evidence of their therapeutic effects is assessed.

Students, practically speaking, are not required to memorise lists of alternative drugs and minor differences between them or arbitrary practical details such as dosage or solution strength, since drugs are now available in adult or pediatric dosage forms and moreover such details should never be required of them in examination. However, more important is the frequency of drug administration to achieve a steady blood level.

It is expected that the students will find this book provides them pharmacological knowledge that is interesting, useful, and manageable in the time period allotted in their curriculum, and to develop a rational, critical attitude to drug therapy during their clinical phase of training.

SL Agarwal
Sunil Agarwal

Contents

Foreword by Dr Arun T Dabke VII
Preface to the Third Edition IX
Preface to the First Edition X

1. Basic Concepts *1–21*

   1.1   Pharmacokinetics 1
   1.2   Pharmacodynamics 6
   1.3   Routes of administration 9
   1.4   Factors modifying drug action 11
   1.5   Drug sources 13
   1.6   Adverse reactions to drugs 14
   1.7   Adverse drug interactions 18

2. Autonomic Nervous System *22–62*

   2.1   The sympathetic nervous system 22
   2.2   Sympathomimetic drugs 26
   2.3   Sympatholytic drugs 37
   2.4   Alpha adrenergic bloking drugs 37
   2.5   Adrenergic neuron blocking drugs 40
   2.6   Ganglionic blocking drugs 40
   2.7   Centrally acting sympatholytics 41
   2.8   Beta adrenergic blocking drugs 41
   2.9   Parasympathetic nervous system 48
   2.10 Parasympathomimetic drugs 49
   2.11 Parasympatholytic drugs 58

3. Central Nervous System *63–179*

   3.1   Anxiolytics and hypnotics 63
   3.2   Analgesics 71

3.3	Nonsteroidal anti-inflammatory drugs	80
3.4	Drugs used for rheumatoid arthritis	93
3.5	Anti gout drugs	101
3.6	Antimigraine drugs	106
3.7	Antiepileptic drugs	109
3.8	Antiparkinsonian drugs	119
3.9	Drugs and mental illness	127
3.10	Emetics and anti-emetics	149
3.11	Local anesthetics	153
3.12	General anesthetics and muscle relaxants	158
3.13	Central nervous system stimulants	173
3.14	Drug dependence (drug addiction)	174

4. Autacoids and Antagonists 180–190

5. Cardiovascular System 191–276

5.1	Cardiac glycosides	191
5.2	Angiotensin converting enzyme (ACE) inhibitors	195
5.3	Diuretics	200
5.4	Drugs used in chronic heart failure	210
5.5	Calcium channel blockers	215
5.6	Drugs used in essential hypertension	221
5.7	Nitrates	232
5.8	Anticoagulants	236
5.9	Antiplatelet drugs	242
5.10	Lipid lowering drugs	246
5.11	Drugs used in angina pectoris	252
5.12	Fibrinolytic (thrombolytics) drugs	257
5.13	Drugs used for acute coronary syndrome	259
5.14	Drugs for cardiac arrhythmia	262
5.15	Hematinics	269

6. Gastrointestinal System 277–300

6.1	Drugs for oropharynx infections	277
6.2	Drugs for dyspepsia and gastroesophageal reflex disease (GERD)	279
6.3	Drugs for peptic ulcer disease	281

6.4	Drugs for inflammatory bowel disease (IBD)	288
6.5	Drugs for irritable bowel syndrome	293
6.6	Purgatives	296
6.7	intestinal sedatives	300

7. Respiratory System   301–313

7.1	Cough preparations	301
7.2	Drugs for bronchial asthma	302

8. Endocrine System   314–360

8.1	Insulin and oral antidiabetic drugs	314
8.2	Thyroid and antithyroid drugs	334
8.3	Corticosteroids	338
8.4	Female sex hormones	349
8.5	Male sex hormones, anti-androgens, anabolic steroids and drugs for impotence	358

9. Prostaglandins and Drugs Acting on Uterus   361–364

10. Parathyroid Hormone and Calcium Metabolism   365–376

11. Antibacterial Drugs   377–427

11.1	Chemoterapeutic antibacterial drugs	380
11.2	Antibiotics	388
11.3	Antituberculous drugs	413
11.4	Antileprotic drugs	423

12. Antifungal Drugs   428–335

13. Antiviral Drugs   436–352

13.1	Antihepatitis agents	450

14. Vaccines, Antisera, Immunoglobulins and Immunotherapy   453–465

15. Drugs used in Malaria — 466–477

16. Antiamebic and other Antiprotozoal Drugs — 478–483
   16.1 Leishmaniasis — 482

17. Antihelmintic Drugs — 484–491

18. Anticancer Drugs — 492–524

19. Vitamins — 525–531

20. Poisons and Management — 532–536

21. Drugs for Skin and Eye — 537–561
   21.1 Skin — 537
   21.2 Eye — 554

Index — 562

1

Basic Concepts

Pharmacology is the study of drugs. The two main areas of pharmacology are pharmacokinetics and pharmacodynamics.

1.1 PHARMACOKINETICS

Pharmacokinetics is the study of drug absorption, distribution, metabolism and excretion.

ABSORPTION

The absorption of a drug molecule depends on its physicochemical properties. To gain access to the site of action, drug molecule must cross one or more barriers—the gastrointestinal mucosa, and the membranes that separate the various aqueous compartments of the body (i.e. plasma, interstitial fluid, intracellular fluid, and transcellular fluid).

In general, there are four main ways by which small drug molecules cross cell membranes:

A. *Diffusion through lipid*

Many drugs are highly soluble in lipids and therefore penetrate cell membranes freely, by diffusion. Lipid solubility is one of the most important pharmacokinetic characteristic of a drug, which determines its site of action.

B. *Diffusion through aqueous channels*

In most parts of the body there are gaps between the endothelial cells of the capillaries, which are large enough to permit small drug molecules to cross by aqueous diffusion, but too small to allow protein molecules to pass through. In central nervous system vascular beds, the capillary endothelium is continuous. In fact, there are tight junctions between adjacent capillary endothelial cells which, together with their basement membrane and a thin covering from the processes of astrocytes separate the blood from the brain tissue.

This **blood–brain barrier** restricts the passage of lipid insoluble substances from the blood to the brain and cerebrospinal fluid. Lipid insoluble (polar) drugs such as penicillin, methotrexate gain little access to the brain.

C. Carrier mediated transport

Many cell membranes possess highly specific transport mechanism, i.e. a protein molecule incorporated in the cell membrane—which binds the drug molecule and ships it to other side of the membrane in the manner of a ferry. The carrier mediated drug transport plays an important role in the transfer of drugs at the renal tubule, biliary tract, and gastrointestinal tract and blood—brain barrier sites.

D. Pinocytosis

It involves the transport of a drug molecule across the cell by formation of vesicles. This is applicable to protein and other macromolecules and rarely to drugs.

FIRST PASS EFFECT (PRE-SYSTEMIC ELIMINATION)

Drugs absorbed from the gastrointestinal tract are carried by portal vein to the liver before reaching the systemic circulation. Many drugs are metabolized as they pass through the liver with the result only a portion (about 30%) of the drug absorbed reaches the circulation. Thus, the **bioavailability** of orally administered drugs is much less as compared to other routes of drug administration. This removal of drug as it passes through liver is called the first pass effect or pre-systemic elimination.

DISTRIBUTION

After absorption a drug passes into the circulation. Many drugs are poorly soluble in plasma and are bound to plasma proteins. It is important to know that the free (unbound) fraction of the drug is pharmacologically active and it is the free fraction of the drug that passes from the circulation into body water (e.g. cerebrospinal fluid, transplacentally to the fetus and into breast milk). The protein bound fraction of the drug acts as a store from where the free drug is released to maintain steady levels of pharmacologically active drug.

The distribution of the drug is an important factor in determining its therapeutic usefulness. The drugs, initially enter the circulation and highly vascular organs, from where, depending on lipid solubility, diffuse out of the circulation into the tissue spaces and some enter the cells and are bound within the tissues.

Thus, the body can be considered a two compartmental system– a central vascular compartment and a larger peripheral extravascular compartment incorporating interstitial fluid, lymph, intracellular fluid, transcellular fluid and fat compartments. The drugs pass in between these compartments, but the entry and elimination is only through the central compartment. The average volume of the distribution space for an adult is–plasma 3 liters, extracellular space 15 liters and total body water 36 liters. When the volume of distribution exceeds the total volume of body water (e.g. with digoxin), there is substantial uptake and binding of the drug within tissues such as heart muscle.

EQUILIBRIUM

After distribution has proceeded to the point where the concentration of drug in plasma is in dynamic equilibrium with that in body tissues, the drug levels in plasma and tissue fall in parallel as the drug is eliminated from the body. This is equilibrium phase or elimination phase. Measurement of drug concentration in plasma provides the best reflection of drug levels in tissues during this phase.

HALF-LIFE

The elimination half-life of a drug is the time taken for the circulating concentration of the drug to fall by half. For most of the drugs, the rate of decline in the plasma concentration is constant and directly proportional to the amount present **(first order kinetics)**. The half-life of a drug is useful in predicting its duration of action and frequency of dosing, for example, twice a day with elimination half-life of about 12 hours.

STEADY STATE PLASMA CONCENTRATION

With repeated dosing, the drug concentration in plasma climbs until a more or less steady level is obtained. During, the steady state, the drug elimination equals the dose administered and the plasma concentration is maintained constant at the optimal therapeutic levels.

In general, it takes around five half lives to reach steady levels for the drugs which follow the first order kinetic clearance.

CLEARANCE

Clearance denotes the volume of blood from which the drug is completely removed per unit time. The systemic clearance takes place through biodegradation of drugs by the action of liver enzymes and/or renal excretion. Majority of drugs follow first order kinetic laws of clearance—the rate of clearance being constant and directly proportional to plasma concentrations.

A few drugs (notably alcohol, phenytoin, salicylates and theophylline) are inactivated by metabolic degradation and do not obey simple first order kinetic laws of clearance. For them the rate of elimination is independent of the plasma concentrations and this mode of clearance is described as **Zero order** or **Saturation kinetics**, in which a constant amount is cleared per unit time, irrespective of plasma concentrations.

METABOLISM (BIOTRANSFORMATION)

The liver is the main site of metabolism for most lipid soluble drugs, where they are broken down or combined with some other chemical so that they are no longer pharmacologically active and become water soluble.

Drug metabolism is often a two phase process. The initial metabolic phase consists of oxidation by a family of enzymes – microsomal or non-microsomal. Microsomal enzymes are mainly found in endoplasmic reticulum of hepatocytes and their primary components are cytochrome P-450 reductase and cytochrome P-450. This enzyme system has been termed a mixed-function oxygenase. Non-microsomal oxidation takes place by soluble enzymes (such as alcohol dehydrogenase, xanthine oxidase, tyrosine hydroxylase and monoamine oxidase) found in the cytosol or mitochondria of cells.

Many drugs also undergo a second step (Phase 2) by conjugation in which an endogenous substance such as glucuronic acid or sulphate is attached to the drug or its metabolite.

PRODRUGS

These are drugs which have been modified so that they are well absorbed or distributed but are pharmacologically inactive. In the body prodrugs are activated by oxidative processes into pharmacologically active form, for example, cortisone to active form hydrocortisone and levodopa to dopamine.

METABOLITES

Although most metabolites (products of drug metabolism) are inactive, some Phase 1 metabolites of drugs such as paracetamol, halothane, sulphonamides are hepatotoxic. Paracetamol in therapeutic doses, does not cause hepatotoxicity, but is fatal in over dosage. It is oxidized by the P-450 system to a reactive quinone (Phase 1), which is removed by conjugation with glutathione (Phase 2). If the dose of paracetamol is large or glutathione is deficient, the quinone binds irreversibly to the proteins of the hepatocytes causing liver damage.

Prodrug metabolites are pharmacologically active.

EXCRETION

The kidney is the most important organ for excretion. Lipid soluble substances are filtered by the glomerulus, but diffuse back into circulation further down the nephron. The extent of back diffusion is less for drugs that are highly ionized or dissociated. Ionization diminishes the lipid solubility and hence tubular reabsorption. This situation can be exploited in the management of poisoning due to certain drugs by altering urinary pH, for example, alkalinization will increase renal excretion of aspirin and barbiturates and acidification that of amphetamine.

Peritubular capillaries of the proximal renal tubule have two non-selective carrier systems—one for acidic drugs (e.g. penicillin, cephalosporins, salicylates, probenecid, and thiazides) and the other for basic drugs (e.g. amiloride, cimetidine, and procainamide) which transport drug molecules into tubular urine. These carrier systems can transport drug molecules even when bound to plasma proteins as well as against electrochemical gradients.

Rarely, drugs are excreted through lungs and this route is important in the case of volatile anesthetics.

1.2 PHARMACODYNAMICS

Pharmacodynamics is the study of pharmacological properties of a drug and its mechanism of action. Drug effects are the results of physiochemical reactions between the drug and functionally important molecules in the body. They interact with the body's natural physiological control systems that include receptors, enzymes, carrier molecules and specialized macromolecules such as DNA. Some of the known mechanisms of drug actions are as follows:

DRUG RECEPTOR

The term 'receptor' is used to mean any clearly defined cellular protein to which a drug binds to initiate its effects. The drug is thought to fit onto a receptor rather as a key fits a lock. It may then either stimulate the receptor or produce effect similar to that of the naturally occurring (endogenous) substances and is called an **agonist** or it may occupy the receptor without producing any effect and block the effect of an endogenous agonist and is called an **antagonist**.

A few drugs have been shown to be **partial agonists** (antagonist at low concentrations and agonists at high), for example, **buprenorphine** and **pidolol**.

Receptors may be viewed to consist of two portions – one which binds the drug (drug binding domain) and the other which propagates (transducers) its regulatory signals (effecter domain) to bring about the drug response. There are four well known transducer mechanisms by which receptors produce a pharmacologic response:

1. Direct regulated ion channels

The receptors enclose ion channels within their molecules. These are confined to excitable tissue (e.g. central nervous system, neuromuscular junctions, and autonomic ganglia).

Most excitatory neurotransmitters cause an increase in sodium and potassium permeability. This results in a net inward current carried mainly by sodium ion which depolarizes the cell and generates an action potential.

2. G protein coupled receptors

The effecter domain of the receptor consists of a group of guanine nucleotide—binding regulatory proteins (G proteins) which occur within cells and act as intermediaries between receptors and enzyme in the synthesis of a second messenger cyclic-adenosine $-3'$, $5'$-monophosphate (cAMP) which regulates many different kinds of cellular activity. G proteins also regulate intracellular calcium concentrations. Some hormone peptide receptors, neurotransmitter receptors and autocoid receptors depend on G proteins to mediate their actions on cells.

3. Intracellular receptors

These are soluble DNA binding proteins that regulate the transcription of specific genes. They are activated by steroid hormones, thyroid hormone, vitamin D and retinoid.

4. Catalytic receptors

These are enzymatic proteins. The extracellular agonist-binding domain is connected to an intracellular catalytic domain through a single stretch of transmembrane stretch of peptide chain. Catalytic receptors regulate cell growth, their differentiation and development and include the receptors for insulin, epidermal growth factor; platelet-derived growth factor and certain lymphocytes.

Receptors exist in a dynamic state. Their number and functional state vary with drug treatment. Continued exposure to an agonist leads to internalization of receptors, thus limiting or reducing efficacy ("down regulation") and development of **tolerance**.

Tolerance, thus is a state of decreased responsiveness seen with the long term use of an agonist and may be a consequence of the down regulation of receptors, a homeostatic adaptive response, or the stimulation of the drug's metabolism.

Tolerance to a selective β_2 adrenoreceptor agonist in asthma is due to down regulation and that of nitrates in angina is due to deficiency of reduced sulphydril groups that nitrates induce in vascular smooth muscle.

Long term treatment with an antagonist will lead to an increase in receptor binding sites ("up regulation"). This phenomenon may explain the syndrome associated with rapid withdrawal of some drugs, for example, rebound angina after withdrawing propranolol.

ENZYME INHIBITION

Interaction between drug and enzyme is in many respects similar to that between drug and receptor. Many important drugs owe their action due to inhibition of the enzyme activity, because they structurally resemble a natural substrate and hence compete with it for the enzyme. Examples of enzyme inhibition include angiotensin converting enzyme inhibitors, carbonic anhydrase inhibitor.

ANTIMETABOLITES

These drugs structurally resemble substances which are used by cells for nutrition and, when absorbed, the cells cannot use them and so fail to multiply. **Methotrexate**, similar in structure to folic acid competes with folic acid for a vital step in the build-up of nuclear material within the cell and blocks the process so that cancer cell dies.

ACTION ON CELL MEMBRANES

General and local anesthetics appear to act on the lipid, protein or water constituents of nerve cell membranes and interfere with the movements of ions and thus, prevent nerve or muscle function.

REPLACEMENT OF DEFICIENCIES

Hormone or vitamin therapy controls the disease in deficiency states.

CYTOTOXIC EFFECT

The drugs kill bacteria or malignant cells without undue change to the patient's cells. The mechanism of action varies between drugs.

CHEMICAL INTERACTION

Drugs, extra-cellularly, react according to simple chemical equation, for example, antacids, acidifying and alkalinizing agents, oxidizing agents and chelating agents.

THE PLACEBO RESPONSE

A placebo or inert treatment may be defined as use of a substance which has no pharmacological action but which, when used, produces a therapeutic effect. In a wide variety of symptoms (e.g. pain, cough, headache) and in some organic disorders (e.g. peptic ulcer, angina), the administration of a placebo will produce satisfactory response in about 30% of patients. The benefit appears to be connected with the powers of suggestion.

1.3 ROUTES OF ADMINISTRATION

Drugs are given in many ways to achieve a systemic response.

ORALLY

The easiest and commonest way to give drugs is by mouth. The absorption of a drug may be delayed by factors which delay emptying of the stomach, for example, food, concomitant disease (migraine), or drug administration (morphine, atropine).

SUBLINGUALLY

Drugs (e.g. glyceryl trinitrate) given sublingually have a rapid onset of action and escape pre-systemic metabolic degradation as they pass straight into the systemic circulation without entering the portal system.

RECTALLY

Certain drugs are absorbed from the rectum and may be given as suppositories or enema.

By injection

Injections may be given intravenously, intramuscularly, subcutaneously, intradermally or into various body cavities such as the pleura or peritoneum or into the spinal theca.

The intravenous route has the advantage of immediate action, 100% bioavailability and can be used for drugs too irritant to be given intramuscularly. However, there is a risk of adverse effects and it is not suitable for oily solutions or insoluble substances

Intramuscular injection is easier and most widely used. It is suitable for moderate volumes, oily vehicles and some irritating substances. Rarely, it may result in abscess formation.

Subcutaneous injection is also widely used. Absorption is slower than intramuscular injection.

Intradermal injection is mainly employed for testing sensitivity to allergens and for immunization.

Intrathecal injection is used for the drugs, which do not penetrate blood–brain barrier.

By inhalation

Volatile and general anesthetics are given by inhalation.

Antiasthmatics, β_2 adrenoreceptor agonists, corticosteroids, and cromoglicate are given as aerosol for local action on bronchi, with minimum systemic effects.

TRANSDERMAL APPLICATION

A number of drugs (e.g. glyceryl trinitrate, hyoscine, estrogens, fentanyl) can be applied to the skin as a plastic patch holding a container, which releases the drug at a constant rate. One patch may be effective for a relatively long period so replacement can be made infrequently. However, absorption may be variable and skin reaction may occasionally occur.

By local application

Drugs are applied locally as solutions, liniments, ointments or creams to the skin, mucous membranes and wound surfaces and produce their action at the site of application.

1.4 FACTORS MODIFYING DRUG ACTION

There are a number of variables that can modify drug response. The main reasons for this variability are pharmacokinetic, pharmacodynamic and a large number of other factors.

PHARMACOKINETIC FACTORS

Children, particularly neonates differ from adults in their response to drugs. Special care is needed in the neonatal period and doses should always be calculated with care. At this age, the risk of toxicity is increased by inefficient renal filtration, relative enzyme deficiencies, differing target organ sensitivity and inadequate detoxifying system.

Old people have a reduction in renal clearances. They excrete drugs slowly, and are highly susceptible to nephrotoxic drugs. Metabolism of drugs by the liver may be reduced in the elderly. The net result of pharmacokinetic changes in the elderly is that the tissue concentration of a drug is commonly increased by over 50%.

PHARMACODYNAMIC FACTORS

Tolerance leads to decrease in drug response of agonists.

Long term treatment with an antagonist leads to an increase in receptor binding sites (upward regulation) which explains rebound angina after withdrawal of propanolol.

The hemostatic and biochemical milieu may also influence the drug response, for example, a depletion of sodium predisposes a patient to lithium toxicity and hypokalaemia to digitalis toxicity.

GENETIC FACTORS

There are a number of inherited variations in the activity of enzymes responsible for the metabolism of drugs (**genetic polymorphism**). Several primary routes of metabolism, such as acetylation and hydroxylation are subject to strong genetic control. This may explain individual susceptibility to enhanced toxicity or poor efficacy with particular drugs.

A poor capacity for hydroxylation helps to explain why some patients develop profound hypotension with debrisoquine and considerable beta blockade with metoprolol.

Throughout the world, there is a much larger variation in acetylation among ethnic group. Fast acetylators are less likely to be cured of tuberculosis by isoniazid. Slow acetylators more often develop peripheral neuropathy when treated with isoniazid and systemic lupus erythematosus when treated with procainamide and hydralazine.

Another example of genetic polymorphism is deficiency in the enzyme glucose-6-phosphate dehydrogenase (G6PD). Quinine, sulphonamides, chloroquine, and chloromycetin cause hemolysis of red cell in G6PD deficient cells. There are many other examples of inherited differences in response to drugs.

PREGNANCY

It affects pharmacokinetics of drugs by decreased gastrointestinal activity, increased blood volume, low plasma albumin, increase in body fat and increase in renal blood flow.

LIFE STYLE

Hepatic microsomal enzymes may be induced by many dietary factors (high protein low carbohydrate diet), alcohol, hydrocarbons in cigarette smoke, and many insecticides (e.g. DDT), which is an important cause of diminished response to a drug.

INTERCURRENT ILLNESS

This may both modify drug elimination and receptor sensitivity and is an important cause of altered response to a drug.

The diseases of liver, kidney and heart are commonly associated with the modification of drug response.

Loss of liver cells (cirrhosis) may result in a dangerous depression of respiratory center with therapeutic doses of morphine due to decreased enzymatic inactivation of the drug.

In renal diseases, therapeutic doses of aminoglycoside antibiotics may result in serious accumulation of the drug leading to ototoxicity.

In addition, there are a number of other situations when the drug response is altered by pathological state of many organs. Drug response of digoxin and morphine is increased in hypothyroids; adrenaline and digoxin in myocardial infarction and morphine in head injury.

INFECTION

Infections, burns and malnutrition are some conditions, which lead to hypoalbuminemia. The concentration of free drug in plasma, especially those that are highly protein bound (e.g. phenytoin, clofibrate) increases the risk of enhanced responses.

DRUG INTERACTION

One drug can modify the response to another drug in a number of ways. This is discussed on page 18.

1.5 DRUG SOURCES

Most drugs are made chemically in the laboratory. Some are extracted from natural sources such as plants or fungi.

Certain naturally occurring substances (such as hormones) are proteins. They are difficult to synthesize chemically and extraction from animals may be unsatisfactory. This problem is now being solved by **genetic pharmacy**. The gene responsible for the production of a complex protein is isolated from human cells and inserted into other vector (carrier) cells (*E. coli* or yeast) which divide rapidly and are manipulated to produce the required protein in large quantities. This method is employed for the production of human insulin and erythropoietin.

1.6 ADVERSE REACTIONS TO DRUGS

In recent years, adverse reactions to drugs have become increasingly common. This is probably due to the enormous increase in the range and number of drugs, now in use.

Though, no drug is completely without side effects, certain group of widely used drugs account for a disproportionate number of reactions–aspirin, digoxin, anticoagulants, diuretics, antibiotics, steroids, antineoplastics, and hypoglycemic drugs account for 90% of reactions.

Adverse reactions can be divided into two categories; an augmented but qualitatively normal response to a drug (Type A) or a bizarre, unexpected response (Type B).

Type A

These reactions occur in patients who are unusually susceptible to the pharmacological effects of the drug. Examples of type A reactions include postural hypotension with antihypertensive drugs, gynecomastia with dopamine antagonists and diarrhea with broad-spectrum antibiotics. These reactions are fairly common and can be predicated from the knowledge of their pharmacological action. They are not usually serious and seldom cause death.

Type B

These reactions are not related to the drug's known pharmacological effects and are usually severe and proportionately more often fatal. Some mechanisms of extra-pharmacologic toxicity include direct cytotoxicity, genetic enzymatic defects, and abnormal immune responses.

CYTOTOXIC REACTIONS

These are caused by the production of reactive metabolites during drug metabolism, which may covalently bind to hepatic protein causing hepatic necrosis. Examples of cytotoxic reactions are isoniazid hepatotoxicity and paracetamol hepatotoxicity. The risk of hepatic necrosis is increased in patients receiving drugs as phenobarbitone or rifampicin, which increase the activity of microsomal enzymes.

GENETIC FACTORS (see Page 12)
Immunological mechanism (allergic reactions)

This type of reaction implies that the patient has been exposed to the drug on some previous occasion. This exposure has resulted in the production of an antibody against the drug. If the drug is given on a second occasion, the drug and the antibody combine in such a way as to cause damage to tissue and produce symptoms of an allergic reaction. Skin, respiratory, gastrointestinal and cardiovascular systems are the main target of allergic reactions. Four types of allergic reactions are:

1. *Immediate type (acute anaphylaxis)*

The antibody (produced in response to a drug) may become attached to the surface of mast cells or leucocytes. On subsequent administration, the drug combines with antibody, destroys the mast cells, liberating local hormones (autacoids) such as histamine, leukotrienes, prostaglandins and platelet activating factor, which cause urticaria, acute anaphylactic reaction and asthma. Treatment includes adrenalin, hydrocortisone, antihistamines, and cardiopulmonary resuscitation

2. *Autoallergy*

The antibody may become attached to the surface of red cells. On second exposure to the drug, the combination occurs leading to destruction of red cells, which cause blood disorders such as hemolytic anaemia, thrombocytopenia, agranulocytosis and aplastic anaemia.

Agranulocytosis is a very rare condition which requires withdrawal of the drug and administration of a bacteriocidal drug (penicillin) to prevent infection.

Chloromycetin is the most important drug that may cause aplastic anaemia.

3. Antigen/antibody/complement combination

Antigens (drugs) and antibodies may combine in the bloodstream to form immune complexes. They may penetrate various organs where they are deposited, together with a further substance called complement, which is present in the blood. The antigen/ antibody/ complement combination stimulates inflammation which may affect the skin, kidneys and other organs and result in serum sickness, glomerulonephrities, vasculities and pulmonary diseases.

4. Delayed type (cell mediated)

Drugs acting as antigens may sensitize lymphocytes which on further contact with the drug leads to a local or tissue allergic reaction, e.g. contact dermatitis.

ALTERATION OF IMMUNOLOGIC STATUS

Alteration in patient's immunologic status may result in adverse reactions to drugs.

Bone marrow transplant patients may experience cutaneous drug reactions.

HIV infected patients run high risk of developing cutaneous reactions to drugs (e.g. co-trimoxazole, dapsone, amoxycillin, clavulanate). They also have a higher risk of the most serious type of allergic reactions (e.g. toxic epidermal necrolysis, Stevens-Johnson syndrome).

IDIOSYNCRATIC REACTIONS

These resemble allergic reactions but have no immunological basis. They are largely genetically determined and are due to release of local hormones (histamine or leukotrienes) by the drug. These pseudo-allergic reactions mimic type 1, 2, and 3 allergic reactions.

MISCELLANEOUS ADVERSE REACTIONS

Apart from vital organs, toxic reactions on eye can occur on long term use of certain drugs like chloroquin, corticosteroids and phenothiazines.

Toxic reactions may be due to the disease during drug treatment. Blackwater fever, a severe and often fatal condition in malaria patients treated with quinine is due to malaria and not quinine.

IATROGENIC DISEASES

These are the diseases caused by drugs. Peptic ulcer after long term use of non-steroidal anti-inflammatory drugs or steroids and Parkinsonism by phenothiazines is common examples.

TERATOGENICITY

Drugs during pregnancy may cross the placental barrier and cause fetal abnormalities. Drugs can produce fetal damage during the first 3 months of pregnancy when cells change into recognizable human beings. Drugs which are known to produce fetal abnormalities are thalidomide, folic acid antagonists, tetracyclines, androgens, danazol, warfarin, diethylstilbestrol, etretinate, lithium and some anticonvulsents.

PREVENTION OF ADVERSE REACTIONS

Though it may not be possible to prevent adverse reactions, certain guidelines may minimize their incidence:
- Drugs to be used only when indicated.
- Patient's history for any allergic or idiosyncratic reactions.
- Cautious use in extremes of life and pregnancy.
- Inform the patient about likely serious allergic reactions.
- Restrict therapy to few familiar drugs.

- Strict vigilance for adverse reactions or any unexpected event with recently introduced drugs.

1.7 ADVERSE DRUG INTERACTIONS

Adverse drug interactions have assumed a great importance with the development of potent drugs, the treatment with multiple drugs, and the increasing usage of drugs in aging population that has various degenerative diseases.

The number of drug interactions described is very large and many of them are of little or no clinical importance. In general those interactions, which are important, occur when the dose of a drug is critical and a small change in blood concentration or the patient's sensitivity to drug results in toxicity or conversely, a lack of therapeutic effect.

Dangerous interactions are particularly liable to occur in patients who take several drugs at the same time as in the case of acute illness or in old age and with drugs which have a narrow margin of safety or are cumulative or have a saturable hepatic metabolism.

The risk of interaction is greatest with drugs like warfarin, chlorpromazine, morphine, verapamil, levodopa, lithium, phenytoin, theophylline, beta-blockers, digoxin, rifampicin and erythromycin.

There are two principal types of interactions between drugs – **pharmacokinetic interactions** resulting from alterations in the delivery of drugs to their sites of actions and **pharmacodynamic interactions** which modify the responsiveness of the target organ or system.

PHARMACOKINETIC INTERACTIONS CAUSING DIMINISHED DRUG DELIVERY

Impaired absorption

Most drugs are absorbed by diffusion through the gut wall. If a well absorbed drug gets attached to poorly or non-absorbed drug, the well absorbed drug will be held in the intestine and its absorption will be decreased. For example, antacids form insoluble complexes with tetracyclines, iron, and prednisolone and anion exchange resins with digoxin, thyroxine, and warfarin and interfere with their absorption.

Enzyme induction

Many drugs increase the synthesis of microsomal enzyme protein that metabolizes drugs. As a result, rate of metabolism of inducing drug and/or other drugs is increased, with a reduction in the circulating concentration of the drug and a reduced effect.

Barbiturates, griseofulvin, most antiepileptics, rifampicin and erythromycin are the most important enzyme inducers in man.

Drugs whose metabolism is significantly affected by enzyme induction are oral contraceptives, warfarin, corticosteroids and cyclosporin.

PHARMACOKINETIC INTERACTION CAUSING INCREASED DRUG DELIVERY

Enzyme inhibition

Most inhibitory interactions also affect hepatic enzymes. Many drugs have the potential for interfering with the metabolism of other drugs, usually by competing for binding sites on the appropriate enzymes. Inhibition of the metabolism of the affected drug results in higher plasma concentration with risk of toxicity.

The most dangerous inhibitors are the antibacterial such as erythromycin and co-trimoxazole, cimetidine, and dextropropoxyphene.

Commonly affected drugs are warfarin, antiepileptics, theophylline and the suphonylureas.

First pass metabolism

Some drugs may suppress the metabolic enzyme activity in the gut wall and liver and increase the oral bioavailability of the affected drug.

The antibiotic chloromycetin is an enzyme suppressor.

The best example of interference with first pass metabolism is "cheese reaction" due to inhibition of tyramine breakdown in the gut wall by non-selective monoamine oxidase inhibitors (MAOIs) such as phenelzine and tranylcypromine that has resulted in severe hypertension.

Displacement of protein binding

Drug displacement from its binding site on plasma protein is normally offset by a compensatory increase in metabolism or excretion, without affecting the free concentration of the drug at the target sites. However, if the displacement is accompanied by metabolic inhibition, toxic reactions would be apparent. This double mechanism explains why phenylbutazone potentiates the effect of warfarin and why the addition of sodium valproate can produce phenytoin toxicity.

Affecting renal excretion

Drugs are eliminated through the kidney both by glomerular filtration and by active tubular secretion. Competition occurs between those which share the same active transport mechanism in the proximal tubule. Thus, probenicid delays the excretion of many drugs including penicillin, some cephalosporins, indomethacin and dapsone. Similarly, thiazide diuretics delay the renal excretion of lithium, which may result in serious lithium toxicity.

Pharmacodynamic Interactions

These are interactions between drugs which have similar or antagonistic pharmacological effects or side effects. They may be due to competition at receptor sites or occur between drugs acting on the same physiological system.

SYNERGISM

Synergism occurs if two drugs with the same effect, when given together produce an effect that is greater in magnitude than the sum of the effects when the drugs are given individually. For example, the effect of a drug depressing the central nervous system (e.g. benzodiazepine) will be enhanced by another depressant (e.g. alcohol).

Synergism of drugs with similar actions may be beneficial also, as with antibacterial components of co-trimoxazole or with combined levodopa and selegiline treatment in Parkinson's disease.

ANTAGONISM

When one drug decreases or inhibits the action of another drug antagonism occurs. A classic example of antagonism is the suppression of the bactericidal activity of penicillin (which acts on dividing bacteria) by tetracycline which reduces bacterial division.

2

Autonomic Nervous System

The autonomic nervous system supplies the viscera. The viscera includes the gastrointestinal tract, the respiratory and urogenital systems, the heart and blood vessels, the intrinsic muscles of the eye and the endocrine and exocrine glands.

The autonomic system consists of two divisions – the sympathetic and the parasympathetic system. The two divisions control homeostatic functions that are primarily involuntary.

The autonomic neurons located in the ganglia outside the central nervous system, give rise to the post-ganglionic autonomic nerves that innervate the viscera. The activity of autonomic nerves is regulated by central neurons. Responses to the sympathetic and the parasympathetic stimulation are frequently antagonistic as exemplified by the opposing effects on the heart rate and gut motility.

NEUROHORMONAL TRANSMISSION

The transmission of the nerve impulse across junctions such as synapses occurs through the release of humoral (chemical) messenger from the prejunctional nerve endings, which bridges the gap at the synapses, and thus activates a receptor in the organ supplied or in another nerve cell. The chemical transmitters involved differ in sympathetic and parasympathetic divisions.

2.1 THE SYMPATHETIC NERVOUS SYSTEM

The sympathetic nervous system consists of a chain of ganglia lying on either side of vertebral column. Preganglionic sympathetic nerve fibers leave the spinal cord between the first thoracic and the second lumbar segments. Sympathetic activity is initiated from the reticular formation of the medulla oblongata and pons and from centers in hypothalamus. The brainstem sympathetic centers, which have an intrinsic activity of their own, are regulated by many stimuli, including impulses from cortex, limbic lobes and hypothalamus, neural afferents that interact at the level of the brainstem centers and at higher centers, and changes in the physical and chemical properties of the extra-cellular fluid, including the circulating levels of hormones and substrates.

NEUROTRANSMITTERS

Nor-adrenalin is the neurotransmitter of postganglionic sympathetic nerve endings, which exerts its effects on the peripheral tissues. In addition, the sympathetic system releases adrenalin from the adrenal medulla, which enters the blood stream producing widespread effects throughout the body.

CATECHOLAMINES

Nor-adrenalin, adrenalin and dopamine are the naturally occurring catecholamines and function as neurotransmitters within the central and autonomic nervous system. Catecholamines are synthesized from the amino acid tyrosine, which is sequentially hydroxylated to form dihydroxyphenylalanine (dopa), decarboxylated to form dopamine and hydroxylated to form noradrenalin.

In the adrenal medulla and in those central neurons utilizing adrenalin as neurotransmitter, nor-adrenalin is N-methylated to adrenalin. Catecholamines are stored in adrenal medulla and sympathetic nerve endings.

METABOLISM

Catecholamines are metabolized by two enzymes: monoamine oxidase (MAO) and Catechol-O-methyltransferase (COMT). MAO causes oxidative deamination of catecholamines and an autacoid 5-hydroxytrypyamine (5-HT or serotonin). COMT causes rapid methylation of catecholamines.

Metabolism does not play an important role in terminating the action of endogenously released catecholamines. The majority of catecholamines released from nerve endings re-enters the nerve endings, thereby terminating the action on the receptors.

ADRENORECEPTORS

Two major types of adrenoreceptors are recognized on the basis of their location – α and β.

Both α and β receptors have been further divided into subtypes that serve different functions and are susceptible to differential stimulations and blockade. The major effects that are produced by these receptors are shown in Table 2.1.

α_1 receptors occur on the effector cells and are stimulated by noradrenalin released at sympathetic nerve endings and by adrenalin, causing constriction of blood vessels, a rise in blood pressure, reflex bradycardia, dilation of the pupil and constriction of the smooth muscle around the neck of the bladder. Phenylephrine and methoxamine are selective α_1 agonists while doxazosine and terazosine are selective antagonists.

α_2 receptors occur on the nerve terminal from where noradrenalin is released, which stimulates the receptors. Some noradrenalin released re-enters the nerve endings limiting further release of noradrenalin, thus acting as a release control mechanism. α_2 receptor agonists like methyldopa and clonidine inhibit noradrenalin release and are used in hypertension and management of opioid dependence.

β_1 receptors occur on the heart and kidney (juxtaglomerular cells) and cause increase in rate and excitability of the heart and release of renin resulting in increased cardiac output.

β_2 receptors occur on the bronchi, blood vessels, uterus, urinary tract, eye and gastrointestinal tract. They have a higher affinity for adrenalin than for noradrenalin and are responsible for bronchial muscle relaxation, skeletal muscle vasodilation and uterine relaxation.

β_3 receptor is a novel and distinct adrenoreceptor, which is likely to regulate noradrenalin induced changes in energy metabolism. They are also present on adipocytes and mediate lipolysis. β_3 receptors are present in cardiac muscle and depress the rate and force of contraction of the heart. The advent of β_3

Autonomic Nervous System

Table 2.1: Effects mediated by adrenoreceptors subtypes

Type	Tissue	Action
α_1	**Blood vessels:** Skin, mucosal, splanchnic and renal	Contraction
	Gastrointestinal: Sphincters	Contraction
	Smooth muscles	Relaxation
	Genitourinary: Urinary bladder—Trigone and sphincter	Contraction
	Non-pregnant uterus	Contraction
	Seminal vesicles and prostate	Activation (ejaculation)
	Eye: Pupillary dilator muscle	Contraction (dialates pupil)
	Aqueous humor	Increases flow (decrease in I.O. pressure)
	Pilomolor smooth muscle	Contraction (erects hair)
α_2	**Nerve-terminals:** Adrenergic and cholinergic (some)	Inhibition of transmitter release
	Brain	Decreased sympathetic outflow
	Coronary blood vessel	Dilation
	Pancreas–Insulin secretion	Diminution (Hyperglycemia)
	Platelets	Aggregation
β_1	Heart	Increase force, rate and automaticity
	Juxtaglomerular cells	Renin release
β_2	Respiratory–Uterine and gastrointestinal muscle	Relaxation
	Coronary blood vassels	Dilation
	Heart	Glycolysis
	Liver and skeletal muscles	Glycogenolysis
	Pancreas—Glucagon	Secretion increased
β_3	Fat cells	Lipolysis
D_1	Smooth muscles	Dilates renal blood vessels
D_2	Nerve endings	Modulates transmitter release

receptor antagonist may provide useful addition to the drugs for the treatment of heart failure. So far no drug is available for β_3 receptor.

DOPAMINE RECEPTORS

Dopamine receptors are distinct from adrenoreceptors and are particularly important in the brain, splanchnic and renal vasculature. There are mainly two types—two D_1-like receptors (D_1 and D_5) and three D_2-like (D_2, D_3 and D_4) receptors. Dopamine also has important action on β_1 receptors in the heart.

RECEPTOR SELECTIVITY

Many clinically available adrenergic agonists have selectivity for α_1, α_2, β_1 or β_2 adrenoreceptors. The selectivity is not usually absolute, as at higher concentrations a drug may also interact with related classes of receptors. The term relative receptor affinity may be more appropriate in dealing with the pharmacology of autonomic drugs.

2.2 SYMPATHOMIMETIC DRUGS

Sympathomimetic drugs have effects similar to those produced by activity of sympathetic nervous system. However, drugs differ quantitatively in responses on the two adrenergic receptors. The sympathomimetic drugs on the basis of mode of action can be classified into three groups.

DIRECT ACTING SYMPATHOMIMETIC

These are the most commonly used drugs for actions on organs innervated by sympathetic nervous system.

Non-selective aplpha and beta receptors agonists
Adrenalin and noradrenalin.

Selective alpha$_1$ receptor agonists
Phenylephrine, midodrine, methoxamine, naphazoline, oxymelazoline and xylometazoline.

Autonomic Nervous System

Selective alpha$_2$ receptor agonists
Clonidine, α-methyeldopa and dexmedetomidine.

Non-selective beta receptor agonist
Isoprenaline

Selective beta$_1$ receptor agonists
Dopamine and dobutamine

Selective beta$_2$ receptor agonists
Salbutamol (albuterol), orciprenaline (metaproterenol), terbutaline, salmeterol, formoterol and ritoderine.

Drugs acting on β$_3$ receptors are still in experimental stage.

Fenoldopam, a synthetic drug, is a selective D$_1$ agonist.

NON-SELECTIVE ALPHA AND BETA RECEPTORS AGONISTS

ADRENALIN (Epinephrine)

Adrenalin, the circulating hormone of adrenal medulla, acts on both α and β receptors.

Pharmacokinetics

Adrenalin is not available for oral administration as it is rapidly conjugated and oxidized. It is given by parenteral routes. The liver is the main organ for its degradation. COMT and MAO metabolize the majority of the dose and the metabolites are excreted in the urine.

Pharmacological actions

Cardiovascular system

Adrenalin, in large doses causes vasoconstriction in the subcutaneous, mucosal, splanchnic, and renal vascular beds by α-receptor mediated mechanism. The venous tone (α$_2$ mediated response) is increased, resulting in increased venous return to the heart. Vasoconstriction in coronary and cerebral circulation is minimal. At low concentrations, it may cause vasodilation, because β receptors are more sensitive to adrenalin than α receptors.

Adrenalin acts on $β_1$ receptors in the heart and causes an increase in heart rate, enhancement of cardiac contractility, and increase in conduction velocity. The cardiac output is increased by enhancing the venous return due to increased venous tone ($α_2$ effect) and more effective ventricular contractions.

Cardiac stimulation increases myocardial oxygen consumption. The systolic blood pressure rises due to increased cardiac output.

The diastolic pressure shows little change as adrenalin produces vasoconstriction only in the skin and the splanchnic area ($α_1$ effect) and vasodilation in the arteries in muscle ($α_2$ effect).

Smooth muscles

Adrenalin relaxes the urinary bladder and intestinal muscles, while the corresponding sphincters are stimulated.

Uterine contractions may be inhibited (β receptor) or stimulated (α receptor), depending on menstrual phase or stage of gestation.

Adrenalin induces bronchodilation by a $β_2$ receptor mechanism.

Metabolism

Adrenalin increases metabolic rate. In a variety of tissues, adrenalin stimulates the breakdown of stored fuel with the production of substrate for local consumption, glycogenolysis in the heart. It accelerates fuel metabolism in liver, adipose tissue, and skeletal muscle, liberating substances (glucose, free fatty acids, and lactate) into the circulation for use throughout the body.

Adipose tissue lipolysis and skeletal muscle glycogenolysis is a β-receptor mediated and hepatic glycogenolysis and gluconeogenesis is both α and β receptor mediated effects of adrenalin.

Adrenalin inhibits the secretion of insulin (α receptor mediated response).

Therapeutic uses

Adrenalin is the life saving drug of choice in the treatment of anaphylactic shock and related acute hypersensitivity IgE mediated reactions. The syndrome of bronchospasm, mucous membrane congestion, angioedema, and severe hypotension responds rapidly to intramuscular injection of adrenalin 0.3 to 0.5 mg of 1:1000 adrenalin solution.

Glucocorticoids and antihistamines (both H_1 and H_2 receptor antagonists) are useful as second-line therapy in anaphylaxis.

Adrenalin is also available as parenteral auto injector (Epipen) for self-administration by patients at risk for insect hypersensitivity, severe food allergy, or other types of anaphylaxis.

Adrenalin is given as an intravenous bolus in a dose of 1 mg (10 ml of 1:1000 solution) to restore cardiac activity in cardiac arrest.

Other uses of adrenalin include, along with local anesthetics (with the exception of cocaine) to prolong the duration of infiltration anesthesia, for pharmacologic hemstasis as nasal packs (for epistaxis) or in a gingival string (for gingivectomy) and topically in the eye to facilitate aqueous drainage in chronic open angle glaucoma (α_1 effect).

Adverse effects

Adrenalin can cause anxiety, tremor, headache, and in overdoses arrhythmias, cerebral hemorrhage and pulmonary edema.

NORADRENALIN (Norepinephrine)

Noradrenalin is the neurotransmitter of the postganglionic sympathetic neurons. Its most important action is to produce widespread vasoconstriction leading to a rise in both systolic and diastolic blood pressure.

Noradrenalin is rarely used for the treatment of hypotension during anesthesia, because of its potent vasoconstrictor action which reduces the blood flow in essential organs, particularly in the kidney, need of regular monitoring of blood pressure and rapid inactivation by the body (given only as intravenous infusion).

Noradrenalin is the drug of choice for treatment of hypotensive patients due to tricyclic antidepressant poisoning, who do not respond to alkalinization.

Its use is contraindicated in absence of facilities for monitoring blood pressure and in pregnancy.

SELECTIVE ALPHA$_1$ RECEPTOR AGONISTS

Phenylephrine

Phenylephrine is a selective α_1 agonist that raises blood pressure by increasing peripheral resistance and causes reflex bradycardia. It is used in the treatment of hypotension and paroxysmal supraventricular tachycardia and as a topical nasal decongestant and in conjunctivitis. It is used for fundus examination when cycloplegia is not required. It can cause adverse effects like that of noradrenalin. Chronic use as a nasal decongestant may lead to rebound nasal congestion.

Midodrine

Midodrine is an orally selective α_1 agonist. It is mainly indicated in the treatment of orthostatic hypotension due to impaired autonomic nervous system function.

Adverse effects include supine hypertension, piloerection and urinary retention.

Methoxamine

Methoxamine has actions like phenylephrine. It is available for parenteral use.

Naphazoline and **oxymetazoline** are direct acting α_1 agonists and are used as topical mucous membrane decongestants to reduce the discomfort of hay fever and is a lesser extent, the common cold by decreasing the volume of the nasal mucosa. Rebound hyperemia may follow the use of these agents, and repeated topical use of high drug concentrations may result in ischemic changes in the mucous membrane, probably as a result of vasoconstriction of nutrient arteries.

SELECTIVE ALPHA$_2$ AGONISTS

Alpha$_2$ receptors are present on the sympathetic nerve terminals in the brain. Systemic administration of therapeutic doses of alpha$_2$ receptors decreases the central sympathetic outflow, which leads to inhibition of sympathetic tone and fall in blood pressure.

Clonidine and **α-methyldopa** are used as sympatholytics in the treatment of hypertension (Chapter 5). These drugs also have a vasoconstrictor action on local application to blood vessels, or when given by I.V. infusion, which may initially cause hypertension followed by a more prolonged hypotension (central alpha$_2$ agonist action).

Alpha$_2$ agonists have a variety of effects on the CNS that are not fully understood.

DEXMEDETOMIDINE, a centrally acting alpha$_2$ agonist, is used for its sedative action in ventilator-dependent patient in intensive care units (ICU). It also reduces the requirements for opioids in pain control.

TIZANIDINE, a congener of clonidine, has significant muscle relaxant action in relieving muscle spasm and is used as a muscle relaxant (Chapter 3).

NON-SELECTIVE BETA AGONISTS

Isoproterenol (Isoprenaline)

It is related to adrenalin but stimulates only β-receptors with little or no effect on α-receptors. It is rarely used in heart block or severe bradycardia because over dosage can cause dangerous cardiac arrhythmias.

SELECTIVE BETA$_1$ AGONISTS

Dopamine

It is a naturally occurring catecholamine with an important role as neurotransmitter in the CNS. It is a direct agonist acting on β$_1$ receptors and releases noradrenalin in the cardiac muscle, thus resulting in increased contractility with little effect on the rate.

Dopamine stimulates peripheral alpha$_1$ receptors and dopaminergic receptors in renal, splanchnic, and other vascular beds.

The effects of dopamine are dose dependent. At dosage of <5 mcg/kg/min, dopamine primarily acts as a vasodilator, increasing renal and splanchnic blood flow. At doses of 5 to 10 mcg/kg/min, dopamine increases cardiac contractibility and cardiac output via the activation of cardiac beta$_1$ receptors. At higher doses (> 10 mcg/kg/min), dopamine increases the blood pressure by activation of peripheral alpha$_1$ receptors.

Dopamine is preferred in patients with cardiogenic shock with an systolic BP less than 80 mm Hg. Addition of noradrenalin or phenylephrine may be required in markedly hypotensive patients (systolic BP<70 mm Hg).

Dobutamine

Dobutamine is similar to dopamine but has no dopaminergic effects on renal and other vascular beds. It is a selective β_1 agonist with powerful selective inotropic effects than chronotropic effects without any significant change in peripheral resistance.

Dobutamine is the inotrope of choice for patients of cardiogenic shock with relatively preserved systolic blood pressure (>90 mm Hg), as it increases myocardial contractility and decreases ventricular after load.

SELECTIVE BETA$_2$ AGONIST

Beta$_2$ selective drugs are most useful in the treatment of respiratory disorders and are discussed in Chapter 7.

RITODRINE is a uterine relaxant and has been used to suppress premature labor with the idea to ensure adequate maturation of the fetus. However, Beta agonist therapy does not have significant benefit on prenatal infant mortality and may increase maternal morbidity.

MIXED-ACTING SYMPATHOMIMETICS

Ephedrine

It is an alkaloid obtained from Ephedra vulgaris. It is absorbed orally and is long acting since it is resistant to COMT and MAO.

Ephedrine is a mixed acting sympathomimetic, that is, it has both direct and indirect action. It causes release of noradrenalin from storage in nerve terminals and also produces direct stimulation of α and β receptors. It crosses the blood brain barrier and causes CNS stimulation.

Tachyphylaxis occurs with repeated administration.

Therapeutic uses

Ephedrine is rarely used intravenously for hypotension due to spinal or epidural anesthesia.

PSUDOEPHEDRINE an isomer of ephedrine is used in nasal congestion in several oral decongestant mixtures. It is occasionally used in the treatment of stress incontinence.

Ephedrine is less suitable and less safe for use as a bronchodilator because it is likely to cause arrhythmia, insomnia, anxiety and restlessness.

PHENYLPROPANOLAMINE was a common component of anorexitant. Its use has been banned because of its potential toxicity for hemorrhagic strokes in young women.

A. INDIRECT-ACTING SYMPATHOMIMETICS

These are centrally acting sympathomimetic and act by two different mechanisms:
- By displacing noradrenalin from the sympathetic nerve endings. These are *amphetamine-like drugs*.
- By inhibiting the *reuptake of noradrenalin* into neurons leading to its increase at the nerve receptors.

AMPHETAMINE-LIKE DRUGS

Amphetamine acts indirectly by releasing noradrenalin in the central nervous system. It produces euphoria, reduces appetite, abolishes fatigue and increases both mental and physical activity. It is no longer used because it causes dependence (drug addiction) and psychotic states. It has no place in the management of depression or obesity.

Methamphetamine has more prominent CNS actions and is a drug of abuse.

Methylphenidate (Ritalin) has actions like amphetamine and is used in low doses (5 mg) in children with attention-deficit hyperactivity disorder (ADHD), a behavioral syndrome consisting of short attention span, hyperkinetic physical behavior, and learning problems.

Modafinil is a non-amphetamine derivative that differs in neurochemical profile. It increases the concentration of noradrenalin, dopamine, serotonin and glutamate while decreasing GABA levels at the junction between neurons in the brain. It is the drug of choice for treatment of narcolepsy, a disorder that is characterized by sleep attacks particularly during the day time, vivid nightmares and sudden loss of reversible muscle tone (cataplexy). It is better tolerated than amphetamine.

REUPTAKE OF NORADRENALIN INHIBITORS

Atomoxetine is a selective inhibitor of noradrenalin reuptake and is a preferred drug for the treatment of attention deficit disorders (ADHD). It is better tolerated and has little cardiovascular effects. It may, however, cause orthostatic tachycardia by inhibiting noradrenalin reuptake in the heart. It should not be used concurrently with selective serotonin reuptake inhibitors (SSRIs).

Sibutramine is the only appetite suppressant, which is approved for long-term treatment of obesity. It blocks the neuronal uptake of mainly noradrenalin (but also of dopamine and serotonin) at the hypothalamic site that regulates food intake. It can be used in severely obese patients with other risk factors such as diabetes and dyslipidemia.

Cocaine, a local anesthetic, inhibits transmitter reuptake at noradrenalin synapse and is a drug of abuse (*see* Chapter 3).

DOPAMINE AGONISTS

Fenoldopam is a selective peripheral dopamine receptor (D_1) agonist. It has no α or β receptor agonist activity. It causes vasodilation in coronary, renal and mesenteric arteries and natruresis.

Fenoldopam has poor oral bioavailability, a short elimination half life ($T_{1/2}$ 5 min) and a rapid onset of action. It is given by IV infusion (0.1 to 1.5 mg/kg/min) for the short-term management of hypertensive emergencies, especially associated with impaired renal function, because unlike sodium nitroprusside, urine output, creatinine clearance, and Na^+ excretion are increased by fenoldopam.

Therapeutic uses of sympathomimetic drugs

The major area of applications of the sympathomimetic drugs is cardiovascular and pulmonary conditions.

Cardiovascular

- **Acute hypotension:** Sympathomimetic drugs are only used in a *hypotensive emergency* to preserve cerebral and coronary blood flow. The treatment is of short duration while the appropriate intravenous fluids or blood is being administered.

  Direct-acting $alpha_1$ antagonists such as noradranalin, phenylephrine, and methoxamine have been used in the setting when vasoconstriction is required.

- **Shock:** In most forms of shock, reflex sympathetic nervous system activation is present and the aim should be to reduce peripheral resistance (sympathetic activity) to improve cerebral, coronary and renal perfusion.

  In cardiogenic shock and acute heart failure usually due to myocardial infarction positive inotropic agents such as dopamine or dobutamine may provide short-term relief of heart failure symptoms in patients with advanced ventricular dysfunction.

  The goal of therapy in shock should be to optimize tissue perfusion, not blood pressure.

- **Chronic orthostatic hypotension.** Impairment of autonomic reflexes that regulate blood pressure can lead to chronic orthostatic hypotension. This is more often due to medication that interfere with autonomic function (e.g., imipramine and other tricycline antidepressants, α blockers for treatment of urinary retention, and diuretics), diabetes and other diseases causing peripheral sympathetic neuropathies. Increasing peripheral resistance is one of the strategies to treat chromic orthostatic hypotension, and drugs activating α receptors can be used for this purpose. Midodrine, an orally active $α_1$ agonist, is frequently used for this indication.

Cardiac applications

Adrenalin is used for temporary emergency management of complete heart block and cardiac arrest pending the implantation of electronic pacemakers.

Local vasoconstriction

Sympathomimetics are largely used for their local vasoconstrictor action to achieve hemostasis in facial, oral, and nasopharyngeal surgery, for prolongation of the actions of the local anesthetics and as mucous membrane decongestants.

Pulmonary applications

One of the most important use of sympathomimetic drugs is the use of $β_2$ selective agonist in the therapy of bronchial asthma.

Anaphylaxis

Anaphylactic shock is another major indication of sympathometics (adrenalin).

Ophthalmic applications

Topical sympathomimetics are rarely used for mydriasis (phenylephrine for examination of retina), as conjunctival decongestant or for lowering the intraocular pressure in glaucoma.

Genitourinary applications

Oral sympathomimetic therapy (ephedrine or pseudoephedrine) is occasionally useful in the treatment of stress incontinence.

Central nervous system applications

Sympathomimetics have limited applications in CNS disorders. Modafinil is useful in narcolepsy and methylphenidate in attention–deficit hyperactivity disorder (ADHD). Centrally acting α_2 agonist sympathomimetics are used in hypertension (clonidine), for sedation under intensive care circumstances and during anesthesia (dexmedetomidine) and as a muscle relaxant (tizanidine).

2.3 SYMPATHOLYTIC DRUGS

Sympatholytic drugs are mainly used for their actions on the blood vessels and heart in the treatment of hypertension and to decrease the work of the heart where they diminish the oxygen demand of the myocardium in coronary insufficiency The sympathetic nervous system can be blocked at different sites, and according to the site of action, sympatholytics can be divided into following groups:

- α adrenergic blocking drugs.
- Adrenergic neuron blocking drugs.
- Ganglion blocking drugs.
- Centrally acting sympatholytics.
- β adrenergic blocking drugs.

2.4 ALPHA ADRENERGIC BLOKING DRUGS

These drugs block the vasoconstrictor action of noradrenalin on vascular smooth muscle and cause a lowering of peripheral vascular resistance and blood pressure. They often cause orthostatic hypotension due to failure of the contraction of veins (venous pooling) in the upright position and dilation of arterioles in the legs due to the blockade of α receptors. Reflex tachycardia is marked with drugs that also block α_2 presynaptic receptors in the heart leading to release of noradrenalin.

Alpha$_1$ receptors are expressed in the base of the bladder and the prostate and their blockade decreases resistance to the flow of urine.

Phenoxybenzamine

Phenoxybenzamine is a noncompetitive and non-selective α blocker. It antagonizes both α_1 and α_2 receptors. Its action is prolonged and irreversible and is associated with many side effects, such as profound postural hypotension. It is rarely used with a β blocker in the short term management of severe hypertensive episodes associated with pheochromocytoma.

Phentolamine

Phentolamine is a competitive, non-selective α blocker. Because of its rapid action and short duration, phentolamine is preferred to phenoxybenzamine for the diagnosis and treatment of pheochromocytoma.

Prazosin

Prazosin, a selective blocker of postsynaptic α_1 receptors, causes vasodilation of both the arteries and veins. Unlike non selective α blockers, prazosin does not usually produce reflex tachycardia.

Prazosin does not increase plasma renin activity, does not affect adversely insulin sensitivity or blood lipids. Selective α_1 blockers antagonize the contraction of the sphincter at the bladder trigone.

Prazosin undergoes significant first pass metabolism and has a bioavailability of about 60%. It is extensively metabolized and is excreted in the feces and bile.

Therapeutic uses

Prazosin is used to treat mild to moderate hypertension. It is also used in the treatment of acute congestive heart failure as an afterload reducing agent. However, it is less effective than diuretics, ACE inhibitors, β blockers, calcium channel blockers, when used as monotherapy.

Selective α_1 adrenergic blocking drugs may improve lipid profile by decreasing total cholesterol and triglyceride levels and

Table 2.2: Salient features of some commonly used alpha-adrenoceptors antagonists

Drug	Main use	Comments
Non-selective α_1 and α_2 blockers		
Phenoxybenzamine	Pheochromocytoma (rarely used)	Irreversible block Significant tachycardia and postural hypotension
Phentolamine	Pheochromocytoma	
Selective (only α_1 blocker)		
Prazosin, Terazosin	Hypertension (add on therapy if BP not controlled with combination therapy consisting ACE inhibitor, CCB and diuretic).	Negligible tachycardia and insignificant postural hypotension
Doxazosin	Benign prostatic hyperplasia	
Tamsulosin	Benign prostatic hyperplasia	Relatively more selective for prostate

increasing HDL cholesterol. They can improve the negative effects on lipids induced by thiazide diuretics and β blockers.

Prazosin is used in benign prostatic hyperplasia to increase urinary flow rate and relieve obstructive symptoms.

Adverse effects

Prazosin may cause sedation, dizziness, postural hypotension and syncope, which often disappear with continued therapy. Other side effects include weakness, dry mouth, urinary frequency and incontinence.

Doxazosin and **terazosin** are long acting selective α_1 blockers and are used in the treatment of hypertension and benign prostatic hyperplasia.

Tamsulosin is a long acting selective α_1 antagonist, which has a greater potency in inhibiting contraction in prostate smooth muscle than vascular smooth muscle as compared to other α_1 selective antagonists. The incidence of orthostatic hypotension, therefore, is the least. Tamsulosin is commonly used in combination with 5 α-reductase inhibitor (**dutasteride**) which stops the conversion of testosterone to more potent dihydrotestosterone in the prostate and may cause prostate to shrink in the management of benign prostatic hyperplasia.

2.5 ADRENERGIC NEURON BLOCKING DRUGS

Guanethidine and **debrisoquine** prevent the release of noradrenalin from postganglionic neurons. Guanethidine also depletes the nerve endings of noradrenalin. These drugs do not control supine blood pressure and may cause postural hypotension. They are no longer used because of their significant adverse effects.

Reserpine, a rauwolfia alkaloid, is no longer used because of serious side effects which include psychic depression that can lead to *suicidal* tendencies and possible an increase risk of breast carcinoma.

2.6 GANGLIONIC BLOCKING DRUGS

These belong to different chemical groups and cause either competitive or depolarizing block and include **hexamethonium, mecamylamine** and **trimethaphan**. They block both the sympathetic as well as parasympathetic ganglia. Their therapeutic application lies in blockade of sympathetic ganglia (sympatholytic acion) while blockade of parasympathetic ganglia constitutes adverse effects.

Trimethaphan is only available for clinical use. It blocks the action of acetylcholine competitively, has a very short duration of action and is rarely used by intravenous infusion for the treatment of hypertensive crisis, in the management of autonomic hyperreflexia, and to provide controlled hypotension during surgery. The drugs of choice for hypertensive crisis are IV sodium nitroprusside and IV esmolol. Adverse effects include atropine like actions due to blockade of parasympathetic ganglia.

2.7 CENTRALLY ACTING SYMPATHOLYTICS

These are potent antihypertensive agents that act by stimulating presynaptic α_2 adrenergic receptors in CNS, resulting in decrease peripheral sympathetic outflow which reduces sympathetic vascular resistance and causes fall in blood pressure and bradycardia.

Methyldopa is rarely used in the treatment of hypertension because of its side effects. Its main use is in the treatment of pregnancy related hypertension, since the first-line antihypertensive drugs tend to adversely affect the growth and functional development of the fetus or have toxic effects on fetal tissues.

Side effects are common. Drowsiness, depression, psychological disorders, and parkinsonism are some of CNS disorders. Hypersensitivity reactions, hemolytic anemia, bone marrow depression and hepatitis have also been reported.

Clonidine is used as an oral loading agent in patients with hypertensive crisis when immediate reduction in blood pressure is not indicated. It is also used to prevent unpleasant withdrawal symptoms that occur during treatment of opioid dependence.

The side effects are similar to those seen with methyldopa except it does not cause hemolytic anemia.

2.8 BETA ADRENERGIC BLOCKING DRUGS

This group of drugs, which block the β adrenoreceptors in the heart, peripheral vasculature, bronchi, pancreas, and liver, is widely used and constitutes a more important group of drugs than are the alpha blocking drugs.

Many β blockers are available and in general they are all equally effective but mainly differ in their cardioselective action, lipid solubility, and duration of action and routes of elimination (Table 2.3).

CARDIOSELECTIVITY

Cardioselective β-blockers predominantly block $β_1$ (cardiac) receptors and have less effect on $β_2$ (bronchial) receptors and therefore called relatively cardioselective, but they are not cardio-specific. Cardioselective β blockers are used for cardiovascular disorders, while nonselective β blockers (e.g. propranolol) are used to control widespread effects of adrenergic stimulation, which occurs in thyrotoxicosis and anxiety.

PARTIAL AGONIST ACTIVITY

β blockers possessing intrinsic sympathomimetic activity (ISA) show partial agonist activity. The implication is that β-blockers with partial agonist activity are associated with fewer cardio-respiratory side effects because of a compensatory agonist activity (PAA).

LIPID SOLUBILITY

This largely determines the pharmacokinetic behavior of an individual β blocker.

Highly lipid soluble β blockers (e.g., metoprolol, propranolol) are well absorbed, undergo extensive presystemic elimination (first pass effect), cross the blood–brain barrier, eliminated by liver and are short acting.

Water soluble (e.g. atenolol, sotalol, nadolol) β-blockers are poorly absorbed, undergo little (if any) presystemic elimination, excreted unchanged in the urine and are long acting. They are less likely to enter the brain and may therefore cause less sleep disturbances and nightmares. Water soluble β-blockers do not interact with drugs that influence liver metabolizing capacity.

β blockers that are partly lipid soluble (e.g. acebutolol, pindolol, timolol) are eliminated by renal and hepatic routes and are less likely to accumulate in patients with liver or kidney disease.

Table 2.3: Properties of beta receptor-blocking drugs (all β blocker ends with "lol")

Drug	Dose (mg)	Partial agonist activity	Local anesthetic action	Lipid solubility	Elimination half-life (hours)	Bioavailability	Renal vs hepatic elimination
Cardio selective (β₁ < β₂) blockers							
Metoprolol	50–200	No	Yes	Moderate	3–4	50	H
Atenolol	25–100	No	No	Low	14–22	90	R
Esmolol	10 mg/ml IV	No	No	Low	10 minutes	0	H > R
Acebutolol	200–1200	Yes	Yes	Low	3–4	50	H > R
Celiprolol		Yes	No	Low	4–5	70	H > R
Betaxolol	10–40	No	Slight	Low	14–22	90	H > R
Bisoprolol	5–10	No	No	Low	9–12	80	R = H
Non-selective (β₁ + β₂) blockders							
Propranolol	40–640	No	Yes	High	3.5–6	30	H
Timolol	10–60	No	No	Moderate	4–5	50	H > R
Sotalol	80–200	No	No	Low	12	90	H > R
Nadolol	25–320	No	No	Low	14–24	33	R
Pindolol	10–60	Yes	No	Moderate	3–4	90	H > R
Mixed (α and β) blockers							
Labetalol	200–2400	Yes	Yes	Low	5	30	H
Carvedilol	12.5–50	No	No	Moderate	7–10	25–35	H > R

MEMBRANE STABILIZING ACTIVITY (MSA)

Certain β blockers, notably propranolol, possess MSA, which implies that these drugs exert a local anesthetic, lignocaine like effect on cardiac conduction, but this action is only seen in doses in excess of those which produce β blockade and does not contribute to any anti-arrhythmic properties.

However, MSA inhibits the conversion of T_4 to T_3, which makes propranolol a very useful drug for symptomatic treatment of Grave's disease, in which the hyperthyroid state is associated with widespread effects of adrenergic over stimulation.

Pharmacological actions

Heart

β blockers have prominent action on the heart and are very valuable in the treatment of angina, chronic heart failure, and following myocardial infarction.

Myocardial oxygen demand, particularly during stress or physical exertion, is reduced as a result of slowing the heart rate (negative chronotropic action) and a decrease in the force of contraction (negative ionotropic action) due to blockade of $β_1$ receptors.

All β blockers have antiarrhythmic properties. They increase atrial refractoriness by prolonging sinus node recovery and increase the period of conduction at the A–V node.

Blood pressure

β blockers lower blood pressure due to the reduction in cardiac output, reduction in plasma renin and aldosterone activity, release of vasodialatory prostaglandins and possibly due to CNS mediated antihypertensive action. These drugs do not lower blood pressure in healthy individuals with normal blood pressure.

Labetalol further reduces peripheral vascular resistance due to their combined α and β adrenoreceptor blocking properties.

Celiprolol has in addition, a direct vasodialating action on the arterioles.

Lung

β blockers cause an increase in airway resistance, particularly in patients with asthma. Cardioselective β-blocker possessing PAA (celiprolol) are preferred in asthmatic patients. However, no cardioselective β blockers is sufficiently specific to completely avoid interaction with $β_2$ adrenoreceptor and are best avoided in patients with asthma. The patients with chronic obstructive pulmonary disease (COPD) generally tolerate these drugs quite well and can be used in patients with concomitant ischemic heart disease.

Endocrine/metabolic

Hypoglycemia and impaired glucose tolerance may arise as a result of blockade of $β_2$ receptors in the liver. Non-selective β blockers may interfere with recovery from hypoglycemia and thus mask symptoms of hypoglycemia in insulin-dependent diabetic patients. β blockers are much safer in type 2 diabetic patients who do not have hypoglycemic episodes.

β blockers are associated with increased triglyceride levels and a reduction in the ratio of high density to low density lipoprotein cholesterol. Cardioselectives are less likely to cause dyslipidemia.

Eye

β blockers reduce intraocular pressure in glaucoma due to decreased aqueous production.

Central nervous system

Lipid soluble β blockers may cause adverse effects such as sleep disturbances and other psychotic changes.

Therapeutic uses

β blockers are widely used drugs in cardiovascular disorders which include:

Angina pectoris

β blockers play a major role in the prophylaxis of angina and are widely used alone or in combination with long acting nitrates or calcium antagonists. Their antiarrhythmic action may confer additional protection on ischemic myocardium. In theory, non-selective β blockers may aggravate coronary vasospasm by blocking the coronary artery $β_2$ adrenoreceptors and so a once-daily cardioselective preparation is used.

Hypertension

β blockers are no longer used as first-line antihypertensive therapy except in patients with another indication for the drug (e.g. angina). **Atenolol** amongst others has been increasingly used.

Celiprolol, a new generation cardioselective β-blocker has the advantage of possessing selective $β_2$ partial agonist activity and direct vasodilator action, causing less impairment of glucose tolerance or hypoglycemia or dyslipidemia.

Cardiac arrhythmias

All β blockers are class II antiarrhythmic drugs. They are used in stress or exercise induced sinus tachycardia and paroxysmal atrial tachycardia. These drugs can also reduce ventricular ectopic beats, particularly, if the ectopic activity has been precipitated by catecholamines.

Sotalol has antiarrhythmic effects involving ion channel blockade in addition to its β blocking action.

Cardiac failure

Bisoprolol, carvedilol and metoprolol reduce the morbidity and mortality and are considered to be amongst the first line of drugs for treatment of chronic heart failure.

Myocardial infarction

Intravenous β blockers (e.g. atenolol, metoprolol, propranolol, sotalol) are strongly indicated in the acute stage of myocardial infarction, as they suppress ventricular fibrillation, reduce infarct size and limit early mortality and morbidity. Their routine oral use has been found to reduce mortality in myocardial infarction.

Thyrotoxicosis

Nonselective β blockers (propranolol, nadolol) relieve the symptoms such as fine tremors, excessive sweating, palpitation, which are due to catecholamine excess in thyrotoxicosis.

Portal hypertension

Propranolol and other nonselective β blockers reduce portal pressure and prevent recurrent bleeding from varices or gastric erosions.

Other cardiovascular disorders

β blockers are found to be beneficial in obstructive cardiomyopathy due to slowing of ventricular ejection and decreased outflow resistance. They are also useful in dissecting aortic aneurysm by reducing aortic pulsations.

Glaucoma

β blockers reduce aqueous humor production as a result of their effects on sympathetic innervations in the ciliary epithelium. Timolol is the most active and is used as 0.25% eye drops in open angle glaucoma.

Migraine

β blockers without PAA (e.g. propranolol, metoprolol, timolol, nadolol) are effective in preventing migraine headache. They are less effective, once the headache has begun.

Anxiety

β blockers, in particular propranolol and oxprenolol are very effective in anxiety resulting from an acute stress (situational anxiety) such as that provoked by an examination or public performances.

Adverse effects

β blockers should not be withdrawn abruptly because this may have a rebound effect and precipitate dangerous arrhythmias, worsening of angina or MI—the β blocker withdrawal syndrome.

The major potentially dangerous or even life-threatening adverse effects are likely to occur if used in asthmatics, patients with heart failure or diabetes.

Central nervous system effects include mild sedation, vivid dreams and rarely, depression. Hydrophilic drugs nadolol or atenolol would be more appropriate in a patient who experience unpleasant central nervous system effects.

β blockers can cause adverse effects on lipid profile. Non-selective β blockers may cause an increase in triglyceride levels and decreased HDL cholesterol, which generally do not occur with β blockers possessing PAA.

β-blockers are contraindicated in severe, symptomatic or "brittle" asthma, uncontrolled heart failure, and cardiogenic shock.

2.9 PARASYMPATHETIC NERVOUS SYSTEM

The parasympathetic preganglionic neurons are located in cranial and sacral portions of the spinal cord. The ganglia lie close to the innervated organ, so that the preganglionic nerves are long and postganglionic nerves are short. The parasympathetic nervous system innervates the heart, the gastrointestinal tract, the genitourinary system, iris and the salivary glands.

NEUROTRANSMITTER

Acetylcholine (Ach)

Ach serves as the neurotransmitter at the postganglionic parasympathetic nerve endings. Ach is also the neurotransmitter at all autonomic ganglia, i.e. in both the sympathetic and parasympathetic nervous systems. In addition to autonomic nervous system, Ach is the neurotransmitter at the somatic nerves supplying the skeletal muscles (neuromuscular junction).

Nerves that release Ach are said to be cholinergic.

Acetylcholinesterases

Ach is hydrolyzed and inactivated by the enzyme acetylcholinesterase at cholinergic synapses. This enzyme (also known as specific or true cholinesterase) is present in the neurons and is concerned with the termination of the effects of Ach.

A non-specific type of enzyme, butyrocholinesterase (serum cholinesterase or pseudocholinesterase) is present in plasma and non-neural tissues, whose physiological functions are not known.

Cholinergic receptors

Two classes of receptors for Ach are recognized—muscarinic and nicotinic.

Muscarinic receptors

These are located primarily on parasympathetic effector cells in smooth muscle, cardiac muscle, and the glandular epithelium. They are selectively stimulated by muscarine and blocked by atropine.

The muscarinic (M) receptors are further divided into M_1, M_2, and M_3 receptors. These subtypes of M receptors are only of physiological importance with little role in pharmacotherapy.

Nicotinic receptors

Nicotine receptors are found mainly in the spinal cord, the autonomic ganglia, adrenal medulla and skeletal muscle end plates.

Nicotine, the classic agonist, first stimulates and then blocks autonomic ganglia and skeletal muscle end plates. d-tubocurarine blocks nicotinic receptors, particularly in skeletal muscles and autonomic ganglia, whereas hexamethonium preferentially blocks autonomic ganglionic receptors.

2.10 PARASYMPATHOMIMETIC DRUGS

These are the drugs which produce actions similar to that of Ach, either by directly interacting with cholinergic receptors or by preventing the hydrolysis of Ach by acetylcholinesterase (anticholiesterase drugs). These are:

Directly acting		Indirectly acting anticholiesterases	
Choline esters	Alkaloids	Reversible	Irreversible
Acetylcholine	Muscarine	Physostigmine	Organophosphates
Methacholine	Pilocarpine	Neostigmine	Dyflos (DFP)
Carbachol	Arecholine	Pyridostigmine	Echothiophate
Bethanechol		Ambenonium	Parathion
		Endrophonium	Malathion
		Demecarium	
		Distigmine	
		Donepezil	
		Rivastigmine	
		Galantamine	

Pharmacological actions

Central nervous system

Ach plays an important role in cognitive functions, especially memory. Presenile dementia of the Alzheimer type is reportedly associated with a profound loss of cholinergic neurons.

Cardio vascular system

Ach reduces the rate of spontaneous depolarization of the sinoatrial node and decreases the heart rate.

Ach delays impulse conduction within the atrial musculature and shortening of the effective refractory period. Delay in impulse conduction and shortening of the effective refractory period of the atrial musculature may initiate or perpetuate atrial arrhythmias.

At the A-V node and His-Purkinje fibers, Ach reduces conduction velocity, increases the effective refractory period, and thus diminishes the ventricular rate during atrial flutter or fibrillation.

Ach markedly reduces the force of atrial contraction, but has no effect on ventricular muscle.

Ach causes generalized vasodilation, though only few (skin) receive cholinergic innervations. Vasodilation is primarily mediated through the release of endothelium dependent relaxing factor (EDRF), which in all probability is nitric oxide (NO). Ach, as such, is not involved in the regulation of peripheral resistance.

Gastrointestinal tract

Ach increases the tone of GIT smooth muscle, enhances peristaltic activity, and relaxes GIT sphincters. Ach stimulates and enhances the secretion of gastrin, secretin, and insulin.

Genitourinary and respiratory systems

Ach increases ureteral peristalsis, contracts the urinary detrusor muscle, and relaxes the trigone and sphincter and plays an important role in the co-ordination of urination.

Ach increases tracheobronchial secretions and causes bronchial constriction.

Eye

Ach produces contraction of the circular muscle of iris, causing pupillary constriction (miosis) and that of ciliary muscle causing spasm of accommodation.

Ach facilitates the out-flow of aqueous into the canal of Schlemn, by pulling the root of the iris centrally and thus relieving the obstruction, if any, imposed by trabecular meshwork.

Exocrine glands

Ach stimulates the salivary, sweat, and lacrimal glands

Nicotinic actions

Ach stimulates both sympathetic and parasympathetic ganglia.

Ach stimulates the skeletal muscles resulting in muscle twitching and fasciculation.

Therapeutic uses

Directly acting parasympathomimetic drugs are seldom used for systemic actions, because of their widespread effects are particularly dangerous on the heart and bronchi.

Acetylcholine

Ach itself has no therapeutic role because of its rapid hydrolysis by acetylcholinesterase and plasma cholinesterase.

Methacholine

Methacholine is hydrolyzed only by acetylcholinesterase and therefore has a longer duration of action than Ach. It exerts purely muscarinic effects and not used in therapy.

Carbachol

Carbachol is not hydrolyzed by cholinesterases and its actions are more prolonged. It has both muscarinic as well as nicotinic actions. It is generally avoided for therapeutic uses because of its longer component of nicotinic action.

Bethanechol

Bethanechol is resistant to hydrolysis by cholinesterase and has only muscarinic action and is devoid of nicotinic action. It stimulates the GIT and genitourinary smooth muscles with minimal effects on CVS. It is the only directly acting parasympathomimetic, which is used for urinary retention in absence of outflow obstruction and less commonly, in GIT disorders, such as postvagotomy gastric atony.

Of the choline esters, bethanechol is the most widely used.

Pilocarpine

Pilocarpine has prominent muscarinic actions like methacholine and is only used as eye drops in glaucoma, especially before operation for angle closure glaucoma in combination with a cholinesterase inhibitor physostigmine.

Muscarine

Muscarine is found in poisonous mushrooms and is of toxicological importance.

Arecoline

Arecoline is found in betel nut Areca catachu. It has nicotinic as well as muscarinic actions and prominent CNS effects. It has no therapeutic use.

ANTICHOLINESTERASE DRUGS

These drugs prevent the breakdown by cholinesterase of Ach produced at nerve endings throughout the body. Except for quantitative differences, their actions are similar to Ach. Lipid soluble drugs (physostigmine and organophosphates) have more marked muscarinic and CNS effects, while lipid insoluble drugs (neostigmine and related other quaternary amines) have marked actions on the skeletal muscles (nicotinic effects).

All anticholinestrases produce similar adverse effects (muscarinic effects) due to the prolongation of the actions of Ach, such as intestinal colic and diarrhea, sweating and salivation, constricted pupil, bradycardia and hypotension. IV atropine blocks the muscarinic actions of anticholinesterases.

Physostigmine (Eserine)

Physostigmine is a tertiary amine alkaloid, is lipid soluble, is well absorbed and penetrates into CNS and the cornea.

Physostigmine has predominant effects on muscarinic receptors, autonomic ganglia and CNS. Being highly toxic, it has only limited use.

Physostigmine has been used as eye drops, especially for simple and secondary glaucoma and parenterally for the reversal of intoxication by drugs with a central anticholinergic action such as atropine, phenothiazines and tricyclic antidepressants.

Neostigmine (Prostigmin)

Neostigmine, a quaternary ammonium compound, is poorly absorbed, does not penetrate CNS and has prominent action on skeletal muscles, which is both a direct action as well as due to blockade of acetylcholiesterase. Of the cholinesterase inhibitors, neostigmine is the most widely used for GIT and urinary tract disorders (muscarinic effects).

Neostigmine is used as an alternate to pyridostigmine in long-term therapy of myasthenia gravis (nicotinic effects) where it is combined with atropine to prevent muscarinic actions such as colic, excessive salivation or diarrhea. The actions on eye and cardiovascular system are less marked than physostigmine.

Neostigmine is also used to reverse the actions of non-depolarizing muscle relaxants.

Pyridostigmine

Pyridostigmine is similar to neostigmine in all respects except that it is less potent and has a longer duration of action (3–6 hours as compared to 0.5–2 hours with neostigmine). It is preferable to neostigmine in myasthenia gravis because of its smoother action and the need of less frequent dosage.

Endrophonium

Endrophonium has a very brief action (5–15 minutes) and is used mainly for the diagnosis of myasthenia gravis and also to determine over dosage or under dosage of anticholinesterase drugs in myasthenia gravis. A single test dose of endrophonium causes substantial improvement in muscle power in myasthenia gravis (**myasthenic crisis**), while if the treatment with cholinergic drugs is excessive, an injection of endrophonium will intensify symptoms of the disease (**cholinergic crisis**).

Distigmine

Disticmine is a longer acting neostigmine analogue and may be used for the treatment of myasthenia gravis and urinary retention.

Ambenonium

Ambenonium is approximately six times more potent than neostigmine, with marked direct stimulant action on skeletal muscles. It is mainly used in the treatment of myasthenia gravis.

Demecarium

Demecarium is more potent and has a longer duration of action than neostigmine and is mainly indicated in the treatment of glaucoma.

Donepezil, rivastigmine and galantamine
These newer oral cholinesterase inhibitors, have adequate penetration into central nervous system, and are much less toxic and exclusively used in Alzheimer's diseases. Although evidence for the benefit of cholinesterase inhibitors is statistically significant, the clinical benefit from these drugs is modest and temporary.

MYASTHENIA GRAVIS (MG)

Myasthenia gravis is characterized by progressive fatigable weakness, particularly of the ocular, neck, facial and bulbar muscles. The underlying defect is a decrease in the number of available acetylcholine receptors at neuromuscular junction due to an antibody-mediated autoimmune attack. Additionally, cellular immune activity against the receptor is found. There are no sensory signs or signs of involvement of the CNS.

Myasthenia gravis occurs at all ages, sometimes in association with a thymic tumor or thyrotoxicosis, as well as in rheumatoid arthritis and lupus erythematosus.

The principles of treatment are:
- To maximize the activity of acetylcholine at remaining receptors in the neuromuscular junctions, by the use of anticholinestenase drugs.
- To limit or abolish the immunological attack on motor plate by immunological treatment.

Anticholinesterase medication
Prolongation of the action of acetylcholine by inhibiting its hydrolyzing enzyme, cholinesterase produces partial improvement.

Pyridostigmine is the most widely used anticholinesterase drug, which is given in a dosage of 30–120 mg, usually 6-hourly. Muscarinic side-effects, including diarrhea and colic, may be controlled by diphenoxylate/propantheline or loperamide.

Over dosage of anticholinesterase drug may cause a cholinergic crisis due to depolarization block of motor and plates, with muscle fasciculation, paralysis, pallor, sweating, excessive salivation and small pupils. This may be distinguished from severe weakness due to exacerbation of myasthenia (myasthenic crisis) by clinical features, and, if necessary by the injection of a small dose of endrophonium.

Immunological treatment

The immunological treatment of myasthenia includes thymectomy, plasma exchange, intravenous immunoglobulin, corticosteroids and other immunosuppressant drugs.

Thymectomy

Thymectomy should be considered in any antibody-positive patient less than 45 years. Thymectomy provides improvement in up to 85% of patients and has the advantage of long-term benefit, in some cases diminishing or eliminating the need for continuing medical treatment.

In view of potential benefits and the negligible risk, thymectomy has gained wide-spread acceptance in the treatment of myasthenia gravis.

Plasma exchange

Plasma exchange (plasmapheresis) consists of removal of the antibody from the blood. It may produce marked improvement but, as this is usually brief, such therapy is normally reserved for myasthenia crisis or for preoperative preparation.

Intravenous immunoglobulin (IVIg)

An alternative to plasma exchange IVIg is used for the short-term treatment of severe myasthenia. It has the advantage of not requiring special equipment or large bore venous access. Adverse effects are generally not serious but can rarely lead to aseptic meningitis or renal failure.

IVIg is not a long-term treatment, which is possible only with immunosuppressive therapy.

Corticosteroids

Corticosteroids provide marked improvement in myasthenia weakness in most of the patients. Improvement is commonly preceded by marked exacerbation of myasthenic symptoms and treatment should be initiated in hospital. The initial dose of prednisone is kept low, which is increased stepwise, depending on the patients tolerance, until there is marked clinical improvement or a dose of 50–60 mg/d is reached. The doses are gradually reduced, modified to an alternate-day regimen.

Patients on long-term corticosteroid therapy must be followed carefully to prevent or treat adverse side effects.

Other immunosuppressive drugs

Corticosteroids are only indicated for the intermediate period until the beneficial effects of azathioprine or mycophenolate mofetil begin (as long as a year).

Mycophenolate mofetil has become one of the most widely used drugs in the treatment of myasthenia gravis because of its effectiveness and lack of serious side effects. A dose of 1.5g twice daily is recommended. Its mechanism of action involves inhibition of purine synthesis by the de novo pathway. Since lymphocytes lack the alternate salvage pathway that is present to all other cells, mycophenolate inhibits the proliferation of lymphocytes but not of other cells. Another advantage of the drug lies in lack of serious side effects with rare development of leucopenia and very small risk of malignancy.

Other immunosuppressive drugs particularly cyclophosphamide is reserved for patients' refractory to the other drugs.

Rituximab, a monoclonal antibody that depletes CD20B cell can also be used.

IRREVERSIBLE ANTICHOLINESTERASES

These are organophosphorus compounds, which are not used therapeutically, but are extensively employed as insecticides. They can be absorbed from the skin and lungs, if inhaled, and may result in poisoning. The treatment of poisoning consists of atropine (1 mg) intravenously followed by a cholinesterase reactivator.

Pralidoxime (PAM)

Pralidoxime reactivates cholinesterase by separating it from irreversible anticholinesterase. It is used, as an adjunct to atropine in organophosphate poisoning, to restore neuromuscular transmission.

Adverse effects

The adverse effects of parasympathomimetic drugs are similar. The symptoms include intestinal colic, diarrhea, sweating and salivation. The pupils are constricted, the pulse is slow and the blood pressure is low.

Parasympathomimetic drugs are contraindicated in patients with coronary insufficiency, hyperthyroidism, peptic ulcer and asthma.

2.11 PARASYMPATHOLYTIC DRUGS

These are the drugs, which inhibit the actions of Ach after it has been released from parasympathetic nerve endings and are better known as antimuscarinics. They belong to the belladonna group or are synthetic substitutes.

ATROPINE

Atropine is an alkaloid derived from the plant *Atropa belladonna*. Atropine is well absorbed when given orally. The liver largely breaks it down.

Pharmacological actions

Cardiovascular system

Atropine increases the heart rate and enhances A–V conduction, due to blockade of inhibitory vagal impulses to the SA node. There is no significant effect on blood pressure.

Central nervous system

Atropine has an overall CNS stimulant action, which is not seen with therapeutic doses. It possesses antitremor activity due to blocking of the relative cholinergic over activity in basal ganglia. High doses can produce hallucinations and ultimately coma.

Smooth muscles

Atropine relaxes all smooth muscles. Tone, amplitude and frequency of contraction of stomach and intestines are decreased. It relaxes the ureter and urinary bladder, but increases the tone of the vesical sphincter. Relaxation of biliary tract is less marked. Atropine produces slight bronchodilation.

Exocrine glands

Atropine markedly decreases the sweat, salivary, tracheobronchial and lachrymal secretions. Larger doses decrease gastric secretions.

Eye

Topical instillation of atropine blocks the Ach response of the ciliary muscle and the circular smooth muscles of the iris, producing paralysis of accommodation (cycloplegia) and dilation of pupil (mydriasis). Its action lasts for 7–10 days. The intraocular tension tends to rise, especially in narrow angle glaucoma.

Therapeutic uses

The use of atropine, because of its widespread effects, is restricted to topical instillation or for short-term treatment of certain acute conditions. The principal uses of atropine are:

- For refraction procedures in children and for treatment of uveitis to prevent posterior synechiae (eye ointment 1% or drops 0.5–1%)
- For intestinal, biliary or renal colic (600 microgram parenterally). Synthetic substitutes are more selective and preferred.

- Very low doses of atropine (0.025 mg) in combination with diphenyoxylate (nonanalgesic congener of meperidine) available under Lomotil name are extremely effective for traveler's diarrhea and other mild condition of hypermotility.
- Bradycardia, particularly, if complicated by hypertension after myocardial infarction.
- To reverse muscarinic actions in organophosphorus poisoning (2 mg IM or IV) every 20 to 30 minutes until the skin becomes flushed and dry, the pupils dilate and tachycardia develops.

Adverse effects

These are dose related. Dry mouth, constipation, urinary urgency and retention, dilation of pupil with loss of accommodation, reduced bronchial secretions; flushing and dryness of the skin are common. Higher doses of atropine cause restlessness, hallucinations and delirium.

Parasympatholytics are contraindicated in glaucoma, paralytic ileus, pyloric stenosis and prostatic enlargement.

HYOSCINE (SCOPOLAMINE)

Hyoscine is an alkaloid, has antimuscarinic actions like atropine. Hyoscine has more potent action on the eye and exocrine glands, but is less potent than atropine in its actions on the heart and smooth muscles. Unlike atropine, hyoscine is a CNS depressant. Hyoscine, even in small doses, causes sedation and dry mouth.

Hyoscine is the most effective drug for the prevention of motion sickness. It can be given by injection or by mouth or as a transdermal patch. The patch formulation produces significant blood levels over 48–72 hours. It is often used in children for premedication to allay the apprehension in the preoperative period.

ATROPINE SUBSTITUTES

Many semisynthetic derivatives of belladonna alkaloids and synthetic substitutes are available and in general, they are all capable of producing atropine like side effects. There are, however, differences between them which may affect choice in treating a particular disease.

Atropine substitutes can be grouped according to their clinical indication based on selectivity of action.

1. Antisecretory drugs

Pirenzepine and a more potent analog, **telenzepine** reduce gastric acid secretion with fewer adverse effects than atropine and other less selective antimuscarinic agents. These drugs provide the same rate of healing of duodenal ulcers as the H_2 receptor blockade ranitidine provides. Though, they are used in some countries, they are not the drugs of choice in the treatment of peptic ulcer.

2. Antispasmodics

Gastrointestinal disorders

Dicyclomine and hyoscyamine are rarely used for providing relief of abdominal pain or discomfort because they may cause atropine-like side effect.

Genitourinary disorders

Oxybutynin is selective for blocking muscarinic receptor (M_3) in the urinary bladder and is used for the treatment of renal colic and to relieve bladder spasm after urologic surgery, e.g., prostectomy. It is also valuable in reducing involuntary voiding in patients with neurologic disorders.

Darifenacin and **solifenacin** have greater selectivity for M_3 receptor and have the advantage of once-daily dosing because of their long half-lives. **Tolterodine** and **fesoterodine** are other selective M_3 antimuscarinic drugs. All these new drugs, however, possess atropine like side effects such as dry mouth.

Valethamate, an antimuscarinic antispasmodic drug is very useful especially in delayed dilatation of cervix during delivery.

Bronchial muscle

Antimuscarinic agents have a selective bronchodilator action. **Ipratropium bromide**, a quarternary ammonium derivative of atropine, given by inhalation is poorly absorbed into the circulation and is useful for the treatment of bronchial asthma for patients intolerant to inhaled β_2 agonist agent. In addition, ipratropium enhances the bronchodilation produced by nebulized albuterol in acute severe asthma.

3. Mydriatics and cycloplegics

Mydriatics and cycloplegics and there synthetic substitutes are used for the examination of fundus of the eye (Table 2.4).

Table 2.4: Mydriatics and cycloplegics

Drug	Duration of action	Uses
Atropine	18 days	Most potent, action not reversible by miotics, rarely used
Homatropine	24 hours	Anterior uveitis
Cyclopentolate	4 hours	Refraction procedure in young children
Tropicamide	12 hours	Examination of fundus

Homatropine (1 and 2% eye drops) is much less potent than atropine; mydriasis lasts for 1–3 days while accommodation recovers in 1 day. It is used in the treatment of anterior segment inflammation and is preferred for its short duration of action.

Cyclopentolate (0.5 and 1% eye drops) is a potent and rapidly acting drug. Mydriasis and cycloplegia last for a day. It is preferred for producing cycloplegia for refraction in young children.

Tropicamide (0.5 and 1% eye drops) is a relatively weak and short acting mydriatic and is commonly used for the examination of the fundus of the eye.

4. Antiparkinsonian drugs (see Anticholinergic drugs, page 126)

5. Antiasthmatics (see page 307)

6. For premedication (see page 158)

3

Central Nervous System

3.1 ANXIOLYTICS AND HYPNOTICS

ANXIOLYTICS

Anxiolytics (sedatives) relieve anxiety. Anxiety is a normal reaction but when severe and disabling it becomes pathological. Anxiolytics induce sleep when given at night.

BENZODIAZEPINES

Benzodiazepines are the most commonly used anxiolytics and hypnotics, they posses distinct advantages over older drugs such as meprobamate and barbiturates.

- Benzodiazepines are remarkably free from serious adverse effects and are generally safe.
- Specific antagonist (antidote) flumazenil reverses the effects of high doses of benzodiazepines.
- Dependence (addiction) on benzodiazepines does occur, but the physical withdrawal symptoms are less marked and less severe.
- Benzodiazepines do not induce hepatic microsomal drug metabolizing enzymes.
- Benzodiazepines exhibit amnesia but with no phenomenon of automatism.

Mechanism of action

Benzodiazepines act on the reticular formation and limbic system in the brain. There are specific receptors for benzodiazepines and they appear to enhance the action of GABA (γ-aminobutyric acid), an inhibitory neurotransmitter.

Pharmacokinetics

Benzodiazepines differ markedly in pharmacokinetic behavior which is related to their varying lipid solubility. They are metabolized in liver and some metabolites are themselves sedative which prolong their actions, they cross placenta and are secreted in milk.

Pharmacological actions

Benzodiazepines can be classified according to their pharmacokinetic characteristics (Table 3.1).

Table 3.1: Benzodiazepines

Drug	Anxiolytics Dose (mg)	Half-lite (hours)	Commants
Ultra-short acting (duration < 6 hours)			
Triazolam	0.125–0.25	< 6	Active, metabolite none, can produce confusion and delirium in elderly, used as hypnotic
Midazolam	5	2–4	Mainly used for anaesthesia induction
Short-acting (duration of action 10–20 hours)			
Lorazepam	2–4	10–20	Most suitable for I.V use in states epilepticus
Oxazepam	10–30	6–20	Not too sedating, perfered for elderly or in liver dysfunction
Temazepam	15–30	10–20	Moderately sedating, less day time hangover, used as hypnotic

(Contd.)

(Contd.)

Drug	Anxiolytics Dose (mg)	Half-life (hours)	Commants
Intermediate acting (duration 12 – 18 hours)			
Alprazolam	0.25–0.5	10–15	Not too sedating-may have specific antidepressant and anti panic activity-tolerance and dependence develop easily
Nitrazepam	5–10	20–30	Mainly used as hypnotic
Longer acting (duration 10–24 hours)			
Chlordiazepoxide	10–20	10–30	Moderately sedating
Diazepam	5–15	20–60	Quite sedating
Flurazepam	15–30	40–80	Prodrug, quite sedating, used as hypnotic
Clonazepam	1–2	18–80	Moderately sedating, mainly used as anticonvulsant

Benzodiazepines cause anxiolysis, sedation, amnesia, and hypnosis. They act as skeletal muscle relaxants by selectively depressing supraspinal polysynaptic reflexes involved in the regulation of muscle tone. They do not posses any analgesic action. Toxic doses produce coma without any specific features and cardio-respiratory depression is usually minimal.

Therapeutic uses

Benzodiazepines are widely prescribed drugs. Their main uses are:

Anxiety

Benzodiazepines are used for the short-term relief of severe anxiety. The treatment should be usually for a limited period and intermittent, because continuous use leads to a decrease in efficacy and drug dependence. They should not be used for depression, phobic or obsessional states or chronic psychosis.

In generalized anxiety disorder (GAD), antidepressants (SSRIs and SNRIs), have largely replaced benzodiazepines. The antidepressants are more effective than benzodiazepines in the long-term treatment of these anxiety disorders. Further, antidepressants do not carry the risk of dependence and tolerance that may occur with benzodiazepines.

Insomnia

Benzodiazepines are the hypnotics of choice. Shorter acting (**temazepam** and **triazolam**) are the most suitable for transient insomnia where residual effects are undesirable. Longer acting such as nitrazepam is indicated when early morning waking is a problem.

As anticonvulsant

Diazepam and **lorazepam** given slowly intravenously are very effective in status epilepticus and febrile convulsions.

Skeletal muscle spasm

Diazepam is used for the relief of chronic muscle spasm or spasticity. Sedation and occasionally extensor hypotonus are the disadvantages.

For premedication

Diazepam, temazepam, lorazepam and **midazolam** are used for premedication and as adjuvant during surgical procedures performed under local anesthesia. As a result of their sedative, anxiolytic, and amnesic properties, and their ability to control acute agitation, these compounds are considered to be the drugs of choice for premedication.

Midazolam is water soluble and is benzodiazepine of choice for parental administration. Midazolam is commonly used for medical procedures such as endoscopy.

Acute alcohol withdrawal syndrome
Diazepam and chlordiazepoxide are used as adjuvant.

Adverse effects
Benzodiazepines are remarkably free from serious adverse effects, although continued use can cause fatigue, memory problem, psychomotor impairment and rarely behavior disturbances.

Benzodiazepines are contraindicated in respiratory depression, severe hepatic impairment, myasthenia gravis and sleep apnea syndrome.

Dependence on benzodiazepines is the main problem. Withdrawal symptoms mainly pertain to CNS and include anxiety, depression, insomnia and depersonalization.

Benzodiazepines toxicity is heightened by malnutrition, advanced age, hepatic disease, and concomitant use of alcohol, other CNS depressants, isoniazid, and cimetidine.

Drug interactions

Alcohol and benzodiazepines taken concomitantly may result in greater impairment of psychomotor functions than either agent alone. A large number of drugs such as antibacterial, calcium channel blockers, ulcer healing drugs (cimetidine and omeprazole) inhibit metabolism of benzodiazepines resulting in enhanced sedation.

FLUMAZENIL

Flumazenil is a specific antidote for the reversal of central sedative effects of benzodiazepines, but is rarely required in severe overdose. Its effects last only for about 1 hour, so repeated doses may be required with long acting bezodiazepines. It can also be used in the differential diagnosis of unclear cases of poisoning due to centrally acting depressant drugs.

Flumazenil carries a risk of seizures, and is contraindicated in patients co-ingesting proconvulscent drugs such as TCAs and in those with a history of seizures.

Adverse effects of flumazenil include agitation, confusion and nausea. Flumazenil may cause a severe precipitated abstinence syndrome in patients who have developed physiologic benzodiazepine dependence.

BUSPIRONE

Buspirone has anxiolytic action without possessing any significant hypnotic action. It acts with a group of specific serotonin ($5HT_{1A}$) receptors in the brain. As compared to benzodiazepines, buspirone has the advantage of being less sedative, does not cause dependence, does not interact with alcohol and does not impair mental activity.

Buspirone is not very effective in patients who have not responded to benzodiazepines, and its anxiolytic effects are relatively slow to develop. Its only adverse effects are occasional nausea and headache.

Buspirone has a limited place in the treatment of anxiety because of its slow onset of action; it requires several weeks to become effective.

β-BLOCKERS

Propranolol and **oxprenolol** (*see* page 47) are useful anxiolytics in controlling the autonomic symptoms of anxiety such as palpitations and tremors. They do not reduce non-autonomic symptoms such as mental tension.

ANTIDEPRESSANTS

Antidepressants are the first-line medication for sustained treatment of generalized anxiety disonders, having the advantage of not causing serious physiologic dependency problems. At initiation of treatment, antidepressants can themselves be anxiogenic—thus, an initial dose, in conjunction with a benzodiazepine, is often indicated. **Velafaxine** and **duloxetive** are generally used in the treatment of generalized anxiety disorders.

HYPNOTICS

Hypnotic drugs produce sleep that is comparable to normal sleep. They do not relieve pain. The natural sleep comprises of cycles of deep sleep lasting for about 80 minutes followed by a short phase (about 10 minutes) of rapid eye movement (REM) sleep, which is characterized by dreaming, increased muscle tone, increased heart rate, and rapid eye movements. The cycle of deep and REM sleep lasting for 90 minutes is repeated for about six times per night. Deprivation of REM sleep leads to psychological changes during waking hours. Many centrally acting drugs and alcohol suppress REM sleep and do not produce natural sleep.

BENZODIAZEPINES

Benzodiazepines are the most commonly used hypnotic drugs. They are equally potent and an individual drug mainly differs in its duration of action. The long acting benzodiazepines (**nitrazepam**, and **flurazepam**) may produce a hangover effect the next day.

Benzodiazepine toxicity is increased by malnutrition, advanced age, concomitant use of alcohol, other CNS depressants, isoniazid and cimetidine.

Benzodiazepnes should be given at the lowest recommended doses with intermittent dosing schedule.

ZOLPIDEM

Zolpidem is a very useful hypnotic drug, with few effects the next morning. It has no withdrawal syndrome, rebound insomnia or tolerance and, because of its rapid onset, is useful for initiating and for maintaining sleep. Side effects include drowsiness, headache and nausea. It should be avoided in patients with obstructive sleep apnea and doses should be reduced in cirrhosis.

ZALEPLON

Zaleplon has a half life of approximately 1 hour and is mainly indicated for short-term insomnia, which may be due to anxiety, illness etc. It is not recommended for patients under 18 years of age and should not be repeated the same night. Side effects include headache, drowsiness, dizziness and impaired co-ordination. It causes drug dependence. It is contraindicated in breast feeding and patients suffering from sleep apnea or myasthenia gravis.

ZOPICLONE

Zopiclone is a long acting hypnotic providing sleep for 6–8 hours. It may cause some drowsiness the next morning. Tolerance and dependence to zopiclone generally occurs. Side effects include a bitter metallic taste, nausea and psychological symptoms such as hallucinations. It is contraindicated in pregnancy and in children.

PROMETHAZINE

Promethazine, an antihistamine, produces sleep by blocking the action of histamine in the brain. It is used for insomnia particularly in patients with a history of drug dependence .It is not a good hypnotic drug, because it is not very effective in producing sleep, has a long duration of action with sedation next morning and causes anti-cholinergic (atropine like) actions.

BARBITURATES

Barbiturates are no longer used as anxiolytics and hypnotics as they are dangerous in over dosage, readily cause psychological and physical dependence, and are potent inducers of liver enzymes.

CHLORAL HYDRATE

Chloral hydrate is effective and cheap hypnotic. It has an unpleasant taste, is a gastric irritant and can cause rashes. It is rarely used in children where its derivative **triclofos** is preferred, being less of a gastric irritant. Chloral hydrate should be used with caution in liver or renal failure. Its action is enhanced by heparin.

PARALDEHYDE

Paraldehyde, a volatile liquid, is a potent hypnotic, but is not used because of its pungent smell and disagreeable taste. It is metabolized in liver to acetaldehyde, which is exhaled in breath leading to pungent smell and soreness of trachea and larynx. Paraldehyde is mainly used in status epilepticus (given rectally or intramuscularly). It causes little respiratory depression and is therefore useful where facilities for close monitoring and resuscitation (if needed) are not available.

3.2 ANALGESICS

Analgesics are drugs which relieve pain without loss of consciousness. Pain is a warning signal of the presence of disease and by its nature may help in the diagnosis of the underlying disease. Analgesics cause symptomatic relief of pain without affecting its cause.

Analgesics belong to two distinct groups:

1. **Narcotic analgesics:** This group consists of opium and synthetic drugs with similar actions. They act on the brain and spinal cord and are used to relieve moderate to severe pain, particularly of visceral origin. These drugs are also called opioids.

2. **Non-steroidal anti-inflammatory drugs** (NSAIDs): These drugs act peripherally by reducing the inflammation and are indicated in musculoskeletal conditions accompanied by pain and inflammation.

NARCOTIC (OPIOID) ANALGESICS

Mechanism of action

Opioids act on specific receptors of several types (u, k and sigma) in the nervous system Stimulation of these receptors, by neurotransmitters or neuromodulators, inhibit the transmission of nerve impulses related to pain and the appreciation of pain is suppressed. A number of peptides (encephalin and endorphins) occur naturally in the brain and act as neurotransmitter or neuromodulators at these receptors and regulate pain responsiveness at supraspinal and spinal levels, particularly in the midbrain and posterior horn of the spinal cord.

Opioid drugs react with these receptors and thus relieve pain. Out of the various opioid receptors, u receptors are the most important, because its stimulation by opioids accounts for the major effects of opioids, such as analgesia, respiratory depression, euphoria and physical dependence.

Opioid receptor interaction can be of three types:

1. Stimulation of the receptor — agonist
2. Partial stimulation and partial blockade of receptor — partial agonist
3. Blockade of receptors — antagonist

OPIUM

Opium is obtained from the unripe poppy (Papaver somniferum) capsule. Crude opium is a brownish resinous material and contains two types of alkaloids:

Phenanthrene derivatives	Benzoisoquinoline derivatives
Morphine	Papaverine
Codeine	Noscapine
Thebain	

Only morphine and codeine posses analgesic activity

OPIOID AGONISTS

Morphine

Morphine is the most powerful opium alkaloid and serves as the standard against which other opioid analgesics are compared.

Pharmacokinetics

Morphine is well absorbed orally, but its bioavailability is less than 30% because of extensive hepatic first pass metabolism. It is widely distributed and freely crosses placenta and affects the fetus. It is metabolized in liver; one of its metabolites (morphine-6-glucuronide) has powerful analgesic activity of its own. Metabolites are excreted in urine and bile.

Pharmacological actions

Central nervous system

The most important effects of morphine are on CNS, which are both stimulant and depressant.

Depressant effects

a. Analgesia

Morphine is the most potent analgesic. Consciousness is not lost and the patient can usually locate the source of pain.

b. Euphoria

Morphine causes a powerful sense of contentment and well-being. This action is an important component of its analgesic action, since the agitation and anxiety associated with a painful illness or injury are thereby reduced.

c. Respiration

Morphine is a powerful respiratory depressant. It reduces the responsiveness of the respiratory centre to carbon dioxide. Depressed respiration and increased arterial carbon dioxide retention causes cerebral vasodilatation leading to an increase in intracranial pressure.

d. Cough center

Morphine is a potent cough depressant.

e. Sedation

Morphine is a mild hypnotic and may produce drowsiness and sleep.

Stimulant effects

a. Emesis

Morphine stimulates the CTZ in the brainstem, producing nausea and vomiting.

b. Miosis

Morphine produces miosis by stimulating the nucleus of the third nerve. The pin-point pupils are indicative of morphine poisoning prior to asphyxia.

c. Oliguria

Morphine stimulates the release of ADH, producing oliguria.

Cardiovascular system

Morphine can cause fall in blood pressure due to vasomotor medullary depression and histamine release.

Gastrointestinal system

Morphine reduces peristalsis and stomach motility. In addition, spasmodic nonpropulsive contractions of GIT smooth muscle are produced. These actions result in constipation. Biliary pressure is increased due to contraction of sphincter of Oddi.

Other systemic effects

Morphine increases detrusor muscle and vesicle sphincter tone leading to urinary retention. It causes histamine release which can cause bronchoconstriction and cutaneous vasodilation.

Therapeutic uses

Opioids are the most potent pain-relieving drugs currently available, of all analgesics. They have the broadest range of efficacy and provide the most reliable and effective method for rapid pain relief. With therapeutic doses nausea, vomiting, pruritis and constipation are the most frequent and bothersome side effects.

Peripherally acting opioid antagonists **alvimopan** and **methylnaltrexone** has virtually no penetration into the CNS. Thus these drugs can reverse the adverse effects of opioid analgesics that are mediated through their peripheral receptors without reversing their analgesic effects. Both the drugs are effective in preventing paralytic ileus following abdominal surgery and opioid-induced bowel dysfunction (constipation) in patients taking opioid analgesics on a chronic basis.

Morphine is still one of the best analgesic for severe pain of a temporary nature such as occurs in surgical emergencies, the postoperative period, following injury, or after myocardial infarction, for not only it relieves pain but also relieves the anxieties and miseries of the patient. It is the drug of choice for the oral treatment of severe pain in terminal cancer on a regular basis.

Morphine is used to control distressing cough in terminal lung cancer.

Morphine, by slow intravenous injection (5–10 mg) is very useful for the treatment of acute dyspnoea of pulmonary edema due to left ventricular failure.

The usual dose of morphine is 10–15 mg by subcutaneous injection, 5–30 mg orally or as a rectal suppository.

Adverse effects

CNS effects include dysphoria, drowsiness and pupillary constriction (pinpoint pupil). Overdose may cause coma.

Respiratory depression is dose related and especially pronounced after IV administration.

Cardiovascular effects include peripheral vasodilation and hypotension.

GI effects. Nausea and vomiting (particularly in initial stage) and constipation are common.

Urinary retention occurs due to increased bladder, ureter and urethral sphincter tone.

Pruritis occurs most commonly with spinal administration.

Hypersensitivity: Patients with respiratory diseases such as chronic bronchitis, asthma and emphysema are very sensitive to opioids and a normal dose may produce signs of overdose.

The fatal dose is variable, but death usually occurs after a dose of 50 mg. Tolerance may develop to the analgesia, the euphoria and the respiratory depression and to a lesser extent to miosis and constipation.

Dependence (addiction) can develop rapidly when opioids are used in a social context.

Opioids are contraindicated in acute disease states such as abdominal pain, head injuries, where the pattern and degree of pain are important diagnostic signs. They are also contraindicated in respiratory depression, acute alcoholism, and chronic rheumatic diseases.

OTHER OPIOID AGONISTS

DIAMORPHINE (HEROIN)

Diamorphine has a greater analgesic potency than morphine. Its action is more rapid and short lasting. It is not used therapeutically but is more popular among addicts.

CODEINE

Codeine has pharmacological effects similar to morphine, but is much less potent and causes less sedation or respiratory depression or GIT effects than morphine. Addiction liability is rare but may occur. Its main useful action is on cough center and codeine is widely used in doses of 15–30 mg as a cough suppressant. In combination with aspirin or paracetamol, it is used as a mild analgesic.

DIHYDROCODEINE

Dihydrocodeine is similar to codeine and is used as a mild analgesic. It causes constipation and occasionally dizziness, low blood pressure and nausea. It is given orally or by intramuscular injection.

DEXTROPROPOXYPHENE

Dextropropoxyphene is a very mild analgesic, somewhat less potent than codeine. It is generally used orally in combination with paracetamol (**co-proxamol**) in painful conditions. It is slightly addictive and like other opioids may cause vomiting. Overdose may result in respiratory depression and acute heart failure due to dextropropoxyphene and hepatic toxicity due to paracetamol.

METHADONE

Methadone is a synthetic opioid. Its analgesic action is as powerful as that of morphine, but is less sedating and euphoric than morphine. It is a drug of dependence. Like morphine, it depresses the cough centre, but the effect on the respiratory center is not so marked. The principal uses of methadone are in severe pain; cough in terminal disease and as an adjunct in treatment of opioid dependence. The usual dose is 5–10 mg orally or by injection.

MEPERIDINE (PETHIDINE)

Meperidine is a synthetic opioid, which is chemically related to atropine. It is less potent and short acting analgesic than morphine and is not suitable for severe continuing pain. It has no effect on cough center, is less depressant to respiratory centre and does not cause constipation. It does not cause constriction of the pupils and can therefore be used in head injuries where observation of the pupil size may be important. It is no longer used for obstetrical analgesia and has been replaced by epidural analgesia to relieve pain in the later stages of labor. Dependence can develop. It is used for moderate to severe pain in doses of 50–100 mg orally or by subcutaneous injection. Its action lasts for 2 to 3 hours.

AFENTANIL, FENTANYL AND REMIFENTANIL

These opioids are very potent and are short acting. They are used by injection for intraoperative analgesia to help maintenance of surgical anesthesia (*see* page 166). They are liable to cause severe respiratory depression. Fentanyl is available in a transdermal drug delivery system as a self adhesive patch which allows slow absorption for up to 72 hours in the relief of terminal pain.

PAPAVERETUM (OMNOPON)

Papaveretum is a mixture of 253 parts of morphine hydrochloride, 23 parts of papaverine hydrochloride and 20 parts of codeine hydrochloride. Its actions are essentially those of morphine and is hardly used any more.

OPIOID PARTIAL AGONISTS

These are mixed narcotic agonist antagonist analgesics. They are powerful analgesics but are less addictive, less likely to depress respiration and are less euphoric. They precipitate withdrawal symptoms, including pain in patients dependent on opioid agonists.

PENTAZOCINE

Pentazocine is an effective analgesic, but exerts adverse effects on the heart and central nervous system and has some potential for causing dependence. It causes hallucinations and thought disturbances. It is not recommended and, in particular should be avoided after myocardial infarction as it may increase pulmonary and aortic blood pressure as well as cardiac work.

BUPRENORPHINE

Buprenorphine is as powerful analgesic as morphine. It seems to be less likely to cause adverse effects, though nausea and vomiting may be troublesome. It has a longer duration of action, but it too seems to have a potential for abuse. Respiratory depression although not so marked as with morphine, is only partially reversed by naloxone.

Buprenorphine is used by injection for postoperative pain in doses of 200–600 micrograms, since orally it is metabolized by liver (first pass effect). Sublingually, it is given in doses of 200–400 micrograms for various forms of chronic pain.

Buprenorphine shows a 'ceiling effect' so that increasing the dose above usual range will not improve its efficacy.

NALBUPHINE

Nalbuphine is as powerful analgesic as morphine and has fewer side effects and less abuse potential. Its action lasts for about 4 hours and has to be given by injection. Nausea and vomiting occurs less than with other opioids but respiration depression is similar to that with morphine. Like buprenorphine, it also shows a "ceiling" effect. It is less suitable than morphine for managing severe pain.

Nalbuphine causes fewer psychotomimetic effects and unlike pentazocine does not exert substantial adverse hemodynamic effects and it may therefore be of value in treating some patients who have heart disease

MEPTAZINOL

Meptazinol is claimed to cause a low incidence of adverse cardiac and respiratory effects. It has a shorter half life than nalbuphine and has therefore been used to treat obstetric pain where its rapid elimination by both mother and fetus is an advantage. It is also useful for breakthrough pain in the postoperative period.

TRAMADOL

Tramadol is a weak opioid. It reduces pain by two mechanisms—an opioid effect and by interfering pain pathways through the spinal cord. It is reported to have fewer opioid side effects, notably less respiratory depression, less constipation and less addiction potential. Its analgesic action is as powerful as meperidine and is given intramuscularly for postoperative pain or orally for chronic pain.

Side effects include nausea and vomiting, dizziness and dry mouth.

OPIOID ANTAGONISTS

These are drugs which occupy the opioid receptors and produce little or no stimulation so that the actions of opioids are reversed. They are used to treat over dosage by opioids.

NALOXONE

Naloxone is a pure opioid antagonist having no stimulant action on opioid receptors. It is given in doses of 0.8–2 mg intravenously at intervals of 2–3 minutes to a maximum of 10 mg in opioid poisoning. It can also be used in doses of 100–200 micrograms to terminate the actions of narcotic drugs in postoperative period.

NALTRXONE

Naltrxone is an orally active opioid antagonist used in the treatment of opioid withdrawal as an aid to relapse prevention since it prevents the euphoric action which is linked to addiction.

3.3 NONSTEROIDAL ANTI-INFLAMMATORY DRUGS

The nonsteroidal anti-inflammatory drugs (NSAIDs) are among the most prescribed analgesic drugs, although their chronic use for anti-inflammatory properties has declined recently because of gastrointestinal, cardiovascular and renal adverse effects.

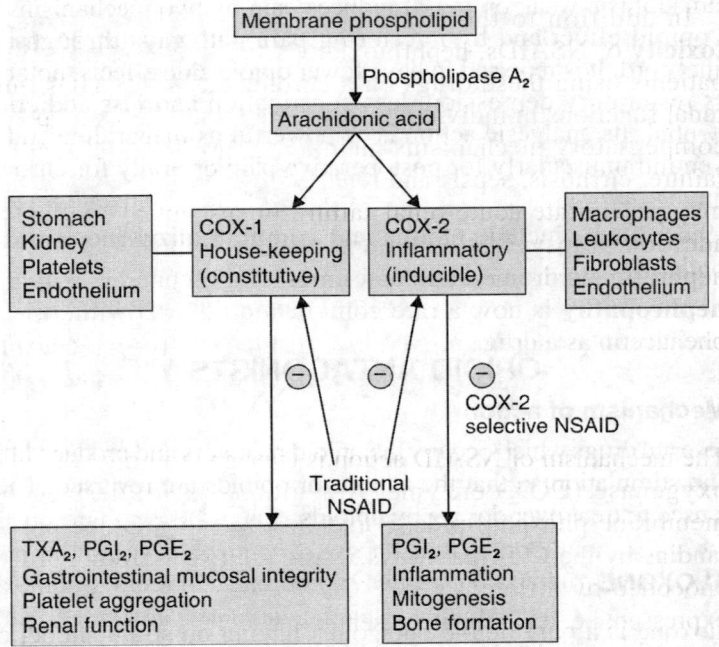

Fig. 3.1: Schematic representation of the steps involved in synthesis of prostaglandin E_2 (PGE_2) and prostacyclin (PGI_2). Characteristics and distribution of the cyclooxygenase (COX) enzymes 1 and 2 are also shown, thromboxane A_2 (TXA_2).

Aspirin, non acetylated salicylates, acetaminophen (paracetamol) and NSAIDs, are considered together because they are used for similar problems and may have similar mechanism of action. All these compounds inhibit the enzyme cyclooxygenase (COX), and except for acetaminophen, have anti-inflammatory action at higher doses. They are particularly effective for mild to moderate headache and pain of musculoskeletal origin.

Occasional uses of analgesics have minimal side effects, but with chronic use, gastric irritation is a common side effect of NSAIDs.

Gastric irritation is most severe with aspirin, which may cause ulceration of the gastric mucosa leading to bleeding, because aspirin, irreversibly, acetylates platelet COX and thereby interferes with coagulation of blood.

In addition to the well known **gastrointestinal disease toxicity** of NSAIDs, nephrotoxicity is a significant problem for patients using these drugs on a chronic basis. NSAIDs impair renal functions in individuals in whom prostaglandin-dependent compensatory mechanisms maintain renal function (e.g. heart failure, cirrhosis, sepsis and renal impairment of any type), and may precipitate acute renal failure in susceptible patients. In addition, idiosyncratic immune reactions may occur, causing nephrotic syndrome and acute interstitial nephritis. **Analgesic nephropathy** is now a rare complication due to withdrawal of phenacetin as a drug.

Mechanism of action

The mechanism of NSAID action is through inhibition of cyclooxygenase (COX) enzyme. Arachidonic acid, derived from membrane phospholipids, is metabolized to produce prostaglandins by the COX pathways. There are two isoforms of COX, enocoded by different genes. COX-1 enzyme is constitutively expressed, i.e. it is always present in most of the cells and fulfills a 'housekeeping' function in the gastric mucosa, platelets and kidneys.

The COX-2 enzymes is largely induced at sites of inflammation, producing prostaglandins that cause local pain and inflammation.

Traditional NSAIDs such as ibuprofen, diclofenac and naproxen inhibit both COX enzymes, whereas newer NSAIDs such as celecoxib and etoricoxib selectively inhibit COX-2.

Whilst NSAIDs have anti-inflammatory activity, they do not reduce peripheral cytokine production, acute phase reactants or ESR, and are not thought to have a disease-modifying effect in osteoarthritis or rheumatoid arthritis.

Antipyretic action

The reduction of fever by lowering of the elevated hypothalamic set point is a direct function of reducing the level of PGE_2 in the thermoregulatory center. The synthesis of PGE_2 depends on the constitutively expressed enzyme cyclooxygenase. The substrate for cyclooxygenase is arachidonic acid released from the cell membrane, and this release is the rate-limiting step in the synthesis of PGE_2. Therefore, inhibitors of cyclooxygenase are potent antipyretics. The antipyretic potency of various drugs is directly correlated with the inhibition of brain cyclooxygenase. **Acetaminophen** is a poor cyclooxygenase inhibitor in peripheral tissue and *lacks noteworthy anti-inflammatory activity*; in the brain, however, acetaminophen is oxidized by the P-450 cytochrome system, and the oxidized form inhibits cyclooxygenase activity. Moreover in the brain, the inhibition of another enzyme, COX-3, by acetaminophen may account for the antipyretic effect of this agent. However, COX-3 is not found outside the CNS.

Oral aspirin and acetaminophen are equally effective in reducing fever in humans. Nonsteroidal anti-inflammatory drugs (NSAIDs) such as ibuprofen and specific inhibitors of COX-2 are also excellent antipyretics. Chronic high-dose therapy with antipyretics such as aspirin or any NSAID does not reduce normal core body temperature. Thus, PGE_2 appears to play no role in normal thermoregulation.

Pharmacokinetics

All NSAIDs except nabumetone are weak organic acid.

NSAIDs are well absorbed orally and food does not substantially change their bioavailability. They are highly metabolized, undergo enterohepatic circulation and finally excreted by kidneys. In fact the degree of lower gastrointestinal tract irritation correlates with the amount of enterohepatic circulation. They are highly protein bound.

NSAIDs are present in synovial fluid after repeated dosing. Drug with short half-lives, remain in the joints for longer periods, which account for their longer duration of action.

Pharmacodynamics

NSAIDs, which inhibit both COX-1 and COX-2 enzymes are non-selective and produce analgesic, anti-inflammatory and antipyretic actions. In addition, possible mechanisms of their actions include inhibition of chemotaxis, down-regulation of interlenkin-1 production, decreased production of free radicals and superoxide, and interference with calcium mediated intracellular events.

Aspirin irreversibly acetylates and blocks platelet COX.

The NSAIDs decrease the sensitivity of blood vessels to bradykinin and histamine, affect lymphokine production from, lymphocyteT, and reverse the vasodilation of inflammation. Although these drugs effectively inhibit inflammation. there is no evidence that — in contrast to drugs such as methotrexate and other DMARDs, they alter the course of any arthritic disorder.

Adverse effects

Adverse effects generally are quite similar for all the NSAIDs:
- Dose related side effects include tinnitus, dizziness, and hearing loss.
- Dyspepsia, abdominal pain, nausea, vomiting, and rarely, bleeding or ulcers. Traditional NSAID—can damage the gastric mucosal barrier and are an important etiological factor in up to 30% of gastric ulcers. Co-prescription of omeperazole (proton pump inhibitor) reduces but does not eliminate NSAID-induced ulceration and bleeding.
- Hypersensitivity reactions, including bronchospasm, laryngeal edema, and urticaria are uncommon, but patients with asthma and nasal polyps are more susceptible.

- Rarely thrombocytopenia, neutropenia, or even aplastic anemia.
- Hepatic toxicity may be severe with acetaminophen (paracetamol).
- Cardiovascular disorders involving increased risk of thrombosis due to inhibition of COX-2 in the endothelium.
- Fluid retention and renal impairment due to inhibition of renal prostaglandin. Rarely chronic excessive use can result in interstitial nephritis and papillary necrosis.
- Rapid destruction of the head of femur ("indomethacin hip") may occur with potent NSAIDs.

ASPIRIN

Aspirin's long use, without prescription and wide publicity, has been largely replaced by the newer NSAIDs. It is now rarely used for its analgesic, antipyretic and anti-inflammatory actions. Its main use is in its inhibition of platelet aggregation.

Pharmacokinetics

Aspirin is rapidly absorbed from both the stomach and intestinal tract. It is a prodrug, which is rapidly hydrolyzed in liver to acetic acid and active metabolite salicylate.

Salicylate is nonlinearly bound to albumin which may act as antibody and be responsible for allergic responses seen with aspirin. Alkalinization of the urine increases the rate of excretion of free salicylate and its water soluble conjugates.

Mechanism of action

Low doses of aspirin (80–100 mg) irreversibly inhibit TXA_2 production by inhibiting COX-1 of platelets without affecting PGI_2 synthesis in the vascular endothelium. The antiplatelet effects last for 8–10 days (the life of the platelet).

Therapeutic uses

Aspirin in low doses decreases the incidence of transient ischemic attacks, unstable angina, coronary artery thrombosis with myocardial infarction, and thrombosis after coronary artery bypass grafting.

Long-term use of aspirin is associated with a lower incidence of colon cancer. It may be valuable in treatment of pre-eclampsia–eclampsia.

Adverse effects

Main adverse effects at antithrombotic doses of aspirin are gastric upset (intolerance), and gastric and duodenal ulcers. Other toxic effects of NSAIDs rarely, if ever, occur at antithrombotic doses.

The antiplatelet action of aspirin requires its stoppage one week before surgery and its use is contraindicated in hemophilia.

As an NSAID, aspirin is contraindicated for fever, myalgia and malaise in children aged under 15 years, as it may rarely precipitate Reye's syndrome with coma and liver damage, which can prove fatal.

NONACETYLATED SALICYLATES

These drugs include **magnesium choline salicylate, sodium salicylate,** and **salicyl salicylate**. All nonacetylated salicylates are effective anti-inflammatory drugs, although they may be less effective analgesics than aspirin. They do not inhibit platelet aggregation; they may be preferable when COX inhibition is undesirable such as in patients with asthma, those with bleeding tendencies, and even in renal dysfunction.

The nonacetylated salicylates are administered in doses up to 3–4 g a day.

ACETAMINOPHEN (Paracetamol)

Acetaminophen is the most widely used minor analgesic and antipyretic drug. The COX inhibiting action is so weak in the peripheral tissues that it is *devoid of anti-inflammatory action and antiplatelet properties*. Its analgesic action is mediated by raising the threshold to pain perception in the CNS. Its main advantage over other NSAIDs lies in the absence of action on other body systems. It does not cause indigestion or gastric bleeding and Reye's syndrome as seen with aspirin.

Pharmacokinetics

It is given orally, well absorbed and peak plasma levels are achieved within 60 minutes. It is partly bound to plasma proteins and inactivated by metabolism in the liver.

Therapeutic uses

It is the *preferred analgesic* for many types of pain such as headache, musculoskeletal pain, dysmenorrhoea, sore throat, toothache, osteoarthritis etc. It is as potent a analgesic as aspirin. It is not effective in rheumatoid arthritis because of absence of anti-inflammatory action.

It is the *ideal drug* to be used as antipyretic. The usual dose is 0.5–1.0 g given orally 4–6 hourly (maximum dose, 4 g/day).

Adverse effects

Adverse effects are uncommon at normal dosage, but in overdose, it may cause dangerous liver damage.

Hepatic toxicity is due to depletion of hepatic glutathione and subsequent accumulation of a toxic intermediate metabolite, N-acetyl-p-benzoquinonimine. Toxicity usually occurs after ingestion of more than 7.5 g. Acetaminophen toxicity also occurs due to chronic ingestion, especially in alcoholics. IV acetylcystine is specific antidote that acts as glutathione substrate.

There is also evidence that large doses taken over a long period may damage the kidneys.

COX-2 SELECTIVE INHIBITORS

COX-2 selective inhibitors, or coxibs, have analgesic, antipyretic and anti-inflammatory actions without affecting the actions of the constitutively active "housekeeping" COX-1 enzyme found in the gastrointestinal tract, kidneys, and platelets. The COX-2 selective NSAIDs are less likely to cause gastrointestinal toxicity but the benefit is attenuated in patients on low-dose aspirin. Co-prescription of a proton pump inhibitor (**omeprazole**) is recommended with selective COX-2 inhibitors, even through the risk of gastrointestinal events is low.

COX-2 inhibitors have been associated with an increased risk of cardiovascular disease as they have no impact on platelet aggregation, which is mediated by thromboxane produced by COX-1 enzyme. In contrast, they inhibit COX-2 mediated prostacyclin synthesis in the vascular endothelium. As a result, COX-2 inhibitors do not offer the cardioprotective effects of traditional nonselective NSAIDs.

COX-2 is constitutively active within the kidney and COX-2 inhibitors can cause renal toxicities similar to those associated with traditional NSAIDs.

COX-2 inhibitors are contraindicated in patients in the immediate period after coronary artery bypas surgery and should be used with caution in patients with history of or significant risk factors of cardiovascular disease.

CELECOXIB AND ETORICOXIB

Celecoxib is a sulfonamide derivative and may cause rashes, and is contraindicated in patients with allergic-type reactions to sulfonamides. **Etoricoxib** is structurally related to diclofenac, hence hepatic functions require monitoring.

Rofecoxib and **valdecoxib** have been withdrawn because of a high incidence of cardiovascular thrombotic events.

MELOXICAM

Meloxicam preferentially inhibits COX-2 over COX-1, particularly at its lowest therapeutic dose of 7.5 mg/d. It is not as selective as celecoxib and may be considered "preferentially" selective rather than "highly" selective.

Meloxicam is associated with fewer clinical gastrointestinal symptoms and complications than piroxicam, diclofenac, and naproxen. It does not have any impact on platelet aggregation.

NONSELECTIVE COX INHIBITORS

DICLOFENAC

Diclofenac is relatively nonselective COX inhibitor.

Gastrointestinal ulceration may occur less frequently than with some other NSAIDs, but renal adverse effects occur in high-risk patients. Diclofenac appears to impair renal blood flow and glomerular filtration rate. Elevation of serum aminotransferase occurs more commonly with this drug than with other NSAIDs.

Topical preparations are used for prevention of postoperative ophthalmic inflammation after intraocular lens implantation and strabismus surgery. A topical gel is effective for solar keratoses.

DIFLUMISAL

Diflumisal has more potent anti-inflammatory and analgesic action than aspirin, but has no antipyretic action (does not cross blood-brain barrier). It is mainly used for cancer pain with bone metastases and for pain control in dental (third molar) surgery. A 2% diflumisal oral ointment is clinically useful analgesic for painful oral lesions. Its use should be limited in patients with significant renal impairment, because of its renal clearance.

FLURBIPROFEN

It has more complex mechanism of action. Apart from COX inhibiting action, it may also affect tumor necrosis factor-α (TNF-α) and nitric oxide synthesis.

It is also available as topical ophthalmic preparations for inhibition of intraoperative miosis. Intravensously flurbiprofen is effective for perioperative analgesia in minor ENT surgery and in lozenge form for sore throat.

Flurbiprofen in addition to adverse effects of NSAIDs rarely may cause cog wheel rigidity, ataxia, tremor, and myoclonus.

IBUPROFEN

It is commonly used NSAID, which in doses of 2400 mg/d has anti-inflammatory effect equivalent to that of 4 g of aspirin. In lower doses it has analgesic action only.

Ibuprofen is effective in closing patent ductus arteriosus in preterm infants, with much the same efficacy and safety as indomethacin.

Ibuprofen is relatively contraindicated in patients with nasal polyps, angioedema and bronchospastic reactivity to aspirin. Aseptic meningitis and fluid retention have been reported. Interaction with anticoagulants is uncommon. The concomitant administration of ibuprofen and aspirin antagonizes the irreversible platelet inhibition induced by aspirin. Thus, treatment with ibuprofen in patients with increased cardiovascular risk may limit the cardioprotective effects of aspirin. Furthermore the use of ibuprofen concomitantly with aspirin may decrease the total anti-inflammatory effect.

INDOMETHACIN

Indomethacin is a potent non-selective COX inhibitor which may also inhibit phospholipase A and C, reduce neutrophil migration and decrease T-cell and B-cell proliferation.

It differs somewhat from other NSAIDs in its indications and toxicities.

Indomethacin had been used for many conditions, especially for gout, ankylosing spondylitis, closure of patent ductus arterious, and other miscellaneous conditions such as rheumatoid and psoriatic arthritis, pleurisy, nephrotic syndrome, diabetes insipidus, urticarial vasculitis, postepisiotomy pain, prophylaxis of heterotopic ossification in arthroplasty, postlaminectomy pain (epidural injection), topical eye drops for inflammation and pain after traumatic corneal abrasion, oral rinse for gingival inflammation.

Adverse reactions to indomethacin are quite common requiring discontinuance. GI effects may include pancreatitis.

CNS effects include headache, dizziness, confusion, and depression. Rarely, psychosis with hallucinations has been reported. Serious toxic effects consist of hematologic disorders, renal papillary necrosis and a number of interactions with other drugs.

KETOPROFEN

It inhibits both COX and lipoxygenase enzymes. Inspite of its dual effect on prostaglandins and leukotrienes, ketoprofen is not superior to other NSAIDs in clinical efficacy.

KETOROLAC

It is mainly used as an analgesic, not as anti-inflammatory drug (although it has typical NSAID properties). It is an effective analgesic and has been used successfully parenterally (IM or IV) to replace morphine in some situations involving mild to moderate postsurgical pain.

Toxicities are similar to those of others NSAIDs, although renal toxicity may be more common with chronic use.

ETODOLAC

It is a preferential COX-2 inhibitor and is more potent than aspirin.

NABUMETONE

It is a preferential COX-2 inhibitor. It has long duration of action and has been reported to cause pseudoporphyria and photosensitivity in some patients.

NAPROXEN

It inhibits leukocyte migration and is useful gout. A topical preparation and an ophthalmic solution are also available. Rare cases of allergic pneumonitis, leukocytoclastic vasculitis, and pseudoporphyria as well as the common NSAID– associated side effects have been noted.

OXAPROZIN

It is a long acting NSAID with the usual therapeutic uses and adverse effects associated with traditional NSAIDs. It is uricosuric and is more useful in gout than other NSAIDs.

PIROXICAM

It is a long acting NSAID that in high concentrations also inhibits polymorphonuclear leukocyte migration, decreases oxygen radical production and inhibits lymphocyte function. It causes highest risk of gastrointestinal disorders.

SULINDAC

In addition to usual NSAID indications, sulindac may inhibit the development of colon, breast and prostate cancers.

Among the more severe adverse reactions, Stevens-Johnson epidermal necrolysis syndrome, thrombocytopenia, agranulocytosis, and nephrotic syndrome have all been observed.

TOLMETIN

Its toxicities and efficacy are similar to those of other NSAIDs with the following exceptions: it is ineffective in the treatment of gout, and may cause rarely thrombocytopenic purpura.

Other NSAIDs

Azapropazone, carprofen, meclofenamate, and tenoxicam are rarely used.

CHOICE OF NSAID

All NSAIDs are almost equally efficacious with a few exceptions—tolmetin seems not to be effective for gout, and aspirin is less effective than other NSAIDs (e.g., indomethacin) for ankylosing spondylitis.

The choice of NSAIDs depends mainly on the basis of toxicity. For example, the gastrointestinal and renal side effects of ketorolac limit its use. Indomethacin or tolmetin are associated with the greatest toxicity, while salsalate, aspirin, and ibuprofen are least toxic.

For patients with renal insufficiency, nonacetylated salicylates may be best. Diclofenac and sulindac are associated with more liver function test abnormalities than other NSAIDs.

Celecoxib, selective COX-2 inhibitor is probably safest for patients at high risk for gastrointestinal bleeding but may have a higher risk of cardiovascular toxicity.

The choice of an NSAID thus requires a balance of efficacy, cost-effectiveness, safety, and numerous personal factors (e.g., other drugs also being used, concurrent illness, compliance, age of the patient), so that there is no best NSAID for all patients. The relatively expensive, selective COX-2 inhibitors are probably safest for patients at high risk for GI bleeding, but may have a higher risk of cardiovascular toxicity. There may, however, be one or two best NSAIDs for a specific person.

Therapeutic uses

The common uses of NSAIDs are:
1. As antipyretic, acetaminophen is the ideal drug.
2. As analgesic, for headache, migraine, myalgias, arthralgias, gout, neuralgias, toothache and dysmenorrhoea.

    Paracetamol (Ig 6–8 hourly) is the oral analgesic of choice. If an unsatisfactory response is obtained, the lowest dose of one of the safer established NSAIDs (e.g., Ibuprofen) is used, the dose of which is increased if required. A trial with another NSAID (e.g., naproxen, diclofenac) is warranted if the pain is not relieved), but more than one NSAID should never be prescribed at a time.

    In gout, a potent NSAID (e.g., indomethacin) may be required, though toxicity may limit its use.

    Diflunisal for cancer pain and bone metastases and ketorolac as a substitute of morphine in mild to moderate post surgical pain has been used.

Topical preparations

NSAID creams, and gels and **capsaicin** (chilli extract) cream are safe and effective for pain relief from osteoarthritis and superficial periarticular lesions affecting hands, elbows, knees and back. They can be used as monotherapy or as an adjunct to oral NSAIDs.

Solution and gels are often used for ocular and dental inflammatory and painful conditions.

3. As anti-inflammatory, in arthritis and fibromyositis. In rheumatoid arthritis NSAIDs are indicated for initial period

(weeks or months) along with disease-modifying anti-rheumatic drugs (DMARDs) for the relief of clinical signs of inflammation till the symptoms are relieved by DMARDs.

4. As an antiplatelet, aspirin in low doses is used routinely, unless contraindicated, in cardiovascular disease.
5. Miscellaneous uses include in obstetrics (e.g. eclampsia), closure of patent ductus arteriosus, colon cancer protection.

ADJUVANT ANALGESICS

An adjuvant analgesic is a drug with a primary indication other than pain but which is analgesic in some painful condition and may enhance the effects of primary analgesia. The adjuvant analgesics are generally employed for painful conditions for which opioid analgesics and NSAIDs are not appropriate (Table 3.2).

3.4 DRUGS USED FOR RHEUMATOID ARTHRITIS

Rheumatoid arthritis (RA) is a systemic disease of unknown etiology, that is characterized by symmetrical inflammatory polyarthritis, extra-articular manifestations (rheumatoid nodules, pulmonary fibrosis, serositis, vasculitis) and serum rheumatic factor in up to 85% of patients.

Drugs used in the treatment of RA belong to three groups:
- NSAIDs
- Glucocorticoids
- Disease-modifying anti-rheumatic drugs (DMARDs).

NSAIDs

NSAIDs are used as initial therapy for RA as an adjunct to DMARDs to provide symptomatic relief of pain and inflammation. They do not prevent the degenerative changes and tissue damage responsible for the deformity and should be discontinued once a clinical response to a DMARD has been achieved.

Table 3.2: Adjuvant analgesics

Drug	Medication class	Indications	Side-effects*
Dexamethasone	Corticosteroid	Raised intracranial pressure, nerve compression, soft tissue infiltration, liver pain	Gastric irritation if used with NSAID, fluid retention, confusion, candidiasis, Cushingoid appearance, candidiasis hyperglycemia
Gabapentin	Antiepileptic	Neuropathic pain of any etiology	Mild, sedation, tremor, confusion
Carbamazepin	Antiepileptic	Neuropathic pain of any etiology	Vertigo, sedation, constipation, rash
Anitriptyline	Tricyclic antidepressant	Neuropathic pain of any etiology	Sedation, dizziness, confusion, dry mouth, constipation, urinary retention, avoid in cardiac disease
Ketamine	Induction anesthetic**	Severe neuropathic pain	Confusion, anxiety, agitation, hypertension

* In old age, all drugs can cause convulsions
** Only under specialist supervision

GLUCOCORTICOIDS

Glucocorticoids have a very rapid and dramatic anti-inflammatory action and there is evidence that systemic steroids favorably modify the disease outcome in RA, vasculitis and SLE.

Since the adverse effects of glucocorticoids are dose-and duration-dependent, the aim is always to use the smallest amount possible for the shortest time to achieve therapeutic goal.

The main indications for systemic glucocorticoids are:
- Short-term control of inflammatory arthritis whilst awaiting efficacy from DMARDs
- Maintenance therapy in RA that cannot be adequately controlled by DMARD alone.
- Systemic vasculitis.
- SLE with involvement of CNS, renal or cardiovascular systems.
- Polymyalgia rheumatica and giant cell arteritis.
- Control of inflammatory disease during pregnancy.

In RA, steroid therapy is initiated for rapid control of inflammatory disease at the same time as commencing a DMARD, and therapy is reduced and withdrawn as DMARD becomes effective.

Oral therapy

Prednisone is the oral steroid of choice. It should be given as a single morning dose to coincide with peak levels of endogenous cortisol. Potential side effects are numerous but osteoporosis, infection, diabetes, hypertension and cardiovascular disease are the major concerns. Patients on long-term oral glucocorticoids (> 7.5 mg for more than 3 months) should be given prophylactically bisphosphonates (**alendronate**) to prevent osteoporosis.

Oral administration of prednisone 5 to 20 mg daily usually is sufficient for the treatment of synovitis, whereas severe constitutional symptoms or extra-articular disease may require up to 1 mg/kg orally daily. Although alternate-day steroid therapy reduces the incidence of undesirable side effect, some patients do not tolerate the increase in symptoms that may occur on the off day.

Parenteral therapy

Parenterally steroids are used in the treatment of inflammatory arthritis, SLE and vasculitis. A single intramuscular injection of **methylprednisolone** (80–120 mg) provides immediate and effective control of inflammation for 2–6 weeks. Intravenously, it is used in high doses (500–1000 mg) along with cyclophosphamide in the treatment of SLE and vasculitis.

Local injections

Intra-articular administration may provide temporary symptomatic relief when only a few joints are inflamed. The beneficial effects of intra-articular steroids may persist for days to months and may delay or negate the need for systemic glucocorticoid therapy.

DISEASE-MODIFYING ANTIRHEUMATIC DRUGS

Disease-modifying antirheumatic drugs (DMARDs) alter the natural history of rheumatoid arthritis (RA) by reducing the progression of bony erosions and cartilage loss. Since, RA leads to long-term disability (and is associated with increased mortality), treatment with DMARDs should be initiated early and the effective drug is usually continued indefinitely at the lowest dosage to prevent relapse.

The main indications for DMARDs are:
- Rheumatoid arthritis
- Persistent inflammatory synovitis (> 6 weeks)
- systemic vasculitis
- Systemic lupus erythematosus (SLE) with cardiac, renal or CNS involvement
- As an adjunct to costicosteroid therapy in polymyalgia rheumatica and myositis

- Seronegative spondyloarthritis
- Connective tissue disease

METHOTREXATE

Methotrexate, a purine inhibitor and folic acid antagonist, is often the *first-choice* DMARD for RA. It is given as a single oral dose once week starting with 7.5 to 10 mg. Clinical response is usually noted in 4 to 8 weeks. The doses can be increased by 2.5 to 5 mg every 2 to 4 weeks to a maximum of 25 mg/week or until improvement is observed or toxicity develops.

Minor adverse effects include GI intolerance, stomatitis, rash, headache and alopecia.

Bone narrow suppression is the major side effect particularly with higher doses. Folic acid supplementation may reduce the toxicity without attenuating efficacy.

Long-term use may cause cirrhosis. Alcohol increases the risk of methotrexate hepatotoxicity. Hypersensitvity pneumonitis is a rare complication and requires withdrawal of the drug. Teretogenicity and severe liver or kidney impairment are other contraindications to its use.

SULFASALAZINE

Sulfasalazine has a good benefit-to-risk profile and is used for treatment of synovitis in the setting of RA and the seronegative spondyloarthropathies. The usual oral daily dose is 500 mg, with 500 mg increments weekly until a total daily oral dose of 2,000 to 3,000 mg is reached. Clinical response usually occurs in 6 to 10 weeks. Nausea is the principal adverse effect. Hematologic toxicity including aplastic anemia rarely occurs. Periodic monitoring of blood and platelet counts is, however, recommended.

Sulfasalazine is contraindicated in patients with glucose-6-phosphate dehydrogenase deficiency or sulfa allergy.

HYDROXYCHLOROQUINE

This antimalarial is used to treat dermatitis alopecia and synovitis in systemic lupus erythematosus (SLE) and mild synositis in RA.

It is given in 200–400 mg oral daily doses. It is also used for RA, usually in combination with other DMARDs, but has relatively weak activity and a slow onset of action (2–4 months).

The most common side effects are allergic skin eruptions and nausea. Serious ocular toxicity occurs but is rare with currently recommended dosages (200 to 400 mg). Hydroxychloroquine is contraindicated in patients with prophyria, glucose-6-phosphate dehydrogenase deficiency, or significant hepatic or renal impairment.

AZATHIOPRINE

Azathioprine is most commonly employed as a steroid sparing agent and to prevent relapse in patients with SLE and vasculitis. It is metabolized to 6-mercaptopurine (6-MP), which is then converted intracellularly to active purine thioanalogues, which inhibit DNA and RNA biosynthesis.

Nausea, diarrhea and mouth ulcers are common side effects, but hepatitis and narrow depression may also occur.

CYCLOPHOSPHAMIDE

Cyclophosphamide is mainly used as pulse therapy in the treatment of systemic vasculitis and in SLE where there is renal, cardiac or CNS involvement. It is an alkylating agent that binds DNA, RNA and proteins and is both mutagenic and teratogenic. It is inactive until converted by the cytochrome P-450 oxidase system to phosphoramide mustard and acrolein. It is usually given as pulse intravenous injections weekly or monthly. The risk of hemorrhagic cystitis can be minimized by good hydration and ingestion of **mesna**, which binds urotoxic metabolites of cyclophosphamide. Nausea, GI upset, alopecia, myelosuppression, azoospermia and anovulation are other side effects.

MYCOPHENOLATE MOFETIL

Mycophenolate mofetil (MMF) is an alternative to cyclophosphamide in inducing remission in SLE and vasculitis and is also used as maintenance therapy to prevent relapse. MMF works by inhibiting purine synthesis, but its effects are relatively specific for lymphocytes because the molecular target (inosine monophosphate dehydrogenase) plays a critical role in production of guanine nucleotides in lymphocytes. Other cells use purine salvage pathways for nucleotide production. Adverse effects include myelosuppression, diarrhea, vomiting, ulceration and hepatitis. Glucocorticoids are administrated with MMF.

LEFLUNOMIDE

Leflunomide, a pyrimidine inhibitor is indicated in the treatment of RA in patients who show poor response or in presence of contraindications to methotrexate. It is given orally in daily doses of 10 to 20 mg and clinical response is generally seen within 4–8 week.

Diarrhea is the most common side effects. Skin rash and alopecia may occur.

It is teratogenic and is contraindicated during pregnancy, in patients with significant hepatic dysfunction or on therapy with rifampin.

Gold, penicillamine and **cyclosporin** A are reserved DMARDs because of their low potency-high toxicity profile.

BIOLOGICAL DMARDs

The treatment with biological DMARDs is very expensive (about Rs 7, 50,000 annually) and because of high cost, the treatment is only indicated in active RA, failing to response to two other DMARDs (including methotrexate).

The main adverse effects of biological DMARDs include:
- Risk of serious infections
- Reactivation of latent tuberculosis
- Possible increased risk of malignancy

Cardiovascular, liver, kidney function are usually monitored with the use of DMARDs.

Anticytokine therapies directed at specific cytokine have been developed.

TNF inhibitors are used for the treatment of RA and seronegative spondyloarthropathies and vasculitis. These agents are used in patients who have failed to respond to earlier DMARDs. The effects of these agents may be dramatic in relieving the symptoms within 1 to 2 weeks. In addition to their symptomatic benefits these agents retard joint damage significantly. Three preparations are available with similar efficacy and toxicity profiles. Methotrexate is commonly used with TNF inhibitors as it results in additive efficacy and a decrease in the formation of HACAs (human autochimeric antibodies) against the TNF blocker. They are given parentally.

ELAMERCEPT is a fusion protein that consists of the ligand-binding portion of the human TNF receptors linked to Fc portion of human immunoglobulin G (IgG). It binds to TNF, blocking its interaction with cell surface receptors, thus inhibiting the inflammatory and immunomodulatory properties of TNF.

INFLIXIMAB is a chimeric monoclonal antibody that binds specifically to human TNF-α blocking proinflammatory and immunomodulatory effects.

ADALIMUMAB is a recombinant human IgG-1 monoclonal antibody that is specific to human TNF-α.

The important side effects of TNF-blocking drugs are severe infections and sepsis. Upper respiratory and sinus infections are most common. Reactivation of dormant tubercular infection may occur and tuberculosis should be ruled out by a tuberculin skin test and chest radiograph before starting the therapy. Other side effects may include injection site reactions, induction of antinuclear antibodies and rarely, a lupus-like illness. A demyelinating disorder has been described as well as exacerbations of pre-existing multiple sclerosis. Frequency of occurrence of lymphomas may be increased. There is also evidence of a possible increased risk of malignancy.

TNF inhibitors are contraindicated in patients with acute or chronic infection and in CHF.

INTERLEUKIN INHIBITORS

ANAKINRA is a recombinant IL-1 receptor antagonist, thus inhibiting the proinflammatory and immunomodulatory actions of IL-1 in RA.

TORCILIZUMAB is antagonist of soluble and membrane bound IL-6 receptors and is useful in RA. Adverse effects include injection site reaction and increased frequency of infections.

B-CELL-DIRECTED THERAPY

RITUXIMAB is a monoclonal antibody directed against CD 20, cell surface receptor found on B cells. It depletes B cells from peripheral blood. Methotrexate is generally used as background therapy. It is a toxic drug and is only indicated in patients, who fail to response to other biological DMARDs. Infusion reactions are common and antihistamine, IV steroids, and paracetamol are routinely given prior to infusion.

Rituximab rarely causes reactivation of JC virus leading to clinical syndrome of progressive multifocal leukoencephalopathy, which is uniformly fatal.

ABATACEPT

Abatacept is a fusion protein comprising the CTLA4 molecule and the Fc portion of IgG1. It blocks selective costimulation of T cells and is indicated in patients with inadequate response to biologic or non-biologic DMARDs.

Combination therapy including two biologic agents in contraindicated because of increased infection complication.

3.5 ANTI GOUT DRUGS

Gout is a metabolic disease of a heterogeneous nature and is characterized early by a recurring acute arthritis. The characteristic lesion is the tophus, a nodular deposit of monosodium urate monohydrate crystals with an associated foreign body reaction.

Tophi are found in cartilage, subcutaneous and periarticular tissues, tendon, bone, the kidneys, and elsewhere. Urates have been demonstrated in the synovial tissues (and fluids) and the acute inflammation of gout is believed to be activated by the phagocytosis by polymorphonuclear cells of urate crystals with the ensuing release from the neutrophils inflammatory mediators.

The acute attack

NSAIDs (except aspirin), colchicine or glucocorticoids are the main drugs for treatment of an acute attack of gout.

NSAIDs

These are the drugs of choice for treatment of acute gout. The effective drugs are any of NSAID with a short half-life and include indomethacin, naproxen, ibuprofen and diclofenac. Acute peptic ulcer disease, impaired renal function, and a history of allergic reactions to NSAIDs are contraindications.

COLCHICINE

Colchicine given orally is a traditional and effective treatment for acute gouty arthritis if used early in the attack.

Colchicine is an alkaloid isolated from the autumn crocus, *Colchicum autumnale*.

Pharmacokinetics

Colchicine is readily absorbed after oral administration with peak plasma level within 2 hours and a serum half-life of 9 hours. Metabolites are excreted in the intestinal tract and urine.

Pharmacodynamics

Colchicine is not an analgesic drug. It only relieves pain and inflammation of gouty arthritis without influencing the uric acid metabolism. Its anti-inflammatory effects in gout are due to inhibition of the proliferation of neutrophils and release of inflammatory mediators.

Indications

Colchicine is not commonly used to treat gout, but is useful when NSAIDs or glucocorticoids are contraindicated or not tolerated.

In acute gout colchicine is most effective if given in the first 12 to 24 hours. The dosage during acute attack is 0.6 mg tablet given every 6 hours with subsequent tapering. This is generally better tolerated than the formerly advised hourly regimen. The drug must be stopped promptly at the first sign of loose stools. It is no longer used by intravenous route.

In chronic gout colchicine (0.6 mg once or twice daily) can be used prophylactically for acute attacks and for a few days before manipulation of the uric acid level to prevent precipitation of acute attack.

Aspirin (uricoretentive), diuretics, large alcohol intake and food high in purines should be avoided.

Adverse effects

Colchicine often causes diarrhea and may occasionally cause nausea, vomiting and abdominal pain. Hepatic necrosis, acute renal failure, disseminated intravascular coagulation, and seizures have been observed.

Colchicine, rarely, may cause alopecia, bone narrow depression, peripheral neuritis, myopathy, and in some case even death.

GLUCOCORTICOIDS

Glucocorticoids are useful when NSAIDs are contraindicated. They often give dramatic symptomatic relief in acute episodes of gout and control most attacks.

Prednisone 30–50 mg/d is the initial dose which is gradually tapered with the resolution of the attack in polyarticular gout.

For a single joint or a few involved joints intra-articular **triamcinolone acetonide** 20–40 mg or **methylprednisolone** 25–30 mg has been effective and well tolerated.

ANAKINRA

Pathophysiologic events occurring in a gouty joint involves the role of interleukin-IB inflammatory mediator. Anakinra a biological agent is interleukin-1 receptor antagonist and has efficacy for the management of acute gout.

Long-term management

Once an acute attack has settled, uric acid lowering drugs are used to bring the serum uric acid level at or below 5 mg/dl, which allows existing crystals to dissolve and prevents new ones forming.

Urate lowering therapy should be initiated in patients with:
- Recurrent attacks of acute gout
- Tophi
- Evidence of bone or joint damage
- Associated renal disease or nephrolithiasis
- Gout with greatly elevated serum uric acid

The drugs which lower the serum uric acid belong to following two groups:
- The uricosuric drugs
- Xanthine oxidase inhibitors

URICOSURIC DRUGS

Uricosuric drugs block the tubular reabsorption of filtered urate and reduce the metabolic urate pool. The formation of new tophi is prevented and the size of the existing tophi is reduced. When administered concomitantly with colchicine, they may lessen the frequency of recurrences of acute gout. The indication for uricosuric treatment is the increasing frequency or severity of acute attacks.

Uricosuric drugs are ineffective in patients with an estimated glomerular filtration rate of <60 ml/min.

Probenecid and **Sulfinpyrazone** are uricosuric drugs employed.

Uricosuric therapy should be initiated in gouty underexcretion of uric acid when xanthine oxidase inhibitors are contraindicated or when tophi are present. Therapy should not be started until 2–3 weeks after an acute attack.

Adverse effects

Both probenecid and sulfinpyrazone cause adverse effects like gastrointestinal irritation, rash and rarely aplastic anemia. Nephrotic syndrome may occur after the use of probenecid. It is essential to maintain a large urine volume to minimize the possibility of stone formation.

Uricosuric drugs are contraindicated in over-producers, in those with renal impairment and in urolithiasis (they increase stone formation).

BENZBROMARONE

Benzbromarone can be effective and safe uricosuric in mild to moderate renal impairment but can rarely cause hepatotoxicity.

XANTHINE OXIDASE INHIBITORS

Inhbitors of xanthine oxidase are of special value in uric acid overproducers; in tophaceous gout; in patients unresponsive to the uricosuric regimen; and in gouty patients with uric acid renal calculi. Asymptomatic hyperuricemia requires no treatment.

Uric acid synthesis inhibitors drugs commonly provoke acute attacks, so prophylaxis with colchicine or NSAID is required for the initial 6 months.

ALLOPURINOL

Allopurinol, the uric acid synthesis inhibitor, is the drug of choice. It is a xanthine oxidase inhibitor, which reduces the conversion of hypoxanthine and xanthine to uric acid. It is long-acting and given only once a day in doses of 100 mg, which is gradually, increased in 100 mg increments until the therapeutic target of serum uric acid is achieved (maximum 900 mg/daily). In most cases the therapy will need to be continued indefinitely.

Allopurinol is well tolerated and is widely used, especially in patients with renal impairment or with urate stones, where uricosuric drugs cannot be used.

Adverse effects

Hypersensitivity to allopurinol occurs in 2% of cases and can be life-threatening. Allopurinol in patients allergic to penicillin and ampicillin are the most vulnerable to serious side effects such as epidermal necrolysis, vasculitis, bone marrow depression, granulomatous hepatitis and renal failure. It should be used with caution during pregnancy, in elderly and in children.

FEBUXOSTAT

Febuxostat is nonpurine xanthine oxidase inhibitor that is useful in patients in whom allopurinol is not tolerated or contraindicated.

Febuxostat is well absorbed orally, extensively metabolized in the liver and less than 5% is excreted in the urine as unchanged drug. Since it is highly metabolized to inactive metabolites, no dosage adjustment is necessary for patients with renal impairment.

Adverse effects

The most frequent treatment-related adverse events are liver function abnormalities, diarrhea, headache and nausea.

Febuxostat may be associated with a slightly higher rate of fatal and non-fatal cardiovascular events than allopurinol.

PEGLOTICASE

Pegloticase is a new urate lowering biologic drug that can be effective in patients allergic to or unresponsive to xanthine oxidase inhibitors.

3.6 ANTIMIGRAINE DRUGS

Migraine headache

Migraine in its 'classic' form is characterized by an aura, which may involve nausea; vomiting and visual scotomas followed by a severe throbbing unilateral headache that lasts for a few hours to 1–2 days.

Migraine involves the trigeminal nerve distribution to intracranial arteries. These nerves release peptide neurotransmitters especially calcitonin gene-related peptide (CGRP), an extremely powerful vasodilator. Substance P and neurokinin A may also be involved.

Management of migraine consists of avoidance of any precipitating factor, together with prophylactic or symptomatic pharmacologic treatment.

Symptomatic treatment

The mainstay of pharmacologic therapy is the judicious use of one or more of the many drugs that are effective in an acute attack of migraine. The drugs that are effective in the treatment of migraine belong to three major pharmacologic classes: NSAIDs, 5-HT receptor agonists and dopamine receptor antagonists.

NSAIDs

NSAIDs significantly reduce both the severity and duration of a migraine attack. They are most effective when taken early in the migraine attack. However, NSAIDs are less effective in moderate or severe migraine attack. The combination of aspirin and metoclopramide is as effective as a single dose of sumatriptan. The most commonly used NSAID is naproxen which has a longer duration of action. Important side-effects of NSAIDs include dyspepsia and gastrointestinal irritation.

5-HT$_1$ RECEPTOR AGONISTS

Stimulation of 5-HT$_1$ receptor can stop an acute migraine attack. Ergotamine and dihydroergotamine are non-selective receptor agonists, while the triptans are selective 5-HT receptor agonists.

A variety of triptans, 5-HT$_1$ receptors agonists—**naratriptan, rizatriptan, eletriptan, sumatriptan, zolmitriptan, almotriptan, and frovatriptan** are useful in migraine. Each drug in the triptan class has similar pharmacological properties but varies slightly in terms of clinical efficacy.

Rizatriptan and eletriptan are the most efficacious of the triptans.

Clinical efficacy appears to be related more to the t_{max} (time to peak plasma level) than to the potency, half-life or bioavailability.

Zolmitriptan has high bioavailability after oral absorption and is effective for the immediate treatment of migraine.

Triptans may cause nausea and vomiting. They should be avoided during pregnancy, in patients with hemiplegic or basilar migraine, and in patients with risk factors for stroke (such as hypertension, prior stroke or transient ischemic attacks, diabetes mellitus, hypercholesterolemia, obesity). Triptans are contraindicated in patients with coronary or peripheral vascular disease. Combination therapy with triptan and naproxen provide greater benefit. Unfortunately, monotherapy with a selective oral 5-HT$_1$ agonist does not result in rapid, consistent, and complete relief of migraine in all patients.

Side effects are common, though often mild and transient. Recurrence of headache is important limitation of tirptan use. Combination of a longer-acting NSAID (naproxen 500 mg) with sumatriptan augments the initial effect of sumatriptan and, more importantly reduces rates of headache recurrence.

Ergotamine is quite effective and oral formulation contains caffeine (theoretically to enhance ergotamine absorption) which possibly adds additional analgesic activity. In general ergotamine appears to have a higher incidence of nausea than triptan, but less headache recurrence.

Nasal

Nasal preparations of dihydroergotamine and zolmitriptan or sumatriplan are fast acting (nonparenteral) and give substantial blood levels within 30–60 minutes. Inhaled dihydroergotamine produce rapid onset of action with good tolerability.

Parenteral

Parenteral administration of dihydroergotamine and sumatriptan produce immediate relief, peak plasma being achieved within 3 minutes after IV dosing.

DOPAMINE ANTAGONISTS

Oral

Oral dopamine antagonists serve as adjunct therapy in migraine. **Metoclopramide** is indicated with oral NSAIDs and/or triptan to enhance gastric absorption in severe attacks. Metoclopromide has the added advantage of decreasing nausea/vomiting and restoring normal gastric motility.

Parenteral

Dopamine antagonists are of significant value in refractory cases of acute migraine. Intravenous administration of **prochlorperazine** and **dihydroergotamine** is used in severe migraine.

OTHER DRUGS

Opioid analgesics are sometimes required when other therapies fail. Intravenous **propofol** in subanaesthetic doses may help in intractable cases.

Preventive therapy

Preventive therapy is indicated in patients having migraine attacks frequently more than two or three times a month or with attacks that are unresponsive to abortive treatments. Significant side effects are associated with the use of many of these agents. The commonly used drugs for prophylaxis are listed in Table 3.3. The mechanism of these drugs is unclear but may involve alteration of central neurotransmitters.

Other drugs have also been used before the headaches are brought under control. These include cardiovascular drugs **candesartan, timolol, selective serotonin reuptake inhibitors** (SSRIs) and **botulinum toxin A** injection. If the patient remains headache-free, the dose may be tapered and the drug is eventually withdrawn.

3.7 ANTIEPILEPTIC DRUGS

Epilepsy is characterized by recurrent unprovoked seizures. Antiepileptic drugs are used with the goal of preventing further attacks and are continued until there have been no seizures for at least three years. In 80% of patients, whose epilepsy is controllable, only the use of a single drug is recommended. The combination of additional drug is required in refractory cases. Patients who have focal epilepsy related to an underlying structural lesion or those with multiple seizure types and developmental delay are particularly likely to require multiple drugs. There are

Table 3.3: Prophylactic treatment of migraine

Drug	Pharmacologic class	Significant adverse effects
First-line drugs		
Amitryptiline	Antidepressant	Drowsiness, weight gain
Propanolol	Beta blocker	Fatigue, hypotension, contraindicated in asthma
Topiramate	Antiepileptic	Paresthesia, cognitive symptoms, weight loss, glaucoma
Valproic acid	Antiepileptic	Drowsiness, alopecia, weight gain, tremor, hepatotoxicity
Gabapentin	Antiepileptic	Sedation
Second line drugs		
Methysergide	Serotogenic	Alopecia, leg cramps, retroperitoneal fibrosis
Phenelzine	MAO inhibitor	Hypotension, drowsiness tremor, sexual dysfunction

currently no clear guidelines for rational polypharmacy although in theory a continuation of drugs with different mechanisms of action may be most useful.

Although, there are now a number of drugs which are useful in controlling epilepsy, the first choice should be one of the established first-line drugs (Table 3.4), with the more recently introduced drug as secondary choice. Carbamazepine, lamotrigine and sodium valproate are preferable to phenytoin as first-line drug because of the side-effect profile and complicated pharmacokinetics of the latter.

Mechanism action

The inhibitory transmitter γ-aminobutyric acid (GABA) is particularly important in limiting hypersynchronous, repetitive discharge from the cerebral cortex in the brain involving large groups of neurons. Drugs that block GABA receptors provoke seizures. Conversely, excessive stimulation by excitatory neurotransmitters, such as acetylcholine, glutamate and aspartate, provoke seizure activity.

Table 3.4: Types of epilepsy (seizures) and choice of antiepileptic drug

Epilepsy type	First-line	Second-line	Third-line
Partial and/or secondary GTCS	Carbamazepine	Lamotrigine Valproate Levetiracetam Topiramate	Tiagabine Pregabalin Gabapentin Clobazam Phenytoin Primidone Phenobarbital Oxcarbazepine Vigabatrin Acetazolamide
Primary GTCS	Sodium valproate	Lamotrigine Topiramate	Carbamazepine Phenytoin Gabapentin Pregabalin Primidone, Phenobarbital Tiagabine Acetazolamide
Absence	Ethosuximide	Valproate	Lamotrigine Clonazepam Acetazolamide
Myoclonic	Sodium valproate	Clonazepam	Piracetam, Levetiracetam Lamotrigine Phenobarbital

GTCS: Generalize tonic-clonic seizures

Most of the antiepileptic drugs act by increasing the activity of the inhibitory neurotransmitter GABA or by inhibition of the activity of excitatory neurotransmitters. Some act by directly blocking sodium and/or calcium channels in the nerve cell membrane.

PHENYTOIN

Phenytoin is the oldest non-sedative antiepileptic drug. Chemically it is diphenylhydantoin.

Pharmacokinetics

Oral absorption is slow but is complete (80–90%). Absorption after intramuscular injection is unpredictable as some drug precipitation in the muscle occurs. Fosphenytoin, a prodrug of phenytoin is water soluble and is well absorbed and is preferred in status epilepticus where parenteral administration is required.

Phenytoin is more than 90% bound to plasma protein, largely metabolized and only a small proportion of the dose is excreted in urine unchanged. It is a potent enzyme inducer. The elimination of phenytion is dose-dependent and follows saturation (mixed order) kinetics. At very low blood levels, phenytoin metabolism follows first-order kinetics. However, as blood levels rise within the therapeutic range, the maximum capacity of the liver to metabolize phenytoin is approached. Further increase in dosage may produce very large changes in blood concentrations leading to development of symptoms of toxicity. Periodic assessment of plasma concentration may therefore be necessary.

The main use of phenytoin (fosphenytoin IV infusion) is in the management of status epilepticus when seizures fail to be controlled by diazepam.

Adverse effects

Diplopia and ataxia are the most common dose-related adverse effects, requiring dose adjustment. Gingival hyperplasia and hirsutism occur to some degree in most of the patients. Long-term use is associated in some patients with coarsening of facial features and mild neuropathy. Long-term use may result in abnormalities of vitamin D metabolism, leading to osteomalacia. Low folate levels and megaloblastic anemia have been reported.

Idiosyncratic reactions and hematological complication (agranulocytosis) are rare.

Lymphadenopathy is another complication with possibility of a causal relationship between phenytoin and Hodgkin's disease.

SODIUM VALPROATE (VALPROIC ACID)

It is the valproate ion, which is the active form and absorbed from GIT, regardless of whether valporic acid or a salt of the acid is administrated.

Mechanism of action

The drug owes its activity to more than one molecular activity, which accounts for its broad spectrum antiepileptic activity.

Its mechanism of action is likely due to:
- Blockade of use-dependent Na^+ channels leading to reduction of sustained high frequency neuronal firing.
- Inhibition of GABA transminase and activation of glutamic acid decarboxylase-both the mechanism increase GABA concentration in the brain.
- Inhibition of Ca^{2+} influx.
- Decrease of the release of excitatory neurotransmitter aspartate in the brain.

Pharmacokinetics

Valproate is well absorbed with bioavailability of greater than 80%. Food delays absorption, but also reduces the toxicity. It is 90% bound to plasma proteins and displaces phenytoin from plasma protein.

It is a potent enzyme inhibitor and inhibits the metabolism of several drugs, including phenobarbital, phenytoin, and carbamazepine, which may result in serious toxicity.

Valproate dramatically decreases the clearance of lamotrigine.

Therapeutic uses

Valproate has a border spectrum of antiepileptic activity. It is very effective against absence seizures and is usually preferred if the patient has concomitant generalized tonic-clonic attacks and myoclonic seizures. The drug is effective in primary generalized tonic-clonic seizures. A few patients of atonic attacks and many cases of partial seizures also respond with valproic acid. It is also a drug of choice for Lennox-Gastaut syndrome and for infantile spasm.

Other uses of valproate include management of bipolar disorder, trigeminal neuralgia and migraine prophylaxis.

Therapy is guided by clinical assessment rather than valproate plasma levels.

Adverse effects

The most common side effects are gastrointestinal disorders. Other reversible adverse effects include tremor, weight gain, increased appetite and hair loss.

The most serious adverse effect is idiosyncratic hepatotoxicity, especially in children under 2 years of age, which may be even fatal. Routine liver function tests need monitoring.

CARBAMAZEPINE

It is structurally related to tricyclic antidepressants.

Mechanism of action

The mechanism of action is similar to phenytoin. Carbamazepine blocks the Na+ channels and inhibits high-frequency repetitive firing in neurons. It potentiates the post-synaptic actions of GABA.

Pharmacokinetics

Carbamazepine taken after meals permits the use of full therapeutic doses with minimum side effects. It is mainly distributed in brain, liver, and kidneys. It is completely metabolized. It is however, a poor enzyme inducer.

Therapeutic use

It is the drug of choice for partial as well as generalized tonic-clonic seizures. Its use is contraindicated in absence seizures. Carbamazepine is not sedative in therapeutic doses.

It is also a drug of first choice for trigeminal neuralgia, though older patients may tolerate it poorly, with ataxia and unsteadiness. It is also effective in some patients with mania (bipolar disorder).

Drug interactions

The increased metabolic capacity of the hepatic enzymes may cause a reduction in steady-state carbamazepine concentration and an increased metabolism of several other antiepileptic drugs.

Adverse effects

The overall incidence of toxicity of carbamazepine seems to be fairly low. The most common dose-related adverse effects are diplopia and ataxia. Other effects include GIT upsets and drowsiness. The drug can cause allergic reactions such as rashes and fever.

Carbamazepine may cause serious idiosyncratic blood dyscrasias including fatal cases of aplastic anemia and agranulocytosis especially in elderly patients with trigeminal neuralgia.

OXCARBAZEPINE

Oxcarbazepine is closely related to carbamazepine and is less potent in epileptic patients. It is liable to cause fewer hypersensitivity reactions and less induction of hepatic enzymes.

ETHOSUXIMIDE

Ethosuximide has a very narrow spectrum of activity, being effective against only absence (petitmal) seizures. If other type of epilepsy is present; it can be combined with other suitable antiseizure drug. It is comparatively less toxic, has a lesser degree of teratogenic effect and drug interaction as compared to other antiepileptic drugs. Valproic acid inhibits ethosuximide metabolism and results in its higher steady state plasma concentration.

Ethosuximide inhibits low threshold (T types) Ca^{2+} channels in thalamic neurons responsible for generating the rhythmic cortical discharge of an absence attacks.

Ethosuximide is completely absorbed after oral administration, is not protein bound and is uniformly distributed in CNS, milk, saliva and fetal tissues but not in fat. It is completely metabolized in liver and its inactive metabolites are excreted through urine.

Adverse effects

The most common adverse effects of ethosuximide are gastrointestinal. Other dose related adverse effects are transient lethargy and, much less commonly, headache, dizziness, hiccup, and euphoria. Behavioral changes are usually in the directions of improvement.

Idiosyncratic adverse effects are extremely uncommon.

LAMOTRIGINE

Lamotrigine is a broad spectrum antiepileptic drug being effective in partial, generalized tonic-clonic, secondary generalized, absence and myoclonic seizures. It directly blocks sodium and calcium channels in the nerve cell membrane. Lamotrigine also decreases the synaptic release of glutamate.

Lamotrigine is well absorbed orally and metabolized in the liver. Enzyme inducers decrease, while enzyme inhibitors (e.g., valproic acid) increase the half life of lamotrigine.

Adverse effects include dizziness, headache, ataxia, diplopia and skin rash (more common in children below 16 years).

CLONAZEPAM

Clonazepam is one of the most potent antiseizure benzodiazepine. It is a long-acting drug effective against absence seizures, myoclonic seizures and in some cases of infantile spasm. Treatment is started with small doses, as sedation is prominent on initiation of therapy.

TOPIRAMATE

Topiramate, a broad spectrum antiepileptic drug, acts by multiple mechanisms, which includes blockade of voltagegated sodium channels, potentiation of the inhibitory effects of GABA at sites different from benzodiazepine or barbiturate, and inhibition of kainate receptors for glutamate.

Topiramate is effective against generalized tonic-clonic, partial and absence seizure as well as for Lennox-Gastaut syndrome and West's syndrome.

Adverse effects include CNS depression, somnolence, amnesia and urolithiasis. Acute myopia and glaucoma requires drug withdrawal.

LEVETIRACETAM

Levetiracetam is used specifically for treating partial seizures. It is also effective against myoclonic seizures of juvenile epilepsy as an alternative to major antiepileptic drugs because of a better pharmacokinetic profile.

Its exact mechanism of action is uncertain, but may be related to modification of the synaptic release of glutamate and GABA.

Adverse effects include somnolence, asthenia, ataxia, and dizziness.

OTHER DRUGS

Third-line antiepileptic drug are rarely used and their main adverse effects are given below:

Tiagabine	Confusion, sedation, depression, paresthesias, psychosis
Pregabalin	Somnolence, dizziness, ataxia
Gabapentin	Somnolence, dizziness, ataxia, fatigue, weight gain, edema
Clobazam	Sedation
Primidone	Sedation, confusion, depression, alaxia, hyperactivity
Phenobarbital	Sedation, confusion, depression, alaxia, hyperactivity
Vigabatrin	Drowsiness, dizziness, psychosis, visual field loss
Acetazalomide	Metabolic acidosis, renal stones, hyperammonemia in cirrhotics

STATUS EPILEPTICUS

Status epilepticus is a medical emergency. An intravenous bolus of **lorazepam** 6 mg is given and repeated once after 5 minutes, if necessary: Alternatively diazepam 10 mg can be given. There is high risk of thrombophlebitis with diazepam, which is minimized by giving diazepam emulsion (as **Diazemuls**). Diazepam can also be given rectally as a gel.

Regardless of the response to lorazepan or diazepam: phenytoin or better **fosphenytoin** 25 mg/kgis is given intravenously to provide initiation of long-term seizure control.

If seizures continue, **phenobarbital** is given in a loading dose of 10–20 mg/kg intravenously. Respiratory depression and hypotension are especially common with this therapy. Alternatively or additionally intravenous valproate 25 mg/kg is used for status epileptius with success.

If these measures fail, general anesthetics with ventilating assistance may be required.

Intravenous **propofol** or **midazolam** may provide control of refractory status epilepticus.

After status epilepticus is controlled an oral drug program for the long-term management of seizures is started.

ANTIEPILEPTICS AND PREGNANCY

Antiepileptic drugs given during pregnancy are associated with an increased risk of fetal malformations.

Carbamazepine, phenytoin and **valproate** carry the risk of neural tube and other defects. To counteract the risk of congenital defects, women should receive **folic acid** (5 mg) daily throughout pregnancy.

In view of the risk of neonatal bleeding associated with carbamazepine, phenobarbitone and phenytoin, prophylactic **vitamin K** is recommended before the delivery.

Antiepileptic drugs induce liver enzymes and thus increase the rate of breakdown of oral contraceptives, which requires necessary changes in the patient's method of contraception.

ECLAMPSIA

Magnesium sulphate intravenously is the most effective drug to control convulsions in eclampsia. It relieves cerebral ischemia by vasodilation and minimizes brain damage. Diazepam or phenytoin is the alternatives.

3.8 ANTIPARKINSONIAN DRUGS

Parkinson's disease is a chronic, progressive neurodegenerative condition which affects the basal ganglia. It is characterized by differing combinations of slowness of movements (bradykinesia), increased tone (rigidity), tremor and loss of postural reflexes (postural instability).

Idiopathic Parkinsonism is due to atrophic changes in substantia nigra leading to depletion of dopaminergic neurons, which results in a neurohumoral imbalance between acetylcholine and dopamine. The drug therapy aims to correct this imbalance by the use of dopaminergic or anticholinergic drugs.

Drugs which increase dopamine activity (Fig. 3.2) can be classified as:

- Drugs that *replace dopamine*
- Drugs that act as *dopamine agonists* (stimulate) at dopamine receptors or nerves in the corpus striatum normally supplied by dopaminergic nerves form the substantia nigra.
- Drugs that *stimulate the release* of dopamine from dopaminenergic nerve terminals in corpus striatum.
- Drugs that *block the breakdown of dopamine* after it has been released from surviving dopaminergic nerve terminals in the corpus striatum. These are of two main types:
  - Monoamine oxidase inhibitor-B
  - Drugs that block the enzyme COMT (Catechol O-methyl transferase).

LEVODOPA

Dopamine does not cross the blood–brain barrier. Levodopa, the metabolic precursor of dopamine enters the brain, where it is decarboxylated to dopamine.

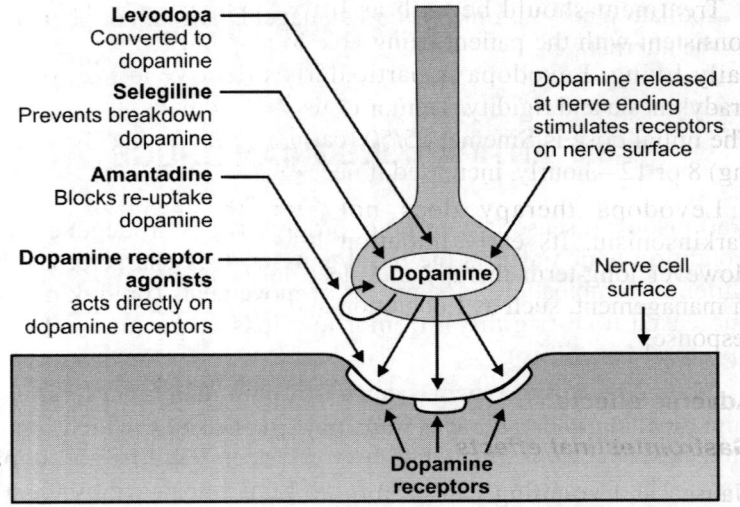

Fig. 3.2: Site of action of dopaminergic drugs used in Parkinson's disease.

If levodopa is administered orally, more than 90% is decarboxylated to dopamine peripherally in the gastrointestinal tract and blood vessels, and only a small portion reaches the brain. This peripheral conversion of levodopa is responsible for the high incidence of side-effects, if it is used alone. The problem is largely overcome by giving a decarboxylase inhibitor, that does not cross the blood brain barrier along with the levodopa.

Two peripheral decarboxylase inhibitors, **carbidopa** and **benserazide** are available as combination preparation with levodopa – **Sinemet** (carbidopa + levodopa) and **Madopar** (benserazide + levodopa).

Therapeutic uses

Levodopa therapy should only be initiated when there is significant disability, to avoid long-term side effects at doses that were well tolerated initially. It may be advisable to initiate treatment with a dopamine agonist, or a slow release preparation (oral sustained – release Sinemet (R).

Treatment should be with as little medication as possible consistent with the patient being able to perform the activities of daily living. Levodopa is particularly effective at improving bradykinesia and rigidity. Tremor is also helped but unpredictably. The initial dose is Sinemet 25/50 (carbidopa 25 mg, levodopa 50 mg) 8 or 12 – hourly, increased if necessary up to 1000 mg/day.

Levodopa therapy does not stop the progression of Parkinsonism. Its early initiation lowers the mortality rates. However long-term therapy may lead to a number of problems in management, such as fluctuation and unpredictable changes in response.

Adverse effects

Gastrointestinal effects

Nausea and vomiting can be minimized by taking the drug in divided doses, with or immediately after meals, and by increasing the total dose very slowly. Antacids taken 30–60 minutes before the drug may be helpful. A peripheral dopamine antagonist such as domperidone may offset the gastrointestinal symptoms.

Antiemetic such as phenothiazines should be avoided as they may exacerbate the disease.

Cardiovasular effects

Postural hypotension is common, but often asymptomatic, and tends to diminish with continuing therapy.

Dyskinesias

Dose-related involuntary movements, particularly orofacial dyskinesias and limb and axial dystonias occur in up to 80% of patients receiving levodopa therapy for long periods.

Behavioral effects

A wide variety of adverse mental effects have been reported, including depression, hallucinations, delusions, change in personality with increased (sometimes pathological) gambling, hypersexuality and drug (levodopa)-seeking behavior. They are precipitated by incurrent illness or operation. It may be necessary to reduce or withdraw the medication.

Several atypical antipsychotic agents that have low affinity for dopamine D_2 receptors (clozapine, olanzapine, quetiapine and risperidone) are now available and may be particularly helpful in counteracting such behavioral complications.

Fluctuations in response

Patients receiving long-term levodopa therapy commonly experiences a 'wearing off effect', which means that the duration of benefit usually shortens with each dose of levodopa as the therapy progresses.

Patient can also develop sudden, unpredictable fluctuations between mobility and immobility characterized by 'on-off phenomenon'. In the 'on state' the patient enjoys normal mobility, which is followed by the 'off state' wherein the patient may be unable to rise from the chair on which he had set down a few minutes ago.

Levodopa has a very short half life (1–2 hrs), which causes such fluctuations in its plasma concentration. The 'on-off' phenomenon is difficult to treat, but sometimes subcutaneous injections of apomorphine, (a dopamine agonist) are helpful to 'rescue' the patient rapidly from an 'off' period.

Miscellaneous adverse effects

These are rare, and include blood dyscrasias, aggravation or precipitation of gout, and abnormalities of smell or taste.

Contraindications

Levodopa should not be used alone, but is given combined with carbidopa. It is contraindicated in psychotic patients because it may exacerbate the mental disturbances. It should not be given in patients with angle closure glaucoma and should be used with care in patients with a history of melanoma or with suspicious skin lesions, because it is a precursor of skin melanin and may activate malignant melanoma.

DOPAMINE RECEPTOR AGONISTS

Large numbers of these drugs are available. They all have slightly different activity at the various dopamine receptors in the brain.

Apomorphine

Apomorphine hydrochloride (Apoky), a potent dopamine agonist, is effective for the temporary relief ("rescue") of off-periods of akinesia associated with prolong use of levodopa.

The most common side-effect of the drugs is marked vomiting and the drug has to be given parenterally. The vomiting can be overcome by concomitant use of domperidone, and parenteral administration achieved through continuous subcutaneous infusion form a portable pump, or by direct injection as needed.

Ergot derivatives

Ergot derivatives (**bromocriptine, lisuride, pergolide** and **cabergoline**) and non-ergot derivatives (**ropinirole** and **pramipexole**) can be taken orally, and **rotigoline** which can be administered as a transdermal patch.

Ergot derivative dopamine agonists have been found to be associated with development of fibrotic reactions and thickening of heart valves and their use is no longer advised.

Dopamine receptor agonists are less powerful than levodopa in controlling symptoms of Parkinsonism, but they are much less likely to cause dose fluctuations or dyskinesia, though they will certainly exacerbate the latter once these have developed.

Dopamine agonists have an important role as first-line therapy for Parkinson's disease. In consequence, dopaminergic therapy may best be initiated with a dopamine agonist. Alternatively, it can be used with low doses of levodopa (Sinemet – 25/100 thrice daily). The dose of dopamine agonist is subsequently increased gradually depending on response and tolerance.

Dopamine agonists are effective in patients who are resistant to treatment with levodopa. However, the response to dopamine agonists is disappointing in patients who have never responded to levodopa.

Newer dopamine agonists

The newer dopamine agonists **pramipexole** (prefential D_3 agonist) and **ropinirole** (pure D_2 agonist) are used as monotherapy for mild Parkinsonism and are also useful in patients with advanced disease, in lowering the dose of levodopa and smoothing out response of fluctuations. They also have a neuroprotective action on dopaminergic neurons. Orally administered, pramipexole is excreted largely unchanged in urine while ropinirole is mainly metabolized by liver.

Rotigotine is administered as a transdermal patch for mild Parkinsonism, but is no longer recommended because of crystal formation on the patches, affecting the availability and efficacy of the agonist.

Adverse effects

Gastrointestinal and cardiovascular effects and dyskinesias, similar to those introduced by levodopa may occur, which can be reversed by reducing the total dose being taken.

Confusion, hallucinations, delusions, and other psychiatric reactions are potential complications and are more common and severe with dopamine agonists then with levodopa.

Contraindications

Dopamine agonists are contraindicated in patients with a history of psychotic illness or recent myocardial infarction or with active peptic ulceration.

AMANTADINE

Amantadine, an antiviral drug, stimulates the release of dopamine and blocks its re-uptake by dopaminergic nerve terminals in the corpus striatum. This results in an increased concentration of endogenously released dopamine at the receptor site. It is not as effective as levodopa, but has the advantage of being relatively free from side effects.

Amantadine can be particularly useful in controlling the dyskinesias produced by dopaminergic treatment later in the disease.

Adverse effects

Nausea, insomnia, convulsions and hallucinations, swelling of the ankles and rarely leucopenia, rashes and livado reticularis are common.

Contraindications

Amantadine is contraindicated in epilepsy, renal disease, pregnancy, breast-feeding and peptic ulcer.

MONOAMINE OXIDASE INHIBITORS

Two types of monoamine oxidase – MAO-A and MAO-B are found in the nervous system. MAO-A metabolizes noradrenalin, serotonin and dopamine while MAO-B metabolizes dopamine selectively.

Selegiline and **rasagiline** are selective inhibitors of MAO-B, and have mild therapeutic effect in Parkinsonism. These selective MAO-B inhibitors enhance and prolong the antiparkinsonism effect of levodopa and may reduce mild on-off or wearing-off phenomena. They are used as adjunctive therapy, which permits the use of smaller doses of levodopa.

CATECHOL-O-METHYLETRANSFERASE (COMT) INHIBITORS

COMT metabolizes catecholamine including dopamine and its precursor levodopa, producing the inactive metabolite 3–0-methyldopa. The therapeutic block of dopamine by decarboxylase inhibitor carbidopa activates COMT- mediated metabolic pathway of levodopa leading to production of inactive metabolite 3-O methyldopa (3-OMD) with a loss of levodopa. Moreover, 3-MOD competes with levodopa for an active carrier mechanism that governs its transport across the intestinal mucosa and blood brain barrier.

Selective COMT inhibitors **tolcapone** and **entacapone**, not only diminish the peripheral metabolism of levodopa, but also increase its bioavailability in the brain (by reducing 3-OMD and its competition with levodopa for active transport across blood-brain barrier). Thus, COMT inhibitors prolong the availability of dopamine by inhibiting the metabolism of dopamine and levodopa outside the neuron. The levodopa dose can be reduced further and its effects are enhanced or extended in patients who have developed response fluctuations – leading to smoother response with more prolonged "on time".

The pharmacological effects of tolcapone and entacapone are similar. However, tolcapone has both peripheral and central effects, while entaqcapone is a peripheral blocker of COMT. Tolcapone has been occasionally associated with severe hepatotoxicity and death and hence entacapone is preferred as it is devoid of hepatotoxicity. Adverse effects include dyskinesias, nausea, diarrhea, postural hypotension and sleep disturbances.

A commercial preparation **Stalevo** consist of a combination of levodopa with carbidopa and entacapone, which ensures better compliance.

ANTICHOLINERGIC DRUGS

In the absence of the inhibitory control of dopamine, the activity of the intrastriatal cholinergic interneuron becomes dominant. Blockade of central muscarinic receptors by anticholinergic drugs reduces striatal cholinergic activity.

Anticholinergic drugs have a useful effect on tremor and rigidity, but do not help bradykinesia. They are most commonly used to treat:

- Early-stages of the disease before bradykinesia is a problem.
- Late-stage Parkinsonism as an adjunct to levodopa+ carbidopa therepy.
- Drug (antipsychotics) induced Parkinsonism.

Many anticholinergics are available. Some of the more commonly used drugs are listed in Table 3.5.

Adverse effects

Anticholinergics should be avoided in elderly patients in whom they cause confusion and hallucinations, apart from usual atropine like side-effects such as dry month, blurred vision, difficulty with micturition and constipation. Trihexyphenidyl

Table 3.5: Anticholinergics used in parkinsonism

Drugs	Usual daily dose (mg)
Benztropine mesylate	1–6
Biperiden	2–12
Orphenadrine	150–300
Procyclidine	7.5–30
Trihexyphenidyl	6–20

(benzhexol) has been reported to have some abuse potential and parkinsonian patients may display 'fake' parkinsonian signs to obtain the drug.

3.9 DRUGS AND MENTAL ILLNESS

Psychosis and depression are two major mental illnesses, which are linked with the abnormalities of the brain neurotransmitters. Drugs that interfere with the action of brain neurotransmitters have been found to be effective in the treatment of mental illness.

ANTIPSYCHOTIC DRUGS

Psychosis may be defined as any major mental disorder of organic or emotional origin marked by derangement of personality and loss of contact with reality, with delusions and hallucinations, often with incoherent speech, disorganized and agitated behavior or illness.

Antipsychotic drugs are used for the treatment of psychotic symptoms in a wide variety of conditions which are mainly functional disorders without any organic cause like schizophrenia, bipolar mania, delusional disorders (paranoia).

SCHIZOPHRENIA

Schizophrenia is a psychosis characterized by delusions, hallucinations and lack of insight. Symptoms are grouped as positive and negative. Positive symptoms include delusions, hallucinations and disorders of thought while negative symptoms include poor concentration, social withdrawal, poverty of speech and lack of initiative and energy.

Schizophrenia is considered to be neurodevelopmental disorders. This implies that structural and functional changes in the brain are even present in utero in some patients, or that they develop during childhood and adolescence, or both. Thus, schizophrenia is a genetic disorder with high heritability. The children of one affected parent have approximately a 10% risk of developing the illness, but this rises to 50% if an identical twin is affected. The usual age of onset is the mid-twenties.

BIOCHEMICAL FACTORS

Dopamine (DA) hypothesis

The dopamine hypothesis for schizophrenia was the first neurotransmitter-based concept to be developed but is no longer considered adequate to explain all aspects of schizophrenia.

Several lines of evidence suggest that schizophrenia is the result of excessive limbic dopaminergic activity, especially of D_2 receptors.

The fact that several of typical antipsychotic drugs have much less effect on D_2 receptors and yet are effective in schizophrenia has redirected the attention to the role of other dopamine receptors and nondopamine receptors.

Serotonin hypothesis

Serotonin receptors-particularly the $5-HT_{2A}$ – receptors subtype blockade is a key factor in the mechanism of action of atypical antipsychotic drugs, which share the property of weak D_2 receptors antagonism and more potent $5-HT_{2A}$ – receptors blockade. Higher affinity for the $5-HT_{2A}$ – receptor than the D_2 receptors suggests an important role for the serotonin 5-HT system in the etiology of schizophrenia.

Glutamate hypothesis

The GABAergic neuronal loss observed in the hippocampus suggest a role of GABA. The role of the excitatory amino acid, glutamine has also been implicated.

CLASSIFICATION

A number of antipsychotic drugs are available. These may be divided into neuroleptics and newer or atypical drugs.

A neuroleptic (typical, first generation) is a subtype of antipsychotic drug that produces high incidence of extrapyramidal side effects (EPS) in clinically effective doses.

The atypical (novel or second generation) antipsychotic drugs dissociate antipsychotic action and EPS and are the most commonly used.

Neuroleptics (typical/first generation)

- Phenothiazines

Aliphatic derivatives	Chlorpromazine
Piperidine derivate	Thioridazine
Piperazine derivatives	Trifluoperazine, perphenazine, fluphenazine

- Thioxathene derivatives — Thiothixene
- Butyrophenone derivative — Haloperidol
- Miscellaneous — Pimozide, Molindone

Atypical (novel/second generation)

Loxapine, paliperidone, clozapine, risperidone, asenapine, olanzapine, ziprasidone, quetiapine, aripiprazole, sulpiride.

Pharmacokinetics

Most antipsychotic drugs are readily absorbed and undergo variable significant first-pass metabolism. They are highly lipid-soluble and protein-bound. They are metabolized mostly by hepatic microsomal oxidase system and at the typical clinical doses do not usually interfere with metabolism of other drugs.

Pharmacodynamics

Antipsychotic drugs have a wide variety of central nervous system, autonomic and endocrine effects. Though their efficacy has been related to D_2-receptors and $5\text{-}HT_{2A}$ blockade, their adverse pharmacologic effects are also as a result of blocking of the major brain neurotransmitters including acetylcholine and α adrenoreceptors, histamine, 5-HT and dopamine.

Psychological effects

Most antipsychotic drugs cause impaired psychomotor performance in nonpsychotic individuals.

Endocrine effects

Neuroleptics or typical antipsychotics, as well as resperidone and paliperidone produce marked elevations of prolactin by blocking dopamine receptors.

Newer antipsychotics such as olanzapine, quetiapine, and aripiprazole cause no or minimal increase in prolactin and reduced risks of extrapyramidal system dysfunction and tardive dyskinesia, reflecting their diminished D_2 antagonism.

Cardiovascular effects

Phenothiazine frequently causes orthostatic hypotension and tachycardia due to their autonomic effects.

Abnormal ECGs have been recorded with thioridazine, but are readily reversed by withdrawing the drug.

Haloperidol, which does not cause QTc prolongation, is associated with increased risk of torsade.

Among the newest atypical antipsychotics, prolongation of the QTc has received much attention, because of an increased risk of dangerous arrhythmias.

Asenapine, aripiprazole, paliperidine, quetipine and ziprasidone increase QTc prolongation which suggests a possible risk of arrhythmia.

Metabolic effects

Weight gain, hyperlipidemia, new-onset diabetes mellitus have been found fairly common with atypical antipsychotics such as clozapine, olanzapine, risperidone and quetiapine.

Therapeutic uses

A. Psychiatric indications

Schizophrenia is the primary indication for antipsychotic drugs. They are also extensively used in patients with psychotic bipolar disorder, psychotic depression and treatment resistant depression.

Other indications for the use of antipsychotics include Tourett's syndrome, disturbed behavior in patients with Alzheimer's disease, and, with antidepressants, psychotic depression.

Although typical antipsychotics are efficacious in the treatment of positive symptoms of schizophrenia, such as hallucinations and delusions, atypical antipsychotics are thought to have efficacy in reducing both positive and negative symptoms.

Antidepressants medications may be used in conjunction with neuroleptics if significant depression is present. Resistant cases may require concomitant use of lithium, carbamazepine or valproic acid.

Antipsychotics are not indicated for the treatment of various withdrawal syndromes, e.g. opioid withdrawal.

B. Non-psychiatric indications

Older typical antipsychotic drugs with the exception of thioridazine have a strong antiemetic effect. This action is due to dopamine-receptor blocking action both centrally (in CTZ of medulla) and peripherally (on receptors in the stomach).

Some drugs, such as prochlorperazine and benzquinamide, are used solely as **antiemetic**.

Phenothiazines have considerable H_1-receptor blocking action and have been used for the relief of pruritus or, in the case of promethazine, as a **preoperative sedative**. The butyrophenone droperidol is used in combination with opioid, fentanyl in **neuroleptanesthesia**.

The characteristic properties of some antipsychotics are given in Table 3.6

Adverse Effects

Most of the untoward effects of antipsychotic drugs are extension of their known pharmacological actions, but a few effects are allergic in nature and some idiosyncratic.

- *Effects due to dopamine blockade*
  1. Behavioral effects
     Pseudodepression due to akinesthesia (loss of control of voluntary muscle movement).
  2. Neurological effects
     Parkinsonism, akathisia (motor restlessness), tardive dyskinesia, seizures (very rare)
  3. Endocrine effects
     Hypeprolactinemia

     Women: Amenorrhea – galactorrhea syndrome, infertility, osteoporosis

     Men: Loss of libido, gynecomastia, impotence

- *Effects due to cholinergic blockade*

  Dry mouth, blurred vision, constipation, urinary retention

- *Effects due to α-adrenoreceptor blockade*

  Orthostatic hypotension, impotence, failure to ejaculate

- *Metabolic effects*

  Weight gain, hyperglycemia, hyperlipidemia

- *Hypersensitivity reactions*

  Cholestatic jaundice, photosensitive dermatitis, blood dyscrasias (agranulocytosis with clozapine)

- *Ocular complication* (long-term use)

  Corneal and lens opacities

- *Pregnancy*

  Neurotransmitter effects involved in neurodevelopment.

Table 3.6: Some representative antipsychotic drugs

Drug	Clinical potency	Extrapyramidal toxicity	Sedation	Hypotension	Disadvantages
Antipsychotics (Neuroleptics)					
Chloropromazine	Low	Medium	High	High	Many adverse effects, esp. autonomic.
Fluphenazine	High	High	Low	Very low	Increased tardive dyskinesia
Thiothixene	High	Medium	Medium	Medium	Ocular complication
Haloperidol	High	Very High	Low	Very low	Severe EPS
Atypical antipsychotics					
Clozapine	Medium	Very Low	Low	Medium	Agranulocytosis
Risperidone	High	Low	Low	Low	EPS, hypotension
Olanzapine	High	Very Low	Medium	Low	Weight gain
Quetiapine	Low	Very Low	Medium	Low	Short T ½
Ziprasidone	Medium	Very Low	Low	Very Low	QT prolongation
Aripiprazole	High	Very Low	Very Low	Low	QT prolongation

EPS: extrapyramidal side effects.

Serious adverse effects of antipsychotic drugs include:

- *Neuroleptic malignant syndrome* is rare but serious. It is characterized by fever, tremor and rigidity, autonomic instability and confusion. Characteristic findings are elevated creatinine phosphokinase and leucocytosis. Antipsychotic drugs must be stopped immediately and supportive treatment including hydration and reducing hypothermia should be initiated. Dantrolene and bromocriptine may be helpful.

- *Prolongation of the QT interval* may be associated with ventricular tachycardia, (torsades de pointes) and sudden death. Ziprasidone carries the greatest risk of QT prolongation. Clozapine is sometimes associated with myocarditis. Treatment requires stopping of the drug and treatment of cardiac disorder.

Individual Antipsychotic Drugs

The antipsychotic drugs differ in their clinical potency, sedation, autonomic and extrapyramidal effects (Table 3.6).

PHENOTHIAZINES

Three subfamilies of phenothiazines, based on the chemical structure, were once the most widely used of the antipsychotic drugs. The aliphatic and piperidine derivations are the least potent and produce more sedation and weight gain. They are mainly used for nonpsychiatric conditions.

Prochlorperazine is solely used as antiemetic.

Promethazine is used as H_1-receptor blocking agent in pruritis and as preoperative sedative.

Piperazine derivatives are more potent. Fluphenazine, a piperazine derivative, is as effective as atypical antipsychotic drugs but carries the risk of tardive dykinesia.

THIOXANTHENES

These are potent antipsychotic drugs. Some of them are available as depot preparation for maintenance therapy of schizophrenia.

BUTYROPHENONES

This group, of which haloperidol is the most widely used, tend to be more potent and to have fewer autonomic effects but greater extrapyramidal effects of the typical antipsychotics.

Atypical Antipsychotics

These drugs have complex pharmacology. They have greater ability to block $5\text{-}HT_{2A}$ receptor than D_2 receptors. Some of the newest atypical antipsychotic e.g. aripiprazole appears to be a partial agonist of D_2 receptors. They have the following advantages over the conventional first generation antipsychotic drugs.

- Extrapyramidal toxicities are very low.
- Newer atypical antipsychotic such as olanzapine, queliapine, and aripiprazole cause no or minimal increase of prolactin.
- Effective in patients who fail to respond to conventional drugs.
- More effective than conventional drugs for treating negative symptoms of schizophrenia.
- Superior adverse-effect profile and low to absent risk of tardive dyskinesia make them first line of treatment.

CLOZAPINE

Clozapine is not the drug of choice. At present its use is limited to those patients who have failed to respond to substantial doses of haloperidol.

Clozapine has following disadvantage:

Weight gain, hyperlipedemia, hyperglycemia leading to diabetes mellitus, agranulocytosis, myocarditis, dose related lowering of seizure threshold.

Clozapine is the only atypical antipsychotic drug indicated to reduce the risk of **suicide**.

OLANZAPINE

Olanzapine is similar to clozapine, but is free from the risk of agranulocytosis. It has the least risk of tardive dyskinesia which accounts for its widespread use. Weight gain is very common and requires monitoring of food intake, especially carbohydrates. Hyperglycemia may develop, but whether secondary to weight gain-associated insulin resistance or to other potential mechanism remains to be clarified. Hyperlipemia may occur and may increase the risk of arteriosclerotic cardiovascular disease. It causes dose related lowering of seizure threshold.

QUETIAPINE

It is similar to olanzapine, but may cause less weight gain. Higher doses are required if there is associated hypotension. Short half-life requires twice-daily dosing.

RISPERIDONE

It has broad efficacy. It's superior side-effect profile (compared with that of haloperidol) at doses 6 mg/d or less and lower risk of tardive dyskinesia have contributed to its most commonly used atypical antipsychotic. However, with high doses extrapyramidal dysfunction and hypotension may occur.

ZIPRASIDONE

It is the atypical antipsychotic that causes the least weight gain. It is also available for parenteral administration.

Ziprasidone carries the greatest risk of QT prolongation and therefore should not be combined with other drugs that prolong the QT interval, including thioridazine, pimozide, and group IA or III antiarrhythmic drugs.

ARIPIPRAZOLE

It is highly potent atypical antipsychotic that has very low extrapyramidal toxicity with the least sedative action. It does not raise prolactin levels and has low weight gain liability. Its long half life, high efficacy and superior side-effect profile makes it a very useful antipsychotic.

MOOD STABILIZING DRUGS

Mood stabilizing drugs are used to prevent recurrent episodes in bipolar disorders.

Bipolar disorder is an episodic disturbance with inter-spersed periods of depressed and elevated moods; the latter is known as hypomania or mania when severe. Psychosis may occur in both the depressive and the manic phases, with delusions and hallucinations that are usually in keeping with the mood disturbance. This is described as an affective psychosis.

The main mood stabilizing drugs are lithium, carbamazepine and sodium valproate.

LITHIUM

Lithium is the mainstay of the treatment in bipolar disorder, although sodium valproate and olanzapine are equally effective in acute mama, as is lamotrigine in the depressed state. The response rate to lithium is 70–80% in acute mania, with beneficial effects appearing in 1–2 weeks. Lithium also has a prophylactic effect in prevention of mania and, to a lesser extent, in the prevention of recurrent depression.

Lithium is rapidly absorbed form the gastrointestinal tract and remains unbound to plasma or tissue proteins, 95% of a given dose is excreted unchanged through the kidney within 24 hours.

Pharmacodynamics

The biochemical basis for lithium's mood-stabilizer action is not clearly understood.

Lithium directly inhibits two enzymes involved in signal transduction pathways in the brain. It causes depletion of intra cellular inositol and inhibits glycogen synthase kinase-3 (GSK-3) that appears to modulate energy metabolism, provide neuroprotection, and increase neuroplasticity. The mood stabilizing drugs may also have indirect effects on neurotransmitters and their release.

Mood stabilizing action of lithium may involve inhibition of the enzymes in the brain that may be implicated in long-term neuroplastic events that could underlie long-term mood stabilization.

Lithium, as a prophylactic drug, decreases the frequency and severity of both manic and depressive attacks in bipolar affective disorder in about 70% of patients. In addition to its use in manic states, lithium in sometimes useful in the prophylaxis of recurrent unipolar depressions. It may ameliorate non-specific aggressive behaviors and dyscontrol symptoms.

Most patients with bipolar disease can be managed long-term with lithium alone, although some will require continued or intermittent use of a neuroleptic, antidepressant or carbamazepine.

Unlike neuroleptics or antidepressant drugs, which exert several actions on the central or autonomic nervous system, lithium at therapeutic concentrations is devoid of autonomic blocking effects and of activating or sedating effects, although it can produce nausea and tremor. Most important is that the prophylactic use of lithium can prevent both mania and depression.

Lithium has proved very useful as an adjunct to anti-psychotics in treatment-resistant schizophrenic patients and to tricyclic antidepressants and selective serotonin reuptake inhibitors in patients with unipolar depression who do not respond well to monotherapy with the antidepressants.

Monitoring treatment

Patients using lithium should be monitored closely, since the blood levels required to achieve a therapeutic benefit are close to those associated with toxicity.

In the treatment of acute mania lithium is initiated at 300 mg twice or thrice daily and the dose is then increased by 300 mg every 2–3 days to achieve therapeutic blood levels of 0.8–1.2, mEq/L (may require 7–10 days to achieve) which requires periodic monitoring. Therapeutic overdoses of lithium are more common.

Adverse effects

Serious side effects from lithium are rare but it is important to be alert to adverse effects that might signify impending serious toxic effects.

Neurologic and psychiatric effects

Tremor is one of the most common adverse effects of lithium that may occur with therapeutic doses, other reported neurologic abnormalities include choreoathetosis, motor hyperactivity, ataxia, dysarthria, and aphasia.

Psychiatric disturbances at toxic concentrations are generally marked by mental confusion and withdrawal.

Appearance of any new neurologic psychiatric symptoms or signs is a clear indication of monitoring serum levels and temporary stopping of the treatment.

Decreased thyroid function

Lithium exerts an antithyroid effect by interfering with the synthesis and release of thyroid hormone.

Nephrogenic diabetes insipidus

Lithium causes loss of responsiveness to antidiuretic hormone (nephrogenic diabetes insipidus), which responds to amiloride. Rarely nephrotoxicity may occur.

Cardiac effects

The bradycardia-tachycardia ('sick sinus') syndrome is a definite contraindication to the use of lithium because the ion further depresses the sinus node.

Lithium can be teratogenic inducing cardiac malformations in the first trimester.

Interaction

Thiazide diuretics, tetracycline and NSAIDs increase, while carbonic anhydrase inhibitors, bronchodilators and verapamil decrease blood levels of lithium.

VALPROIC ACID

Valproic acid may be better antimanic than lithium and effective in some patients who have failed to respond to lithium. Moreover, its side-effect profile is such that one can rapidly increase the dosage over a few days to achieve therapeutic range blood levels, with nausea being the only limiting factor in some patients.

Combinations of valproic acid with other psychotropic medications likely to be used in the management of either phase of bipolar illness are generally well tolerated. Valproic acid is an appropriate first-line treatment for mania and combination therapy with lithium is advocated in patients who do not respond to either agent alone. Tremor and weight gain are the most common side effects, hepatotoxicity and pancreatitis are rare toxicities.

CARBAMAZEPINE

Carbamazepine has been found to be effective in acute mania and also for prophylactic therapy and is a reasonable alternative to lithium. It can also be used in combination with lithium or valproic acid in refractory cases. Blood dyscrasias are not a major problem with doses used as a mood stabilizer.

Other drugs

Second-generation antidepressant drugs have also been shown to be effective either alone or in combination with a mood stabilizer.

Lamotrigine has been reported to be useful in preventing the depression that often follows the manic phase of bipolar disorder.

Riluzole, a neuroprotective agent used in amyotrophic lateral sclerosis may prove useful for bipolar depression.

ANTIDEPRESSANT DRUGS

Antidepressant drugs are primarily indicated in the treatment of major depressive disorder (MDD) – a condition characterized by depressed mood for at least 2 weeks and /or loss of interest or pleasure in most activities. In addition, depression is characterized by disturbances in sleep and appetite as well as deficits in cognition and energy. It is a major cause of disability and of **suicide**.

If present with other medical disease, depression magnifies disability, diminishes adherence to medical treatment and rehabilitation, and may even shorten life expectancy. Such comorbid depression may incrementally worsen health more than any combination of chronic diseases with depression.

Pathophysiology of major depression

There is a genetic predisposition to depression.

Associated biological factor include:

- Hypofunction of monoamine neurotransmitter systems (5-HT and noradrenalin) in the cortical and limbic system.
- Loss of nerve growth factors such as brain – derived neurotrophic factor (BDNF) leading to atrophic changes in the hippocampus.
- Abnormal hypothalamo-pituitary-adrenal axis (HPA) regulation leading to elevated cortisol levels that do not suppress with dexamethasone.
- Thyroid dysregulation including blunting of response of thyrotropin to thyrotropin-releasing hormone.
- Sex steroids (estrogen in females and testosterone in males) deficiency.

Pharmacodynamics

Antidepressant act by enhancing monoamine, serotonin and noradrenalin (norepinephrine) levels in the brain either by inhibiting their reuptake by binding the serotonin transporter (SERT) or norepinephrine transporter (NET) or by inhibiting their enzymatic degradation (the MAOIs).

The increased availability of monoamines for binding in the synaptic cleft results in a cascade of events that enhance the transcription of some proteins and inhibition of others.

It is the net production of these proteins, including BDNF, glucocorticoid receptors, β adrenoreceptors, and other proteins that appears to determine the benefits as well as the toxicity of different antidepressants.

The antidepressants on the basis of their pharmacologic profiles are classified as given in Table 3.7.

TRICYCLIC ANTIDEPRESSANTS (TCAs)

TCAs are well absorbed and have long half-lives. They undergo extensive metabolism. Only about 5% of TCA are excreted unchanged in the urine.

The TCAs are now considered to be second or third-line treatment for MDD, because they are potentially lethal in overdose, require titration to achieve a therapeutic dose, have serious drug interactions and have many troublesome adverse effects. As a consequence TCAs are now reserved in the treatment of MDD or anxiety disorders in patients who have been unresponsive to other agents.

Adverse effects of TCAs include weight gain and sedation (H_1 antagonism), anticholinergic effects (most common) like dry month, constipation, urinary retention, blurred vision and confusion, postural hypotension (α-blocking property), lowering of the seizure threshold and cardiotoxicity. The TCAs have a prominent discontinuation syndrome characterized by cholinergic rebound and flulike symptoms. TCAs may be dangerous in overdose and in people having coexisting heart disease, glaucoma and prostatism.

ATYPICAL ANTIDEPRESSANTS

These are second-generation antidepressants. Commonly used atypical antidepressants include **bupropion** and **mirtazapine**.

Bupropion is a selective noradrenalin and dopamine reuptake inhibitor. The most significant effect of bupropion is presynaptic release of catecholamine. It has no effect on any other receptor including the serotonin transporter.

Bupropion may be associated with stimulant-like side effects, may lower seizure threshold, and has an exceptionally short half-life, requiring frequent dosing. An extended-release preparation is available.

Table 3.7: Antidepressants

Drug	ACh M	α₁	H₁	5-HT₂	NET	SERT
Selective serotonin receptor inhibitors (SSRIs) antidepressants						
Fluoxetine	0	0	0	0/+	0	+++
Sertraline	0	0	0	0	0	+++
Paroxetine	+	0	0	0	+	+++
Fluvoxamine	0	0	0	0	0	+++
Citalopram	0	0	0		0	+++
Escitalopram	0	0	0		0	+++
Tricyclic antidepressants (TCAs)						
Amitriptyline	+++	+++	++	0/+	+	++
Nortriptyline	+	+	+	+	++	+
Imipramine	++	+	+	0/+	+	++
Desipramine	+	+	+	0/+	+++	+
Doxepin	++	+++	+++	0/+	+	+
Clomipramine	+	++	+	+	++	+++
Serotonin-norepinephrine reuptake inhibitors (SNRIs)						
Venlafaxine	0	0	0	0	+	++
Desvenlafaxine	0	0	0	0	++	++
Duloxetine	0	0	0	0	++	++
Mirtazapine	0	0	+++	+	+	0
Atypical antidepressants						
Bupropion	0	0	0	0	0/+	0
Amoxapine	+	++	+	+++	++	+
5-HT2 antagonists						
Trazodone	0	++	0/+	++	0	+
Nefazodone	0	+	0	++	0/+	+
Monoamine oxidase inhibitors						
Phenelzine	0	+	0	+	++	++
Tranylcypromine	0	+	0	+	++	++
Isocarboxazid	0	+	0	+	++	++
Selegiline	0	+	0	0	++	+

Ach M: acetylcholine muscarinic receptor; α₁: alpha₁-adrenoceptor; H₁: histamine receptor; 5-HT₂: serotonin receptor; NET: norepinephrine transporter, SERT: serotonin transporter. 0/−: minimal affinity; +: mild affinity; ++: moderate affinity; +++, high affinity.

Bupropion is generally used as add-on therapy to an SSRI or SNRI to augment antidepressant benefit if monotherapy is unsuccessful. It is also used as a treatment for smoking cessation. Bupropion may mimic nicotine's effects on dopamine and noradrenalin and may antagonize nicotine receptors.

Bupropion has the least association with sexual side effect.

Bupropion is not effective in anxiety disorders.

Mirtazapine antagonizes presynaptic α_2 adrenoreceptor and enhances the release of both noradrenalin and 5-HT. In addition it is an antagonist of $5-HT_2$ and $5-HT_3$ receptors. It is a potent H_1 antagonist which is responsible of its sedative effects.

Mirtazapine has the same uses as that of bupropion.

Amoxapine has actions like tricyclic antidepressants on brain receptors and transporters. Maprotiline has actions like amoxapine except that it does not inhibit SERT.

SELECTIVE SEROTONIN ANTIDEPRESSANT (SSRIs)

SSRIs allosterically inhibit the serotonin transporter by binding the receptor at a site other than the active binding site for serotonin. At therapeutic doses, about 80% of the activity of transporter is inhibited. Functional polymorphisms exist for SERT that determine the activity of the transporter.

Except for paroextine, which has modest muscarinic blocking and NET inhibiting effect, none other SSRIs has any effect on other neurotransmitters.

SSRIs are the most commonly prescribed first-line agents in the treatment of major depressive disorder (MDD) and anxiety disorders including post-traumatic disorder, obsessive-compulsive disorder, social anxiety disorder, generalized anxiety disorder, and panic disorder.

SSRIs are equally effective and perhaps more effective than benzodiazepines in the long-term treatment of anxiety disorders and have the advantage of being free from the risk of dependence and tolerance.

The advantage of SSRIs, apart from relatively free from cardiotoxic, sedative, anticholinergic effects, is that they do not require titration, because of similar starting and therapeutic dose and safety in overdose.

Adverse effects

The adverse effects of SSRIs can be predicted from their potent inhibition of SERT. SSRIs enhance serotonergic tone, not just in the brain but through out the body. Increased serotonergic activity in the gut is associated with gastrointestinal symptoms such as nausea and diarrhea. Increasing serotonergic tone at the level of spinal cord and above is associated with diminished sexual function and interest.

Other adverse effects include headache and insomnia. Some patients may gain weight particularly with paroxetine.

Sudden discontinuation of half-life SSRIs such as paroxetine and sertraline is associated with a discontinuation syndrome characterized by dizziness, paresthesias, and other symptoms which may last for one week or longer after stoppage of the therapy.

SEROTONIN-NOREPINEPHRINE REUPTAKE INHIBITORS (SNRIs)

SNRIs inhibit both serotonin and noradrenalin transporters. They also have a modest affinity for dopamine. The affinity to bind serotonin receptor is much greater than noradrenalin receptor.

SNRIs in addition to serotonergic adverse effects may have noradrenergic effects which include increased blood pressure and heart rate, and CNS activation, such as insomnia, anxiety, and agitation.

Venlafaxine has been rarely, associated with cardiac toxicity and duloxetine with hepatic toxicity.

SNRIs do not possess antihistaminic or anticholinergic effects as seen with TCAs.

SNRIs are indicated in the treatment of MDD, pain disorders including neuropathies and fibromyalgia, generalized anxiety, stress urinary incontinence, and vasomotor symptoms of menopause.

5-HT$_2$ ANTAGONISTS

Trazodone and nefazodone block 5-HT$_{2A}$ receptor leading to antianxiety, antipsychotic, and antidepressant effects.

Nefazodone is also a weak inhibitor of α-adrenoreceptors as well as that of SERT and NET. Its use has been associated with hepatotoxcity.

Trazodone is well tolerated and safe in over dosage. It can cause postural hypotension and priapism due to its α$_1$ blocking effect.

Sedative effects, particularly with trazodone can be quite pronounced making the treatment of insomnia due to depression with or without anxiety as its primary application.

MONOAMINE OXIDASE INHIBITORS (MOIs)

MOIs increase the availability of neurotransmitter at synaptic clefts by inhibiting the metabolism of noradrenalin, 5-HT and dopamine.

There are two forms of monoamine oxidase—MAO-A and MAO-B, which differ in their specificity for neurotransmitters (noradrenalin, 5-HT and dopamine) and on whether effects are reversible or irreversible.

Moclobemide is a reversible and selective inhibitors of MOI-A where primary substrates are noradrenalin, adrenalin and serotonin. In contrast selegiline is an irreversible MAO-B-specific agent at low doses and is useful in the treatment of Parkinson's disease, while at higher doses it becomes a non-selective MAOI similar to other non-selective MAO inhibitors like phenelzine, isocarboxazid and tranylcypromine, which enhance neuronal levels of noradrenalin, dopamine and 5-HT.

MAOIs like TCAs are potentially lethal in overdose require titration to achieve a therapeutic dose, have serious drug interactions and many other troublesome adverse effects.

MAOIs are only used in MDD or anxiety in patients who have been unresponsive to other agents, and whose depression responds to only MAOIs.

The most common adverse effects of the MAOIs are orthostatic hypotension and weight gain, insomnia and sexual dysfunction. They cause potentially dangerous interactions with drugs such as amphetamines, and foods rich in tyramine such as cheese and red wine, which may lead to fatal hypertensive crisis. Sudden discontinuation of MAOIs leads to a discontinuation syndrome manifested in a delirium-like presentation with psychosis, excitement, and confusion.

Moclobemide causes minimal potentiation of the pressure response to dietary tyramine.

MAOIs should not be used concomitantly with SSRIs because of the risk of serotonin syndrome, or with TCAs because of possible hyperadrenergic effects.

Therapeutic uses of antidepressants

- *Depression*

  Treatment of major depressive disorder aims in the remission of all symptoms. Successful treatment requires the patient to take an appropriate dose of an effective drug for at least 8–12 weeks. If an inadequate response is obtained, therapy is often switched to another agent or augmented by addition of another drug like bupropion or mirtazapine.

  Psychotherapy combined with antidepressant treatment may be more effective.

  Severe depression complicated by psychosis, dehydration or suicide risk may require electroconvulsive therapy (ECT).

- *Anxiety disorders*

  Antidepressants are the drugs of choice for anxiety disorders which include phobic anxiety disorder, panic disorder, generalized anxiety disorder and obsessive compulsive disorder.

  Benzodiazepines are useful in the short term but long-term use can lead to dependence.

  A β-blocker such as propronolol can help when somatic symptoms are prominent.

- *Pain disorders*
  Ascending corticospinal monoamine pathways appear to be important in the endogenous analgesic system. SNRIs are useful in the treatment of pain associated with diabetic neuropathy, fibromyalgia, post herpetic neuralgia and chronic backache.

- *Premenstrual dysphonic disorder (PMDD)*
  SSRIs are useful in relieving symptoms of PMDD such as anxiety, depressed mood, irritability, insomnia, fatigue and a variety of other physical symptoms, if given for 2 weeks out of the month in the luteal phase.

- *Smoking cessation*
  Bupropion reduces the urge to smoke. In addition, bupropion appears to experience fewer mood symptoms and possibly less weight gain in patients while withdrawal from nicotine dependence.

- *Eating disorders*
  Antidepressants are useful in the treatment of bulimia but not anorexia. Bulimia is characterized by episodic binge (large amounts of food) eating usually followed by purging behaviors such as vomiting or laxative abuse.

- *Other indications*
  The SNRI duloxetine is used in the treatment of urinary stress incontinence and vasomotor symptoms in premenopause.

DEMENTIA

Dementia is the progressive loss of cognition (power of perceiving, thinking, and remembering) and normal brain function.

Alzheimer's disease is the most common cause of dementia in which neurons and other CNS cells are damaged and killed.

Dementia can also result due to cerebral atherosclerosis, stroke (or infarcts), cerebral injuries, use or abuse of drugs (e.g. alcohol, sedatives, anticonvulscents), lesions affecting subcortical brain structures amongst others.

There are no satisfactory or effective drugs available for dementia. Acetylcholine, the neurotransmitter in the brain, is associated with memory and the anticholinesterases which inhibit the breakdown of Ach at the synapse between neurons may have some palliative role in the alleviation of symptoms.

Donepezil, galantamine, rivastigmine and **tacrine** are the available anticholineserases, which cross the blood brain barrier and preserve Ach in subcortical brain structures. The effectiveness of these drugs is limited to an intact neuro-cholinergic system. These drugs produce adverse effects attributable to the inhibition of cholinergic system (muscarinic actions).

Antidepressants, anxiolytics and atypical antipsychotic drugs are sometimes prescribed for patients with Alzheimer's disease, but these should be given with caution.

3.10 EMETICS AND ANTIEMETICS

EMETICS

Vomiting is a complex series of actions involving the stomach, esophagus and pharynx with the voluntary muscles of the chest and abdomen, and results in the ejection of the stomach contents. Vomiting centre in the medulla of the brain coordinate these actions.

There are four important sources of afferent input to the vomiting center (Fig. 3.3).

1. The "chemoreceptor trigger zone" (CTZ) or area postrema is rich in dopamine D_2, opioid, 5-HT_3 and NK, receptors. It is located outside the blood-brain barrier and is accessible to emetogenic stimuli in blood and cerebrospinal fluid.
2. The vestibular system is rich in muscarimic M_1 and histamine H_1 receptors and plays an important role in motion sickness via carnial nerve VIII.
3. Vagal and spinal afferent nerves from gastrointestinal tract are rich in 5-HT_3 receptors. Irritation of gastric mucosa leads to release of serotonin, which stimulates vagal nerve.
4. Higher brain centers play a role in vomiting due to psychiatric disorders and stress.

Emetics are of very limited value in the treatment of poisoning.

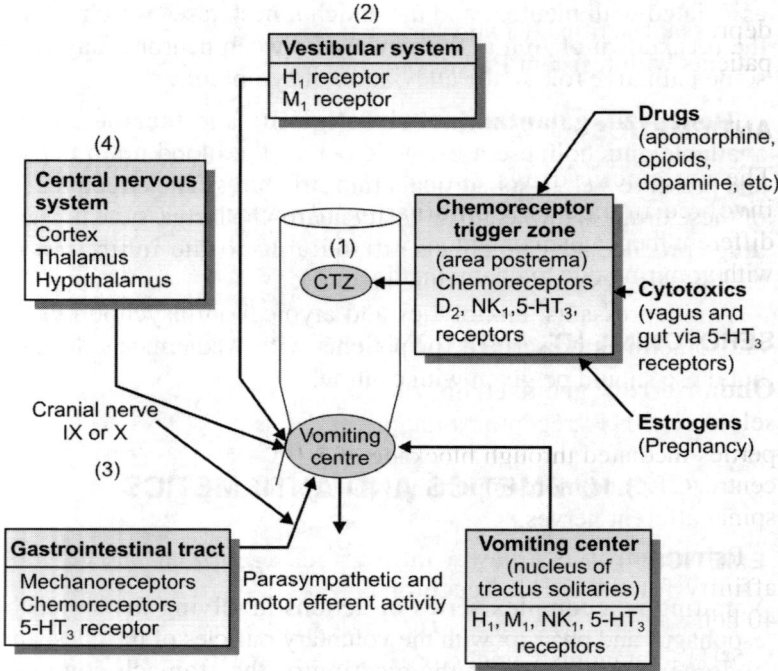

Fig. 3.3: Diagrammatic representation of neurologic pathways involved in pathogenesis of nausea and vomiting.

REFLEX EMETICS

Ipecacuanha is a dried root that contains emetine and induces vomiting reflex by irritating the stomach. It is of very limited value, since there is no evidence that it prevents significant absorption of poison and because of its own toxicity (mucosal damage and cardiac toxicity). Its use should only be considered, if the patient is fully conscious, if the poison ingested is neither corrosive nor a petroleum distillate, if poison is not absorbed by activated charcoal or if gastric lavage is inadvisable or refused.

CENTRAL EMETICS

Apomorphine is a semisynthetic derivative of morphine. It stimulates dopamine receptors in the CTZ and has some central depressant action. It is no longer used in poisoning except for patients with resistant Parkinson's disease.

ANTIEMETICS

The antiemetic drugs antagonize the different transmitters involved in emesis. Combination of antiemetic agents with different mechanism of actions is often used, especially in patients with vomiting due to chemotherapeutic agents.

SEROTONIN 5-HT$_3$ ANTAGONISTS

Ondansetron, granisetron, dolasetron and **palonosetron** are selective 5-HT$_3$ receptor antagonists that have antiemetic properties mediated through blockade of 5-HT$_3$ receptor in vomiting centre, CTZ and more importantly on extrinsic intestinal vagal and spinal afferent nerves.

Palonosetron is a newer intravenous agent that has greater affinity for the 5-HT$_3$ receptor and a long serum half-life of 40 hours.

5-HT$_3$ antagonists undergo extensive hepatic metabolism and are eliminated by renal and hepatic excretion. They can safely be given in renal insufficiency.

Corticosteroids and NK$_1$-receptor antagonists enhances the antiemetic efficacy of 5-HT$_3$ antagonists and combination therapy is used in chemotherapy inclued nausea and vomiting.

5-HT$_3$ antagonists are increasingly used to prevent or treat postoperative nausea and vomiting as well as following radiation because of their excellent safety profile.

5-HT$_3$ antagonists are well tolerated. Dolasetron is not used in patients with prolonged QT interval.

CORTICOSTEROIDS

Corticosteroids have antiemetic properties, but the basis for these effect is unknown. They are of great value in enhancing the effects of 5-HT$_3$ receptor antagonists for prevention of acute and delayed nausea and vomiting in patients receiving highly emetogenic chemotherapeutic regimens.

NEUROKININ RECEPTOR ANTAGONISTS

Neurokinin 1 (NK_1)—receptor antagonists have antiemetic properties that are mediated through central blockade in the area postrema.

Aprepitant is a highly selective NK_1- receptor antagonist that crosses the blood-barrier and occupies brain NK_1-receptor.

Fosaprepitant is a prodrug that is given intravenously and is converted to aprepitant within 30 minutes. They are used in combination with HT_3 antagonists and corticosteroids for the prevention of acute and delayed nausea and vomiting from highly emetogenic chemotherapeutic regimens.

Aprepitant may be associated with fatigue, dizziness and diarrhea and drugs that inhibit CYP3A4 increase its plasma levels.

DOPAMINE ANTAGONISTS

The phenothiazines, butyrophenones and substituted benzamide have potent antiemetic and sedative properties.

The principal adverse effects of these central dopamine antagonists are extrapyramidal; restless, dystonias and parkinsonian symptoms.

The most commonly used phenothiazine antiemetics are prochlorperazine, promethazine and thiethylperazine. They are used in toxic or metabolic induced emesis.

Droperidol, a butyrophenone, causes QT prolongation leading to ventricular tachycardia (torsades de pointes), hence is no longer recommended as an antiemetic agent.

Metoclopramide, a substituted benzamide, has $5-HT_4$ agonist and antidopaminergic action and is mainly used as a prokinetic agent in gastroparesis.

ANTICHOLINERGICS

Hyoscine is the most effective drug for the prevention of motion sickness. Adverse atropine like effects are not generally prominent at the doses (0.2–0.4 mg) employed. It is also available as a transdermal preparation. Drowsiness and blurring of vision due to paralysis of ocular accommodation can occur.

ANTIHISTAMINES

Antihistamines block the action of histamine and have acetylcholine blocking action. They are slightly less effective in vestibular disorders, but are generally better tolerated. All antihistamines are equally effective, but generally a less sedative such as cyclizine or cinnarizine is preferred for motion sickness.

Promethazine is the preferred drug for vomiting of pregnancy, which is combined with pyridoxine.

OTHER ANTIEMETICS

Nabilone, a synthetic derivative of cannabis indica, is used for vomiting induced by cytototoxic drugs, unresponsive to conventional antiemetic. Side effects include dysphoria and dizziness. It is contraindicated in severe hepatic impairment.

Betahistine. The use of betahistine is only confined to Meniere's disease in which vertigo and vomiting are due to disturbance in the labyrinth of the inner ear. It is believed to lower pressure in the inner ear and thus relieves symptoms. Side effects include GIT disturbances, headache and rashes.

3.11 LOCAL ANESTHETICS

Local anesthetics act by causing a reversible inhibition of conduction along nerve fibers of both sensory and motor nerves without loss of consciousness.

Pharmacokinetics

Local anesthetics vary widely in their solubility in water, ability to penetrate mucous membranes, duration of action, potency and toxicity. These variations determine their suitability for use by various routes, e.g. topical (direct application to skin and mucous membranes), intradermal injection, local infiltration (into subcutaneous tissues or deeper to involve muscles, other soft tissues or periosteum), local nerve blocks, extradural injection (extradural, epidural or caudal), subarachnoid injection (spinal) and intravenous regional anesthesia (Bier's block).

Local anesthetics used as surface anesthetics (cocaine, lignocaine, prilocaine) are well absorbed from mucous membranes. Absorption can be extremely rapid and has led to deaths from overdose, especially via urethra.

Local anesthetics are either hydrolyzed by liver and plasma esterases or dealkylated in the liver.

Mechanism of action

Local anesthetics block the nerve conduction by interfering with cell membrane permeability to sodium by blocking sodium ion channels.

Use of vasoconstrictors

Most local anesthetics, with the exception of cocaine, cause dilation of blood vessels. The addition of a vasoconstrictor such as adrenalin diminishes local blood flow, slows the rate of absorption of local anesthetics, and prolongs the duration of its action.

Adrenalin must never be combined with local anesthetics given intravenously, as in a Bier's block, because of its obvious dangerous effects on the heart, nor in blocks for digits and appendages as it may produce ischemic necrosis.

An alternative vasoconstrictor is **felypressin** (synthetic vasopressin), which does not affect the heart rate or blood pressure and may be preferable in patients with cardiovascular diseases.

Therapeutic uses

The choice of local anesthetic for infiltration, peripheral nerve blocks, and central neuraxis (spinal/epidural) blockade is usually based on the duration of action required.

Procaine and chloroprocaine are short acting: lidocaine, mepivacaine and prilocaine have an intermediate duration of action, and tetracaine, bupivacaine, levobupivacaine, and ropivacaine are long-acting local anesthetics. Articaine has a fast onset and intermediate duration of action that make it suitable for use in dental procedures.

Satisfactory topical local anesthesia requires an agent capable of rapid penetration across the skin or mucosa, and with limited tendency to diffuse away from the site of application. Cocaine has an excellent penetration and local vasoconstrictor effects, but is no longer used because of several disadvantages — irritating to conjunctiva, cardiotoxicity when combined with adrenalin in otolaryngology surgery, drug of abuse, protoplasmic poison on injection and CNS toxicities.

Topical local anesthesia is often used for eye, ear, nose and throat procedures. The drugs used for topical anesthesia include lidocaine, adrenalin and lidocaine – bupivacine combinations, tetracaine, pramoxine, dibucaine, benzocaine and dyclonine.

Infiltration anesthesia is mainly used for minor procedures like incisions, drainage of an abscess, excision, etc. by injecting the anesthetic solution directly into the tissue. Lidocaine and ropivacaine are generally used.

Field block is generally used for forearm, scalp, anterior abdominal wall and lower extremity where local anesthetic is injected proximal to the site of operation.

Systemic local anesthetics (e.g., intravenous lidocaine and oral mexiletine and tocainide), because of their membrane-stabilizing effects, are commonly used as adjuvant to the combination of a tricyclic antidepressant (e.g, amitriptyline) and an anticonvulsant (e.g., carbamazepine) in chromic neuropathic pain in patients who fail to respond to the combination of antidepressant and anticonvulsant.

LIGNOCAINE (lidocaine, xylocaine)

Lignocaine is the safest and most commonly used local anesthetic. It has a rapid onset of action and duration of action of 1–2 hours. It is a mild vasodilator and is generally combined with adrenalin for a longer duration of action.

Lignocaine suppresses the excitability of the ventricular muscle with only moderate depression of the heart's action. It is not likely therefore to cause cardiac arrest or a fall of blood pressure except in overdose.

Lignocaine is considered to be the first line drug for treating ventricular arrhythmias after acute myocardial infarction and cardiac operation.

BUPIVACAINE

Bupivacaine has a slow onset of action, but has the advantage over other local anesthetics in its longer duration of action. It is more toxic to the heart than other local anesthetics and must never be given for intravenous regional anesthesia (a Bier's block) (Table 3.8).

PRILOCAINE

Prilocaine is similar to lignocaine, although less potent and less toxic. In high doses, it may cause cyanosis due to formation of methemoglobin, which can be treated with intravenous injection of methylene blue.

Table 3.8: Individual local anesthetics

Drug	Main uses	Contraindication
Lignocaine (Lidocaine, Xylocaine)	All types of local anesthesia, ventricular arrhythmias	Complete heart block, Inflamed or infected tissues, traumatized urethra
Bupivacaine	Local infiltration, peripheral nerve block, spinal and sympathetic block	Intravenous regional anesthesia (Bier's block). Pregnancy
Ropivacaine	Lumbar, epidural, thoracic epidural, major nerve block, field block	Bier's block
Prilocaine	Infiltration anesthesia, Bier's block, dental block, nerve block	Anemia, methemoglobinemia
Amethocaine	Topical anesthetic for eye, prior to venepuncture or venous cannulation	Inflamed traumatized or highly vascular surfaces, bronchoscopy
Cocaine	Topical anesthetic for ENT procedures	Systemic use because of toxicity and drug abuse

ROPIVACAINE

Ropivacaine is a recently introduced local anesthetic, which is similar to bupivacaine, but is less cardiotoxic.

ETIDOCAINE

Etidocaine long-acting local anesthetic, is mainly used for epidural, infilteration and regional anesthesia.

AMETHOCAINE

Amethocaine is a vasodilator and is very toxic giving rise to hypersensitive reactions. Its use is limited for surface anesthesia.

MEPIVACAINE and ARTICAINE

These are local anesthetics commonly used in dentistry.

BENZOCAINE

Benzocaine is used as a constituent of proprietary drug mixtures for use in sore throat, mouth ulcers and musculoskeletal conditions.

COCAINE

Cocaine, an alkaloid, is rarely used because of its potent sympathomimetic actions and its liability to cause euphoria and to increase capacity for physical work (misused as a drug of addiction).

Procaine is an old drug that is now rarely used.

Adverse effects

All local anesthetics can cause dangerous side effects, if absorbed. CNS toxicity is common and includes confusion, respiratory depression and convulsions. Hypotension and bradycardia leading to cardiac arrest may occur.

Hypersensitivity reactions rarely occur. Routine tests for allergy or intolerance have been advocated. Reactions are least with lignocaine. Hypersensitivity reactions are more common with ester local anesthetics.

3.12 GENERAL ANESTHETICS AND MUSCLE RELAXANTS

In anesthetic practice large number of drugs, have been used prior to induction of general anesthesia, which constitutes preanesthetic medication.

PREANESTHETIC MEDICATION

Premedication before surgical anesthesia may be needed to allay anxiety, to reduce oral secretions, to reduce the volume and increase the pH of gastric contents, and to relieve pain and discomfort when present. Drugs used for preanesthetic medication include anxiolytics, anticholinergics, prokinetics and analgesics.

Anxiolytics

Benzodiazepines possess useful properties for premedication including anxiolysis, sedation and amnesia. They have no analgesic action. **Temazepam** given orally (10–20 mg) is the usual choice. Its effects last for about 90 minutes.

Anticholiergics

Anticholiergics are used less commonly as premedicants to dry bronchial and salivary secretions which are increased by intubations, by surgery to the upper airways and by some inhalation anesthetics.

Glycopyrronium (0.2–0.4 mg IM or IV) is preferred, because it produces good drying of salivary secretions and produces less tachycardia than atropine. It is widely used with neostigmine for reversal of non-depolarizing muscle relaxants.

Prokinetics

Metoclopramide hastens gastric emptying, thus reduces the risk of vomiting, regurgitation and of subsequent inhalation of gastric contents during general anesthesia. It is commonly used before delivery in obstetric patients or general anesthesia in patients known to have significant gastroesophageal reflex. Sodium citrate or ranitidine raises the pH of gastric content, which also reduces the risk of vomiting in the obstetric patient or general anesthesia.

Analgesics

Opioid analgesics are now rarely used as premedicants as they cause respiratory depression, CVS depression, nausea and vomiting.

NSAIDs do not depress respiration, do not impair GIT motility, do not cause dependence and are useful alternatives to opioids for the relief of pain. Ketorolac is usually preferred and can be given orally or parenterally.

GENERAL ANESTHETICS

The cardinal features of general anesthesia include analgesia, amnesia, loss of consciousness, inhibition of sensory and autonomic reflexes, and skeletal muscle relaxation.

An ideal anesthetic drug should posses a wide margin of safety, induce a smooth and rapid unconsciousness, adequate skeletal muscle relaxation, and prompt recovery after its discontinuation.

No single agent is capable of achieving all of these desirable effects. Hence, in anesthetic practice several different categories of drugs are used concomitantly to produce a "balanced anesthesia", which takes advantages of the favorable properties of each agent while minimizing their adverse effects.

For major surgical procedures, anesthesia requires induction of anesthesia with an intravenous anesthetic (e.g. thiopental or propofol), maintenance of anesthesia with a combination of inhaled (e.g. volatile agents, nitrous oxide) and intravenous (e.g. propofol, opioid analgesic) drugs, and muscle relaxation to facilitate intubation and suppress muscle tone to the degree required for surgery.

Stages of anesthesia

The traditional description of four stages of anesthesia was derived from the observations of diethyl ether, which produced a slow onset of anesthesia owing to its high solubility in blood.

In current clinical anesthesia practice, the stages of anesthesia have lost its relevance because of several factors including use of preanesthetic medication, more rapid onset of action of modern intravenous and inhaled anesthetics, control of ventilatory functions, use of intraoperative analgesics and muscle relaxants.

The attainment of surgical anesthesia is assessed clinically by loss of motor and autonomic responses, loss of corneal reflex and establishment of regular respiratory pattern.

Though monitoring of vital signs is the most common method of assessing depth of anesthesia during surgery, newer techniques "computer assisted monitoring" of vital signs and cerebral functions reduces the anesthetic dose requirements, which contributes to a more rapid recovery from general anesthesia.

INTRAVENOUS INDUCTION ANESTHETICS

Intravenous drugs are usually used to induce anesthesia. Induction is faster than any of the inhaled anesthetics. Intravenous induction drugs act only for a few minutes and anesthesia is then maintained using inhalational anesthetics and other drugs.

Induction anesthetics have also been increasingly used as intravenous anesthetics that do not include any inhaled anesthetics (e.g. total intravenous anesthesia). Their advantage is that do not require specialized vaporizer equipment for their delivery or facilities for the disposal of exhaled gases.

Although induction anesthetic, with exception of ketamine, do not possess analgesic properties, their potency is adequate for short superficial surgical procedures when combined with nitrous oxide or local anesthetics or both.

Adjunctive use of potent opioids contributes to improved cardiovascular stability, enhanced sedation, and perioperative analgesia. However, opioid compounds also enhance the ventilatory depressant effects of the intravenous agents and increase postoperative emesis.

Recent studies suggest that intravenous lidocaine may be useful as an adjuvant for reducing acute pain in the preoperative period. As a result of its opioid-sparing effect, use of intravenous lidocaine has been found to facilitate recovery of bowel function and lead to an earlier discharge after abdominal surgery.

Barbiturates

Thiopental sodium is widely used intravenously for induction but has no analgesic action. Induction is generally smooth and rapid (within 20 seconds). It cannot be used for maintenance of anesthesia throughout surgery because of its narrow therapeutic margin. Overdose causes cardiorespiratory depression.

Accidental intra-arterial injection is dangerous and may result in arterial spasm and permanent ischemic damage to the arm.

Awakening from moderate dose of thiopental sodium is rapid due to redistribution of the drug from the brain into other tissues, particularly muscle or fat.

Etomidate

Etomidate is not a barbiturate. It is metabolized more rapidly and recovery is more rapid without hangover effect. Its use is associated with a high incidence of involuntary muscle movement and pain on injection. It has minimal or no effect on blood pressure and may be preferred for induction in patients with cardiac problems. It is otherwise not commonly used.

Propofol

Propofol has become the most popular intravenous anesthetic. Apart from the rapid onset of action, the notable feature is that the recovery is the most rapid of other IV anesthetics and the patient feels better in the immediate postoperative period because of the reduction in postoperative nausea and vomiting and a sense of well-being.

Propofol is used for both induction and maintenance of anesthesia as part of total intravenous or balanced anesthesia techniques, and is the agent of choice for ambulatory surgery. Pain at the site of injection is the most common adverse effects of bolus administration.

Prolonged use of propofol for sedation or ventilatory management in the ICU should be avoided because it can lead to delay arousal, increase serum lipid level, severe acidosis with possible neurologic sequel, respiratory depression, hypotension, and muscle movements, hypoclonus and rarely tremors.

Ketamine

Ketamine produces a dissociative anesthetic state characterized by catatonia, amnesia, and analgesia, with or without loss of consciousness.

It differs from other induction anesthetic drugs in following respects:
- It is the only induction (intravenous) anesthetic that possesses both anesthetic and analgesic properties.
- It produces cardiovascular stimulation by stimulating the central sympathetic nervous system.
- It markedly increases cerebral blood flow, oxygen consumption and intracranial pressure.
- Its use is associated with postoperative disorientation, sensory and perceptual illusions and vivid dreams (so called emergence phenomena).

Ketamine in small doses is used as an alternative to opioid analgesics in combination with other intravenous and inhaled anesthetics to minimize respiratory depression. It is also very useful for poor-risk geriatric patients and high-risk patients in cardiogenic or septic shock because of its cardiostimulatory properties.

MAINTENANCE OF ANESTHESIA

There are three important group of drugs used for maintenance of anesthesia throughout surgery following induction with intravenous anesthetic drug. These are:
- Inhalation anesthetics
- Short acting opioids
- Muscle relaxants

Inhalation anesthetics

Inhalation anesthetics may be gases or volatile liquids.

Nitrous oxide

Nitrous oxide is a safe anesthetic gas (also called laughing gas because it causes some patients to laugh if used on its own for induction of anesthesia). It is a weak anesthetic and is commonly used in combination with 30% oxygen, as part of a balanced technique in association with other liquid volatile (e.g. sevoflurane) or intravenous (e.g. propofol) anesthetics.

Unlike other inhalation anesthetic, it has a powerful analgesic effect in sub-anesthetic concentrations.

A mixture of nitrous oxide and oxygen containing 50% of each gas (Entonox) is used for pain relief in labor.

Induction and recovery is rapid and nitrous oxide has no adverse effects on CVS, respiratory system, liver or kidney. It has no muscle relaxant action and commonly requires the use of muscle relaxants.

Untoward effects of nitrous oxide are due to anoxia (resulting from unskilled use) or megaloblastic anemia due to inhibition of a vitamin B_{12} co-enzyme necessary for folate metabolism. It may also depress bone marrow leading to leucopenia. The increased incidence of postoperative nausea and vomiting (PONV) however has resulted in a significant decrease in its use.

Volatile liquid anesthetics

These are all halogenated volatile liquids that require a carrier gas, usually oxygen or nitrous oxide-oxygen mixtures, to deliver them. Unlike nitrous oxide, they have no analgesic properties in sub-anesthetic concentrations.

Halothane

Halothane causes cardio-respiratory depression and severe hepatotoxicity. It produces moderate muscle relaxation and is rarely used.

Enflurane

Enflurane is less potent than halothane and is a powerful cardiorespiratory depressant. The risk of hepatotoxicity is less than halothane.

Isoflurane

Isoflurane has a pungent odour. Induction, though unpleasant, is rapid. It does not cause cardiac arrhythmia or damage to liver or kidney. It relaxes the smooth muscles (bronchial and vascular) and also the skeletal muscles. Being a vasodilator it causes hypotension and reflex tachycardia. In patients with coronary artery disorders, redistribution of coronary blood flow to the normal vessels at the cost of poorly perfused ischemic area (**coronary seal phenomenon**) may precipitate myocardial ischemia.

Low concentrations of isoflurane do not increase cerebral blood flow or intracranial pressure. It depresses cortical EEG activity and is preferred for neurosurgery. Emergence from anesthesia is rapid.

Isoflurane is one of the most widely used routine ane-sthetic.

Desflurane

Desflurane has action similar to isoflurane. It is irritant and may cause cough, apnea, laryngospasm and increased secretions. Incidence of postoperative nausea and vomiting is greater than propofol. It is not suitable for induction and in children.

However, it has a very rapid onset and emergence from anesthesia and recovery from psychomotor and cognitive skills with desflurane are more rapid than any other anesthetic. It rarely precipitates malignant hyperthermia and sensitizes myocardium to catecholamine to a lesser extent than halothane. Seizure provoking potential is also negligible.

Desflurane is very popular anesthetic for outpatient surgery, as the patient can be discharged few hours after surgery.

Sevoflurane

Sevoflurane is the latest volatile halogenated anesthetic. Being non-pungent, it does not cause respiratory irritation. Acceptability is better even in children. Induction and emergence are as fast as with desflurane. It has good muscle relaxant properties. Cardiovascular effects are similar to those of desflurane but it does not produce 'coronary seal'.

It may trigger malignant hyperthermia in susceptible patients but risk is much lower than halothane. Though the chances of renal toxicity are minimal, it is best avoided in patients with renal failure. Shivering, nausea and vomiting have been reported in postoperative period.

It makes an excellent choice for inhalation anesthetic in children and for surgical procedures performed on ambulatory (short stay) basis.

Xenon

Xenon, an inert gas, is a potent anesthetic with rapid induction and recovery. It has no effects on CVS, pulmonary, hepatic or renal function. It is not metabolized, and but for the cost, is the ideal anesthetic.

Ether

Ether is no longer used except in rural areas where resources (anesthetic equipment and resuscitation facilities) and skills are limited. It is a fairly safe anesthetic and can be used with simple and portable equipment using room air instead of cylinder oxygen.

Ether has a great margin of safety, is an effective analgesic and causes good muscular relaxation due to a curare like action and depression of synaptic pathways in spinal cord.

The disadvantages of ether are that it is highly explosive and cannot be used with diathermy. It is highly irritant and can cause copious bronchial secretions, the induction is very slow and recovery from anesthesia is associated with a prolonged hangover with nausea and vomiting.

Short acting opioids

Intraoperative opioids in small doses are given before or with induction to reduce the dose requirement of inhalational anesthetics to a minimum.

Alfentanil, fentanyl and **remifentanil** are particularly useful because they act within 1-2 minutes.

High (versus low) dose opioid based anesthetic techniques may be associated with increased postoperative morbidity (e.g. prolonged ventilator support, gastrointestinal and bladder complications) and even increase in mortality after cardiac surgery.

Remifentanil

Remifentanil is of particular interest, because unlike other opioids (which are metabolized in liver), remifentanil is rapidly metabolized by non-specific blood and tissue esterases and its short duration of action allows prolonged administration at high doses without accumulation, and with little risk of residual post-operative respiratory depression. Because of its potency, short action and lack of CVS side effects, remifentanil is the drug of choice in the management of general anesthesia for major operations on patients with heart disease.

Fentanyl and doperidol (an antipsychotic drug) administered together produce analgesia and amnesia and combined with nitrous oxide provide a state referred to as **neuroleptanesthesia**.

If necessary, as with longer acting opioids, the action of short acting opioids may be easily reversed at the end of anesthesia by naloxone.

Muscle relaxants

Muscle relaxants used in anesthesia are neuromuscular blocking drugs, which have greatly revolutionized the anesthesia practice by enabling the use of low doses of general anesthetics for major surgery.

Neuromuscular blocking drugs relax the muscles of the abdomen and diaphragm and vocal chords permitting the employment of light levels of surgical anesthesia and intubation.

Patients who have received muscle relaxants should always have their respiration assisted or controlled until the drug has been inactivated or antagonized.

All the neuromuscular blocking agents are highly polar compounds and inactive orally. They are administered parenterally.

On the basis of their mechanism action they are classified into two groups:

1. Non-depolarizing (competitive) muscle relaxants

These drugs competitively block the access of Ach to the receptor of motor end plate and prevent its depolarization leading to profound skeletal muscle relaxation.

2. Depolarizing relaxant (persistant depolarizer)

The drug produces persistent depolarization at neuromuscular junction and is not amenable to hydrolysis by true cholinesterase present in synaptic cleft.

NON-DEPOLARIZING (COMPETITIVE) MUSCLE RELAXANTS

These are most commonly used along with volatile (inhaled) anesthetic drugs to achieve adequate muscle relaxation for all types of surgical procedures without cardiorespiratory depressant effects produced by deep anesthesia. These groups of drugs occupy the receptor sites at the neuromuscular junction and render acetylcholine ineffective that is released following nerve stimulation.

The neuromuscular blockade action of competitive muscle relaxants can be reversed by anticholinesterases such as neostigmine and pyridostigmine. Recently a unique reversal drug, **sugammadex**, has been developed which can rapidly inactivate commonly used steroidal neuromuscular blockade (e.g. rocuronium and vecuronium) by forming an inactive compound, which is excreted in the urine.

The choice of a muscle relaxant depends on:
- Potency (relative to *d*-tubocurarine)
- Onset of action
- Adverse effects

Pharmacological actions

Tubocurarine, the initial non-depolarizing agent, has been replaced by a number of synthetic drugs, having distinct advantages, with the same mode of action.

The most important properties distinguishing the non-depolarizing muscle relaxants lies in the time of onset and liability to produce cardiovascular effects that are mediated by either autonomic or histamine receptors (Table 3.9). A rapid onset of action determines how rapidly the patient's trachea can be intubated. Of the currently available non-depolarizing drugs, **rocuronium** (60–120 seconds) has the most rapid action.

Gantacurium, currently under clinical trials, has a very rapid onset and short duration of action and may prove to be the muscle relaxant of choice for intubation.

Cardiovasular effects

Vecuronium, pipecuronium, doxacurium, cisatracurium, and **rocuronium** all have minimal, if any, cardiovascular effects. The rest produce cardiovascular effects, that are mediated by either autonomic of histamine receptors.

The intermediate acting muscle relaxants (e.g. vecuronium and cisatracurium) are the most commonly used muscle relaxants in clinical practice.

DEPOLARIZING MUSCLE RELAXANT

Succinylcholine is the only depolarizing muscle relaxant which is rarely used. It has rapid onset of action which is short lasting. It had been used for endotracheal intubation at the beginning of anesthesia and for very short procedure requiring relaxation.

Common side effects include postoperative muscle pain, cardiovascular disorders, apnea and respiratory depression. Prolonged paralysis (suxamethonium apnea) may occur in patients with low or atypical plasma cholinesterase. Other side effects include hyperkalemia in certain diseased condition (e.g. burns, head injury), which rarely may cause cardiac arrest. It may trigger malignant hyperthermia in susceptible patients.

Table 3.9: Characteristic features of common neuromuscular blocking drugs

Drug	Relative Potency to Tubocurarine	Onset (Minutes)	Duration (Minutes)	Autonomic ganglia	Effect on Cardiac Muscarinic Receptor	Histamine Release
		Non-depolarizing (competitive blocking drugs long acting)				
Doxacurium	6	4–8	>35	None	None	None
Pancuromium	6	4–6	>35	None	Moderate	None
Pipecuronium	6	2–4	>35	None	None	None
Intermediate acting						
Atracurium	1.5	2–4	20–35	None	None	Slight
Cisatracurum	1.5	3–6	25–44	None	None	None
Vecuronium	6	2–4	20–35	None	None	None
Rocuronium	0.8	1–2	20–35	None	Slight	None
Short acting						
Mivacurium	4	2–3	10–20	None	None	Moderate
			Depolarizing agent			
Succinylcholine	0.4	<1.5	5–10	Stimulation	Stimulation	Slight

Uses of neuromuscular blocking drugs

1. As an adjuvant to general anesthesia

The most important indication of the muscle relaxants is to facilitate intracavity surgery, especially during abdominal and thoracic surgery. Cisatracurium is the muscle relaxant of choice.

2. For tracheal intubation

Relaxation of pharyngeal and laryngeal muscle facilitates endotracheal intubation and laryngoscopy. Endotracheal intubation ensures an adequate airway and minimizes the risk of pulmonary aspiration during general anesthesia.

3. To control ventilation

In the intensive care unit muscle relaxants are frequently used to eliminate chest wall resistance and ineffective spontaneous ventilation in patients having obstructive airway disease.

CENTRALLY ACTING SKELETAL MUSCLE RELAXANTS

This group of drugs differs in action from the muscle relaxants used in anesthesia which act at the neuromuscular junction. They reduce skeletal muscle tone by a selective action on cerebrospinal axis without affecting consciousness with the exception of dantrolene, which has a peripheral action.

Centrally acting muscle relaxants are used for the relief of chronic muscle spasm or spasticity. Spasticity is characterized by an increase in tonic stretch reflexes and flexor muscle spasm along with muscle weakness. It is often associated with spinal injury, cerebral palsy, multiple sclerosis, and stroke, and involves abnormal function of bowel, bladder and skeletal muscles. The symptoms of spasticity may be controlled by modifying the stretch reflex arc by enhancing the activity of the inhibitory internuncial neurons or by interfering directly with skeletal muscle (i.e., excitation-contraction coupling).

These drugs relax spasm without altering normal muscle function by damping down reflexes in the spinal cord. However, these drugs do not significantly improve meaningful function (e.g., mobility and normal return to work).

Diazepam

Diazepam acts by damping down reflexes in the spinal cord. It is the most commonly used skeletal muscle relaxant in anxiolytic doses for the relief of chronic muscle spasm or spasticity of varied etiology including tetanus.

Sedation and occasionally, extensor hypotonus are the disadvantages.

Baclofen

Baclofen is an orally active GABAmimetic drug which acts as a GABA agonist at GABA receptors. It depresses both monosynaptic and polysynaptic reflexes in the spinal cord.

Baclofen causes less sedation and also reduces pain compared to diazepam in spastic conditions. In addition baclofen does not reduce overall muscle strength as much as dantrolene. Baclofen is used in painful spasticity resulting from disorders such as multiple sclerosis or traumatic partial section of spinal cord. It may also provide relief in intractable low back pain, migraine headaches, trigeminal neuralgia, tardive dyskinesia, and in reducing craving in recovering alcoholics.

Adverse effects include drowsiness, muscle weakness and ataxia. Withdrawal from baclofen must be done very slowly to prevent seizures.

Its use is contraindicated in peptic ulcer, and should be used with caution in psychiatric illness, epilepsy and hepatic or renal impairment.

Tizanidine

Tizanidine, α_2 adrenoceptor agonist, is indicated in spasticity associated with multiple sclerosis or spinal cord injury. It causes drowsiness, nausea and other gastrointestinal disorders, cardiovascular disturbances, hallucinations and insomnia. It is contraindicated in severe hepatic impairment.

Other centrally acting muscle relaxants

A large number of inhibitory neurotransmitters have been found to be useful muscle relaxants in patients with multiple sclerosis. These include:

- Gabapentin, an antiepileptic drug.
- Pregabalin, a analog of gabapentin in painful disorders that involve a muscle spasm component.
- Progabide, a GABAmimetic drug.
- Glycine, an amino acid neurotransmitter.
- Inhibitors of glutamatergic transmission – idrocilamide and riluzole for muscle spasm reducing effects in amyotrophic lateral sclerosis.
- Carisoprodol, cyclobenzaprine, methocarbamol, chlorphenesin, chlorzoxazone and orphenadrine are used in acute muscle spasm caused by local trauma. They are structurally related to the tricyclic antidepressants and possess anticholinergic properties causing sedation. These drugs have limited therapeutic value.

Dantrolene

Dantrolene, a phenytoin analog, differs from centrally acting drugs in acting directly on the skeletal muscle at an intracellular level (but not by blocking the neuromuscular junction).

Dantrolene reduces skeletal muscle activity by interfering with excitation-contraction coupling in the muscle fibers. The normal contractile response which involves release of calcium from its stores in sarcoplasmic reticulum is reduced by dantrolene.

Cardiac and smooth muscles are almost unaffected because calcium release form their sarcoplasmic reticulum occurs by a different mechanism.

The drug also facilitates GABA which results in the depression of brain stem reticular functions. Hence, it produces sedation but has no selective action on polysynaptic reflexes.

Dantrolene is the drug of choice for the treatment of malignant hyperthermia, a rare genetically inherited condition that can be triggered by a variety of stimuli, including volatile anesthetics and succinylcholine. It is not effective in the treatment of heat stroke.

Major adverse effects include generalized muscle weakness, sedation and occasionally hepatitis.

Botulinium toxin

Botulinium toxins are neurotoxins, which prevent the calcium dependent release of acetylcholine at neuromuscular junction and produce a state of denervation leading to muscle relaxation.

Local facial injection of botulinium toxin is widely used for the short-term treatment of wrinkles associated with aging around the eyes and mouth. Local injection is also used for the treatment of strabismus and blepharospasm, and cerebral palsy. Adverse effects include speech disorders, vertigo and dry eyes.

3.13 CENTRAL NERVOUS SYSTEM STIMULANTS

Central nervous system (CNS) stimulants have very little place in therapy and should not be used to treat depression, obesity, senility, and debility or for relief of fatigue.

AMPHETAMINES

These are sympathomimetics, whose main action is on CNS.

Pharmacological actions

Amphetamines are potent CNS stimulants, acting probably by releasing noradrenalin and dopamine. They produce euphoria, abolish fatigue, increase activity and reduce appetite. There is considerable psychic dependence but the withdrawal symptoms are not severe.

Dexamphetamine has a greater central stimulant and less peripheral sympathomimetic action than amphetamine.

METHYLPHENIDATE (Ritalin)

Ritalin is a drug related to amphetamine. It is the only CNS stimulant used in narcolepsy and as an adjuvant in the management of refractory hyperkinetic states in children.

CAFFEINE

Caffeine, one of the naturally occurring methylxanthine, has a weak CNS stimulant action. It has no therapeutic use and its combination with analgesics (aspirin) is unfounded.

RESPIRATORY STIMULANTS (ANALEPTICS)

Respiratory stimulants have a limited place in respiratory failure.

NIKETHAMIDE (coramine)

Nikethamide is an obsolete drug because therapeutic doses are close to toxic doses which may result in convulsions.

DOXAPRAM

Doxapram is the most effective analeptic with greater margin of safety. It stimulates cerebrospinal axis at all levels.

Doxapram is used in postoperative respiratory depression and acute respiratory failure. Its use is contraindicated in severe hypertension, status asthmatics, coronary artery disease, thyrotoxicosis, epilepsy and physical obstruction of respiratory tract.

3.14 DRUG DEPENDENCE (DRUG ADDICTION)

Drug dependence is a condition arising from habitual use of a drug in which the person has a compulsion to continue the use of the drug to have pleasurable psychic effects and feels ill, if deprived of it (abstinence or withdrawal syndrome).

Drug dependence has two characteristic components: psychological and physical dependence.

Psychological dependence on drug leads to euphoria, which is characterized by an exaggerated feeling of physical and mental well-being, especially when not justified by external reality and the patient often resorts to antisocial activities.

Psychological dependence is also called addiction. Drugs of addiction have no therapeutic value (exception opiods) and as a general rule, activate the mesolimbic dopamine system.

Dopamine is considered to be a "pleasure neurotransmitter". Some of the portent drugs of addiction include cocaine, cannabis, ecstasy and gamma-hydroxybutyrate (GHB).

Physical dependence produces biochemical changes in the patient, which results in very unpleasant signs and symptoms, if the drug is withdrawn. Physical dependence is of a temporary nature and lasts for a varying period, which finally disappears.

Central stimulant drugs of addiction, namely cocaine, amphetamines, cannabis, lysergide (lysergic acid diethylamide, LSD) are characterized by the absence of any important physical dependence.

COCAINE

Cocaine is an alkaloid found in the leaves of erythroxyion coca. It is available as a water soluble hydrochloride salt suitable for nasal inhalation (**"snorting"**), or as an insoluble free base (**'crack'** cocaine), which can be smoked. Inhaled crack cocaine gives a more rapid and intense effects.

Cocaine causes addiction in susceptible individuals, in whom it causes intense psychic dependence with a feeling of elation and an increase in physical activity, only after a few exposures to cocaine. Physical dependence is practically absent, withdrawal symptoms being depression, sleepiness and increased appetite. Cravings are very strong and underline the very high addiction liability to cocaine.

Cocaine addicts typically lose their appetite, are hyperactive, and sleep little.

Cocaine toxicity includes ischemic strokes, myocardial infarction, and seizures. Overdose may lead to hyperthermia, coma, and death.

Cocaine does not have any specific antagonist and the management of intoxication remains supportive.

CANNABIS

Cannabis is derived from the dried leaves and flowers of Cannabis sativa. **Marijuana** and **Bhang,** are the dried leaves and flowering heads and **Hashish** or **charas** is the dried black resinous substance obtained from the leaves of the plant. When smoked (except bhang which is taken orally), the onset of action occurs within 10–30 minutes and lasts for 4–8 hours.

Cannabis produces euphoria, perceptual alterations and conjunctival infection, followed by enhanced appetite, relaxation, dream-like state, slurred speech and ataxia. High doses may produce anxiety, confusion, hallucinations and psychosis.

Psychological dependence is common but tolerance and withdrawal symptoms are unusual. Long-term use is thought to increase the lifetime risk of developing schizophrenia. Ingestion or smoking of cannabis rarely results in serious poisoning and supportive treatment is all that is required.

HALLUCINOGENS

D-lysergic acid diethylamide (LSD), **mescaline** and **psilocybin** are the drugs commonly called hallucinogens, because of their ability to cause perceptual effects, such as heightened visual awareness of colors, distortion of images, and sensing of things, which may be pleasurable or horrifying ('bad trip') and associated with panic, confusion, agitation or aggression. Dilated pupils, hypotension, pyrexia and metabolic acidosis may occur and psychosis may sometimes last for several days.

Psychosis like manifestations (depersonalization, hallucinogens, and distorted time perception) have led them to be classified as psychotomimetics, psychedelics or psychodysleptics.

Hallucinogens do not cause dependence or addiction, but repetitive exposure leads to rapid tolerance (tachyphylaxis). They do not stimulate dopamine release, but cause an increase glutamate release in the cortex.

Patients with psychotic reactions or CNS depression are required to be isolated in a quiet, dimly lit room to minimize external stimulation. Diazepam is the drug of choice for sedation. Antipsychotic drugs are contraindicated as they may precipitate cardiovascular collapse or convulsions.

ECSTASY (MDMA)

Ecstasy is the name of a class of drugs that includes a large variety of derivatives of the amphetamine-related compound methylenedioxymethamphetamine (MDMA). Ecstasy is a popular socializing drug and largely used in small quantities in parties, because the main effects of ecstasy appears to be to faster feelings of intimacy and empathy without impairing intellectual capacities.

Like amphetamine, ecstasy causes release of endogenous biogenic amines, such as dopamine and noradrenalin. It has a preferential affinity for the serotonin transporter (SERT) and therefore most strongly increases the extracellular concentration of serotonin.

Ecstasy has several acute toxic effects. Hyperpyrexia, rhabdomyolysis, metabolic acidosis, acute renal failure, hepatocellular necrosis, acute respiratory distress syndrome (ARDS), cardiovascular collapse and even irreversible brain damage have all been described following ecstasy use, though rare, the occasional recreational use of ecstasy cannot be considered safe.

There is no specific antidote and the management is supportive and directed at complications.

GAMMA HYDROXYBUTYRATE (GHB)

GHB is a sedative agent with psychedelic and body-building effects, acting mainly by inhibiting GABA neurons at the concentration typically obtained with recreational use. It is quite popular in social gathering because it is odorless and can be readily dissolved in beverages. It causes euphoria, enhanced sensory perception, a feeling of social closeness, and amnesia.

Toxic features are those of a sedative hypnotic and may end in coma. Coma usually resolves spontaneously and abruptly within a few hours, but can also persist for several days.

OPIOIDS

The most potent and frequently opioid of addiction is heroin. Psychological and physical dependence is severe, tolerance develops rapidly and withdrawal symptoms are severe which include nausea, vomiting and muscle cramps. Injections under nonsterile and sharing conditions can give rise to septicemia and risk of being infected with the virus of hepatitis B or C or the HIV causing AIDS.

Lofexidine is used for the alleviation of symptoms in patients undergoing opioid withdrawal. It prevents the rise of noradrenalin in the brain (responsible for many of the unpleasant withdrawal symptoms) which occurs when opioids are withdrawn. It does not lower the blood pressure.

Naltrexone, an opioid antagonist, blocks the euphoric effect of opioids, which is linked to addiction and is given to former opioid addicts as an aid to prevent relapses.

BARBITURATES

Barbiturates are still used in epilepsy. They are dangerous drugs of addiction and cause very severe physical dependence. Tolerance is less marked than with opioids, but withdrawal symptoms are more severe.

ALCOHOL

Psychological dependence on alcohol is very common and its management is a difficult medical and social problem. Chronic use of alcohol leads to physical dependence. Sudden withdrawal from an addict can precipitate an acute psychotic attack (**delirium tremens**) with agitation, anxiety, excessive sympathetic activity and convulsions.

Disulfiram (antabuse) is used as an adjunct to the treatment of alcohol dependence. It inhibits the breakdown of alcohol, leading to accumulation of acetaldehyde which causes flushing, nausea, vomiting and headache and thus the patient is discouraged from further drinking.

Acamprosate, a centrally acting drug, may be helpful in maintaining abstinence in alcohol-dependent patients. It may cause GIT disorders and occasionally skin rashes. It is contraindicated in renal and severe hepatic impairment

4

Autacoids and Antagonists

Autacoids are circulating or locally acting hormone like substances that originate from diffuse tissues. Their main function is to modulate local circulation and to influence the process of inflammation. Many autacoids have other physiologic and pathologic functions, which are not understood.

Autacoids antagonists have emerged as important drugs for the management of allergic disorders (histamine$_1$ receptor antagonists), peptic ulcer (histamine$_2$ receptor antagonists), CVS disorders (angiotensin converting enzyme inhibitors) and NSAIDs (cyclooxygenase enzyme inhibitors concerned with prostaglandin synthesis).

Autacoids can be divided into three major categories on the basis of their structure:

- **Decarboxylated aminoacids:** Histamine, serotonin
- **Polypeptides:** Angiotensins, kinins, vasoactive intestinal polypeptide, substance P
- **Eicosanoids:** Prostaglandins, lenkotrienes, thromboxanes.

Histamine and antihistamines

Histamine is derived chiefly by decarboxylation of dietary histidine. Large amounts of histamine are found in the lungs, skin and intestinal mucosa. It is stored in the granules of the mast cells and basophils in an inactive form.

Degranulation of the mast cells release histamine which causes capillary leakage, cellular edema, smooth muscle contractions and sensory nerve ending stimulation resulting in anaphylaxis and allergic reactions.

Histamine produces its effects by acting on histamine receptors located on the surface membrane. The four different histamine receptors thus far characterized are designated H_1-H_4.

Receptor subtype	Location
H_1	Smooth muscles, endothelium, brain
H_2	Gastric mucosa, cardiac muscle, mast cells, brain
H_3	Presynaptic–in the brain mesenteric plexus, other neurons
H_4	Eosinophils, neutrophils, CD4 T cells.

H_1 and H_2 receptor antagonists are therapeutically used in the management of allergic disorders and peptic ulcer disease respectively. No selective H_3 or H_4 antagonists are presently available, though they have great therapeutic potential. H_3 receptor antagonists may be of value in sleep disorders, obesity, and cognitive and psychiatric disorders. H_4 blockers have potential in inflammatory conditions such as asthma in which eosinophils and mast cells play a prominent role.

H_1-receptor antagonists (Antihistamine)

Antihistamines are divided into first–generation and second–generation agents. This distinction is based on their relative sedative and anticholinergic effects (Table 4.1).

Pharmacokinetics

Antihistamines are rapidly absorbed after oral administration with peak blood levels within 1–2 hours. They are widely distributed in the body except for second generation antihistamines which do not enter the central nervous system readily.

Antihistamines are metabolized in the liver by microsomal system. Some of the second generation agents (terfenadine and astemizole) are metabolized by specific CYP3A4 enzyme and thus are subject to important interaction (life threatening arrhythmias) when other drugs (such as azoles, erythromycin) inhibit this subtype of P450 enzyme.

Table 4.1: Commonly used antihistamine

Drugs	Dose (oral)	Anticholinergic activity	Comments
\multicolumn{4}{c}{First generation antihistamines (Duration 4–6 hours)}			
Highly sedative			
Dramamine	25–50 mg	+++	Antimotion sickness
Diphenhyramine	25–50 mg	+++	Antimotion sickness
Doxylamine	15–25 mg	++	Sleep Aid
Hydroxyzine	25–50 mg		Antiemetic
Promethazine	10–25 mg	+++	Antiemetic, α-blocker
Moderately sedative			
Pyrilamine	25–50 mg	+	Sleep Aid
Cyproheptadine	4 mg	++	Antiserotonin activity
Mild sedative			
Cyclizine	25–30 mg	++	Antimotion sickness
Meclizine	25–50 mg	++	Antimotion sickness
Chlorpheniramine	4–8 mg	+	Common cold medication
\multicolumn{4}{c}{Second Generaton Antihistamines Long acting (Duration 12-24 hours)}			
Fexofenadine	120–180 mg	–	Non arrhythmogenic
Cetrizine	5–10 mg	–	Inhibitors of histamine release and cytotoxic mediators
Levocetrizine	5 mg	–	Long acting
Loratidine	10 mg	–	Long acting
Deslorotadine	5 mg	–	Long acting and anti-inflammatory

Therapeutics uses

Antihistamines are one of the most widely prescribed drugs because of their relative safety and the prevalence of allergic conditions. The second generation antihistamines because of low incidence (5–7%) of sedation are preferred.

Allergic disorders

Second generation antihistaminics are the drugs of choice to prevent and treat allergic rhinitis (hay fever) and urticaria. For atopic dermatitis (eczema), first generation drugs such as diphenhydramine is preferred because their additional sedative effects reduce the awareness of itching and sleep disorders.

Antihistamines relieve skin symptoms of anaphylaxis but have no immediate effects on systemic allergic reactions; adrenaline (IV), glucocorticoids (IM), antihistamine (IM) are life saving along with supportive measures such as nebulized β_2-agonists, IV fluids and oxygen.

Motion sickness and vestibular disturbances

First generation antihistamines and scopolamine (anticholinergic) are effective for the prophylaxis of the motion sickness. Diphenhydramine and promethazine are the most effective, though cyclizine and meclizine, which are less sedative, also have significant activity in preventing motion sickness. These antihistamines have also been claimed to be effective in Meniere's syndrome. Combination with ephedrine or amphetamine potentiates the effects of scopolamine and antihistamines in preventing motion sickness.

Nausea and vomiting of pregnancy

Some antihistamines have been found to have teratogenic effects in rodents. Doxylamine in combination with pyridoxine had been widely used for "morning sickness", but for its disputed adverse effects in pregnancy, it is safer to avoid antihistaminic drugs during pregnancy.

Miscellaneous uses

First generation antihistamines, because of their sedative and anticholinergic actions, have limited effectiveness in conditions like drug-induced Parkinsonism, insomnia, common cold and in acute dystonia due to antipsychotic drugs.

Adverse effects

Sedation and anticholinergic effects constitute the most common undesirable actions seen with first generation antihistamines.

Less common toxic effects include excitation and convulsions in children, postural hypotension and allergic responses. Drug allergy is relatively common after topical use of antihistamines.

Terfenadine and astemizole are generally avoided because they may induce cardiac arrhythmias and are contraindicated in patients taking azoles or macrolides and in presence of liver disease.

Tolerance to their actions may also develop after prolonged use.

5-HYDROXYTRYPTAMINE

5-Hydroxytryptamine (5-HT, serotonin) is an important chemical neurotransmitter in the central nervous system, a local hormone in the gut, and a component of the platelet clotting process.

The action of 5-HT depends of the class of receptor (seven main type $5\text{-}HT_1$ to $5\text{-}HT_7$ and 14 subtypes of $5\text{-}HT_1$ and $5\text{-}HT_2$ receptors), many of which lack any specific physiological role. It is, therefore, easier to discuss its actions on specific tissue and organ system instead of on receptor basis. Drugs, 5-HT agonists and antagonists, are important in the treatment of abnormalities in the action of 5-HT that are involved in several disorders:

- Brain depression
- Brain and gut: vomiting caused by certain cytotoxic drugs
- Cranial blood flow – migraine
- Carcinoid tumors producing large amounts of 5-HT.

Pharmacological actions

5-HT is an important neurotransmitter at several sites in the CNS and is involved in numerous diffuse functions such as mood, behavior, emotion, sleep, appetite, temperature regulation, perception of pain, regulation of blood pressure and vomiting. 5-HT agonists are used in clinical condition such as depression, anxiety and migraine.

5-HT receptors in GIT and in the vomiting center of the medulla participate in the vomiting reflex. 5-HT antagonists are very important in the prevention of nausea and vomiting associated with surgery and cancer chemotherapy.

Gastrointestinal tract

5-HT is present in large quantities (over 90% of 5-HT in the body) in enterochromaffin cells in the gastrointestinal cells. It has a powerful stimulant action on GIT smooth muscle, which causes a motility-enhancing or **"prokinetic"** effect of selective 5-HT agonists such as **cisapride**. Overproduction of 5-HT in **carcinoid tumors** is associated with severe diarrhea.

Cardiovascular system

5-HT is a powerful vasoconstrictor except in skeletal muscle and heart, where it dilates blood vessels. 5-HT causes aggregation of blood platelets.

Skeletal muscle

5-HT causes contraction of skeletal muscles leading to **serotonin syndrome** seen when MAO inhibitors are given with 5-HT agonists especially antidepressant of the selective serotonin reuptake inhibitors (SSRIs) class.

5-HT AGONISTS

5-HT has no clinical application as drug. However, its receptors agonists, especially 5-$HT_{1D/1B}$ agonists (triptans) have emerged as the most effective first-line therapy for acute severe migraine attacks.

Buspirone, a 5-HT_{1A} agonist is an effective nonbenzodiazepine anxiolytic.

Other 5-HT agonists are **dexfenfluramine**; an appetite suppressant, **cisapride**, a prokinetic agent and **tegaserod**, a drug used for irritable bowel syndrome and constipation are either banned or withdrawn in many countries because of their toxicity.

5-HT_1 (5-$HT_{1D/1B}$) agonists – triptans are used almost exclusively for migraine headache.

Drugs such as fluoxetine and other SSRIs, which modulate serotonergic transmission by blocking reuptake of the transmitter, are the most commonly prescribed first-line agents in the treatment of depression, anxiety and similar disorders (*see* Chapter 3).

5-HT ANTAGONISTS

Cyproheptadine and **ondansetron** are the most commonly used 5-HT antagonists. Cyproheptadine has H_1-receptor blocking as well as 5-HT_2-blocking actions. It prevents the smooth muscle effects of both amines but has no effect on H_2-receptor involved in gastric secretion. It has significant anticholinergic effects and causes sedation.

The major clinical applications of cyproheptadine are in the treatment of the smooth muscle manifestations of carcinoid tumor and in cold-induced urticaria. It is also of some value in serotonin syndrome.

Ondansteron is a 5-HT_3 antagonist. This drug and its analogs are very important in the prevention of nausea and vomiting associated with surgery and cancer chemotherapy.

Partial 5-HT agonist/antagonist

Ergot alkaloids occur naturally in a fungus (Claviceps purpurea) that infests cereal crops.

Ergot alkaloids fall into two major categories – *amine alkaloids* and *peptide alkaloids*.

Lysergic acid diethylamide (LSD), **methysergide** and **ergometrine** are amine alkaloids while **ergotamine, dihydroergotamine and bromocriptine** are peptide alkaloids.

Ergot alkaloids have agonist, partial agonist and antagonistic actions at 5-HT, alpha adrenergic and dopamine receptors. Thus, their actions are complex. Their actions on different neurotransmitters and autacoids are summarized in Table 4.2. Clinically they can be considered as **vasoselective, uteroselective** and **CNS selective**.

Ergotamine is vasoselective. It has mixed partial agonist effects at 5-HT_2 and alpha adrenoreceptors. It causes marked

Table 4.2: Action of ergot alkaloids at receptors

Drug	α-adreno-receptors	Dopamine receptor	5-HT$_2$ receptor	Uterine contraction
Ergotamine	**PA**	–	**PA**	++
Dihydroergotamine	**AG**	–	PA	+
LSD	–	AG	ANT*	+
Bromocriptine*	ANT	**AG**	ANT	–
Ergometrine	AG	ANT	PA	**+++**

Important effects indicated in **bold** type.   * **Agonist in CNS.**   AG: agonist.
PA: partial agonist.   ANT: antagonist.

vasoconstriction and is used in migraine and cluster headache. The vasoconstrictor effect is responsible for gangrene.

Ergometrine (ergonovine) is uteroselective, has same mechanism of action as ergotamine, but selective for uterine smooth muscle.

Lysergic acid diethylamide (LSD) is CNS selective. It is (CNS) 5-HT$_2$ and dopamine agonist and 5-HT antagonist in periphery. It causes hallucinations, is psychotomimetic and is widely abused.

Adverse reactions

Common side effects of ergot derivatives are nausea, vomiting and diarrhea. The most dangerous toxic effect of ergotamine and ergometrine is gangrene which may require amputation.

Other toxic effects of ergot alkaloids include drowsiness and, in case of methysergide central stimulation and hallucinations.

Contraindications include obstructive vascular (peripheral and coronary) and collagen diseases. Ergotamine for migraine is best avoided during pregnancy.

EICOSANOIDS

Prostanoids and leukotrienes are derived from arachidonic acid which is a component of cell membrane phospholipids of all tissues. The term prostanoids encompasses prostaglandins, prostacyclin and thromboxanes.

Cyclooxygenase enzymes promote oxygenation and cyclisation of arachidonic acid to yield PGG$_2$ and PGH$_2$ which are highly unstable, and get converted to prostaglandins (PGE$_2$, PGF$_{2a}$ and PGD$_2$), prostacyclin (PGI$_2$) and thromboxane-A$_2$ by separate pathways as shown in Fig. 4.1.

In platelets, the pathway leads to thromboxame A$_2$ (TXA$_2$), in vascular endothelium it leads to prostacyclin (PGI$_2$). Prostaglandins are formed in mast cells (PGD$_2$); in vasculature, GIT, lungs and other tissues (PGE$_2$), and in smooth muscles of GIT, bronchi, uterus and blood vessels (PGF$_{2a}$).

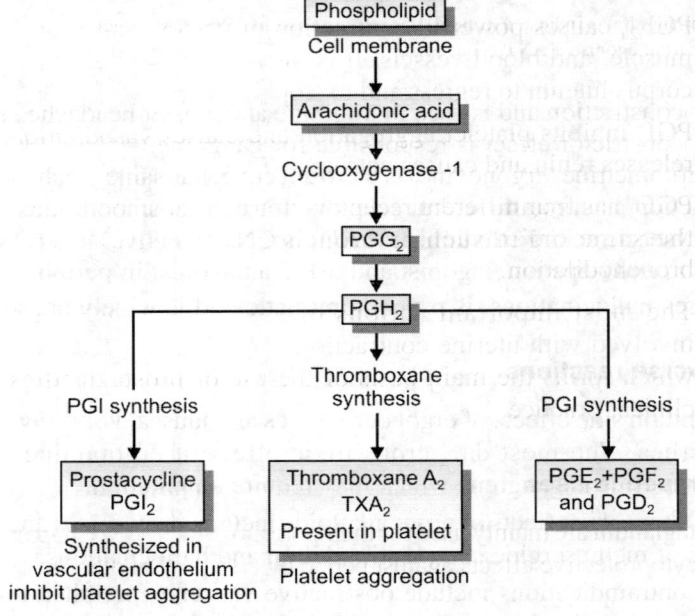

Fig. 4.1: Prostanoids synthesis

Pharmacological effects

Prostanoids have prominent effects on smooth muscle, platelets, kidney, reproductive organs, central and peripheral nervous systems. They are associated with inflammation and immunity, bone metabolism, and regulation of intraocular pressure. There has been significant interest in the role of prostaglandins and in particular the COX-2 pathway, in the development of malignancies.

Prostanoids are unstable, and have limited availability. Stable oral or parenteral long-acting analogs of the naturally occurring prostaglandins have been developed for clinical use.

The important effects of prostanoids are:
- TXA_2 causes platelet aggregation. It is a potent vasoconstrictor and bronchoconstrictor.
- PGD_2 inhibits platelet aggregation. It causes vasodilation and relaxation of GIT and uterine muscle.
- PGF_{2a} causes powerful contraction of uterine and bronchial muscle, and blood vessels. It is luteolytic (i.e., it causes the corpus luteum to regress and to stop producing progesterone).
- PGI_2 inhibits platelet aggregation and causes vasodilation. It releases renin and causes natriuresis.
- PGE_2 has four different receptors with antagonistic effects on the same organ such as bronchoconstriction as well as bronchodilation.

The most important actions of PGE_2 is on the receptor involved with uterine contraction and cytoprotective action, which forms the main basis of the use of prostaglandins in clinical practice.

Therapeutic uses

Prostaglandin are mainly used for their potent oxytocic (*see* Chapter 9) and cytoprotective effects against peptic ulcers (*see* Chapter 6)

Miscellaneous uses

Epoprostenol (PGI_2) is used for pulmonary hypertension. It has extremely short plasma half-life (3–5 min) which necessitates continuous IV infusion. Long-acting prostacyclin analogs **iloprost** (half-life 30 min) and **treprostinil** (half-life 4 hours) are clinically used.

Beraprost (PGI_2) is used for peripheral vascular disease.

Latanoprost (PGF_{2a}) and newer prostaglandins **bimatoprost, travaprost** and **unoprostone** are used in glaucoma as topical ocular drops.

Alprostadil (PGE$_1$) is second line treatment for erectile dysfunction in male. It is also used to maintain the patency of the neonate's ductus arteriosus before corrective surgery.

Adverse effects

Side effects are dose related and broadly consist of vomiting, diarrhea, bronchoconstriction and vasodilation. Long-term use of misoprostol may result in dose-dependent hyperostosis and bone pain in patients having liver disease.

LEUKOTRIENES (LTs)

Leukotrienes are the products of arachidonic acid metabolism synthesized by the lipoxygenase pathway. Leukotriene synthesis takes place chiefly in leucocytes (neutrophils, basophils, eosinophils, and, monocyte-macrophages) and other inflammatory cells such as mast cells and dendritic cells. LTA$_4$ is the precursor from which the various LT$_S$ are derived. LTC$_4$ and LTD$_4$ are potent bronchoconstrictor and are primary component of the slow reaching substance of anaphylaxis (SRS-A), that is secreted in asthma and anaphylaxis.

Leukotriene antagonists reduce bronchospasm and associated symptoms that are mediated through LT$_S$. **Zafirlukast, montelukast** and **pranlukast** are used for prophylactic therapy of asthma mainly as an alternative to inhaled glucocorticoids.

5

Cardiovascular System

5.1 CARDIAC GLYCOSIDES

Cardiac glycosides are the drugs that have inotropic action. They increase myocardial contractility and cardiac output in a hypodynamic heart without an increase in oxygen requirement and thus the overall myocardial efficiency as a pump is increased.

The cardiac glycosides are mainly obtained from the dried leaves of the foxglove plant, though they are also present in stropanthus and squill species and animals.

Digoxin and **digitoxin** are the two principal glycosides obtained from Digitalis purpurea (digitoxin) and Digitalis lanata (digitoxin, digoxin). Digoxin is the only cardiac glycoside which is used and is being produced synthetically (Table 5.1).

Pharmacokinetics

Cardiac glycosides are well absorbed. They are cumulative drugs, because they are bound to heart muscle which accounts for the prolonged action. Digoxin is excreted by the kidneys and accumulation occurs in patients with poor renal functions. Digitoxin is metabolized by the liver.

Table 5.1: Pharmacokinetics of oral digoxin and digitoxin

Drug	Absorption	Protein binding	Maximum effect	Duration of action	Principal metabolic route	Maintenance dose
Digoxin	75%	25%	6 hours	2 days	Kidney	0.125–0.26 mg
Digitoxin	90–100%	97%	17 hours	7 days	Liver	0.1–0.2 mg

Pharmacological actions

Effects on the failing heart.

Positive inotropic action

Digoxin increases the force of contraction of the ventricular muscle by increasing both the velocity of muscle contraction and the maximum force that is developed without causing corresponding increase in the oxygen consumption. Thus overall myocardial efficiency is increased.

Cardiac glycosides do not prolong the duration of the contraction and they do not directly affect myocardial contractile proteins energy for contraction. This action is due to an increase in calcium ions in the heart muscle for interaction with contractile proteins. In large doses, digitalis causes increase excitability of the ventricles. The positive inotropic action of digoxin is observed only on the failing heart.

Heart rate

Digoxin slows the heart rate (*negative chronotropic effect*), partly due to increased activity of the vagus nerve and partly due to a direct action on the sinoatrial (SA) node.

A-V conduction

Digoxin depresses conduction in the atrioventricular (AV) node and the bundle of His. This action does not affect the heart in sinus rhythm, but in atrial fibrillation, it decreases the number of impulses reaching the ventricles and thus decreases the rate of ventricular contraction

The most important of these three actions is slowing of the ventricular rate, particularly in atrial fibrillation where the slower and more regular ventricular contractions allow the heart to function more efficiently leading to an increase in the cardiac output. The positive inotropic effect is less important and if the heart is in sinus rhythm the benefits are minimal.

Extracardiac effects

Digoxin in congestive heart failure causes a drop in peripheral resistance and venomotor tone. Increased cardiac output and renal blood flow has a diuretic effect

Digoxin in higher doses causes stimulation of CTZ resulting in nausea and vomiting.

Therapeutic uses
Low-output cardiac failure

Although the digitalis glycosides were once the mainstay of treatment of congestive heart failure, their use in patients who are in sinus rhythm has declined because they lack the benefits of the neurohormonal antagonists on prognosis and have a narrow therapeutic index.

Digoxin is used only for patients who remain symptomatic even after taking diuretics and ACE inhibitors as well as for patients with heart failure who are in atrial fibrillation and require rate control.

Cardiac arrhythmias

Digoxin has great value in certain cardiac arrhythmias, even if they are unassociated with heart failure.

Atrial fibrillation

Digoxin reduces the ventricular rate by prolonging the refractory period of conduction tissue.

Atrial flutter

Digoxin may convert atrial flutter to atrial fibrillation. If digitalis is then stopped, normal sinus rhythm may be restored.

Paroxysmal atrial tachycardia

It responds to digoxin, presumably as a result of reflex vagal stimulation.

Digitalization

Digoxin is a cumulative drug and treatment is started with a full dose (loading dose) of the drug followed by the maintenance dose to replace the day-to-day loss.

Loading dose Rapid digitalization is done with digoxin 1–1.5 mg in divided doses over 24 hours and for less urgent digitalization 0.25–0.5 mg is given daily.

Maintenance dose is 0.125–0.25 mg daily, according to renal function.

The toxic-therapeutic ratio is narrow and therapy should be followed by monitoring of plasma levels of digoxin, particularly in patients with unstable renal functions.

Adverse effects

Undue slowing of the heart

A pulse rate below 60 indicates that the drug should be omitted for a day or two.

Coupled beats

This are due to ventricular extrasystoles following normal beats (double pulsation followed by a pause) and necessitates omission of the drug. Overdose may lead to paroxysmal tachycardia or even ventricular fibrillation–a fatal complication.

Nausea and vomiting

Digoxin stimulates the vomiting centre in medulla, but heart failure itself can also produce vomiting.

Visual disturbances (color vision), headache, confusion, delirium and hallucinations are other symptoms of digoxin overdose.

Drug Interactions

Drug interactions with digitalis are common. Oral antibiotics such as erythromycin and tetracycline may increase digoxin levels by 10 to 40%. Quinidine, verapamil, flecainide, and amiodarone also increase digoxin levels significantly. Digoxin toxicity may be caused or exacerbated by drug interactions, electrolyte abnormalities (particularly hypokalemia), hypoxemia, hypothyroidism, renal insufficiency and volume depletion.

Contraindications

Cardiac glycosides are contraindicated in intermittent heart block, second degree A-V block, supraventricular arrhythmias caused by Wolff-Parkinson-White syndrome, high output CHF and constructive pericarditis.

Treatment of digoxin intoxication

Lignocaine is the preferred antiarrhythmic drug for ventricular arrhythmias.

Digoxin-specific antibody (**digibind**) is indicated in life threatening digitalis intoxication. Each 4.0 mg of digibind neutralizes approximately 0.6 mg of digoxin.

5.2 ANGIOTENSIN CONVERTING ENZYME (ACE) INHIBITORS

The renin-angiotensin system (RAS) is of primary importance in the control of blood pressure, body fluid volume and myocardial function. Renin controls the formation of angiotensin II. Angiotensin II is one of the most potent vasoconstrictors being 40 times more potent than noradrenalin.

Angiotensin II interacts with the AT_1 receptor (angiotensin II receptor type I) and accelerates numerous cellular processes, which contributes to hypertension and end-organ damage (Fig. 5.1). These include:
- Aldosterone secretion from adrenal gland leading to salt and water retention.
- Vasoconstriction due to (a) peripheral vasoconstriction, (b) vascular hypertrophy, (c) production of superoxide anions and other reactive oxygen species that inactivate nitric oxide,

thereby inhibiting endothelium-dependent vasodilation, and (d) augmentation of both central and peripheral sympathetic nervous system leading to excessive stimulation of adrenergic receptors in peripheral blood vessels.

- Cardiotoxic action due to (a) hypertrophy of cardiac musculature and (b) aldosterone induced collagen deposition leading to cardiac fibrosis.

Mechanism of action

ACE is responsible for converting angiotensin I to angiotensin II and inactivating bradykinin. Angiotensin II causes a rise in blood pressure in several ways – by causing direct vasoconstriction, hypertrophy of vascular smooth muscle and release of aldosterone which causes retention of sodium. Further, angiotensin II is an important stimulus for cardiac growth.

ACE inhibitors inhibit the conversion of angiotensin I to angiotensin II in vascular endothelium, resulting in vasodilation and reversal of vascular changes and inhibition of bradykinin breakdown. This accounts for their role in hypertension.

ACE inhibitors are of great value in heart failure as the main hemodynamic disturbances in heart failure is the angiotensin II mediated increase in systemic vascular resistance, producing increased left ventricular afterload and an increase in left ventricular filling pressure (preload), which in turn is caused by retention of sodium mediated by excess aldosterone. Decrease of angiotensin II concentrations reduces both afterload and preload which in turn reduces cardiac work and raises cardiac output.

Pharmacokinetics

ACE inhibitors are well absorbed orally; they differ in their onset and duration of action. Most of them are prodrugs (except lisinopril) which are converted into active forms in the liver. They are eliminated by the kidneys. Fosinopril is unique in that 50% of the drug is eliminated by the liver under normal conditions, but his percentage increases in the presence of renal inefficiency.

Cardiovascular System 197

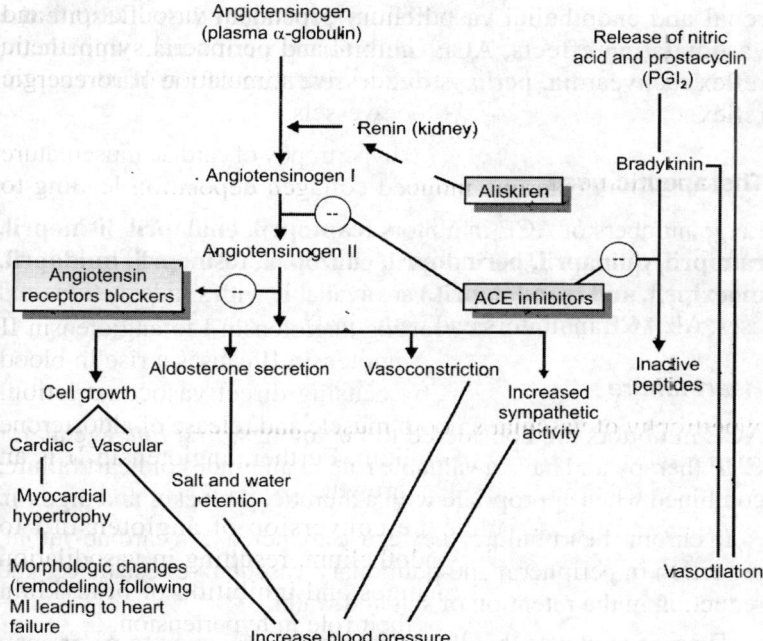

Fig. 5.1: Renin-angiotensin–aldosterone system and site of action of antihypertensive drugs

Pharmacological actions

ACE inhibitors produce beneficial hemodynamic effects by inhibiting the conversion of angiotensin I to angiotensin II. They also inhibit the degradation of bradykinin, resulting in an increase in the levels of vasodilaory bradykinins. These result in a fall of blood pressure.

Hemodynamically, ACE inhibitors increase cardiac output by reducing afterload by decreasing total peripheral resistance, and pulmonary resistance, and preload by decreasing the blood volume due to mild natriuresis, caused by reduction of aldosterone secretion. They decrease K^+ secretion.

ACE inhibitors reduce hypokalemia, hypercholesterolemia, hyperglycemia and hyperuricemia caused by diuretic therapy. Some agents (i.e. catopril) directly stimulate production of renal and endothelial vasodilatory prostaglandins. Despite the vasodialating effects, ACE inhibitors do not cause significant reflex tachycardia, perhaps due to resetting of the baroreceptor reflex.

Therapeutic uses

Large numbers of ACE inhibitors **(captopril, enalapril, lisinopril, ramipril, quinapril, perindopril, cilazopril, fosinopril, imidapril, moexipril, and trandolapril.)** are available with similar actions and uses. All ACE inhibitors end with "pril".

Heart failure

ACE inhibitors are considered to be amongst *first line* agents for CHF therapy and have a valuable role in all grades of heart failure, combined when appropriate with a diuretic, β blocker and digoxin.

In chronic heart failure, they cause an increase in cardiac output, reduction in peripheral and pulmonary vasculative resistance, and reduction in the retention of salt and water.

There is evidence that they not only control symptoms of heart failure but also reduce the *mortality rate* in heart failure (Digitalis does not reduce mortality).

A marked fall in blood pressure occurs occasionally with the first dose of ACE inhibitor, especially if the patient is already taking a diuretic. For this reason the initial dose in heart failure should be low and taken before going to bed.

The starting dose of captopril is 6.5 or 12.5 mg to minimize any hypotensive effect and maintenance dose is 25 or 50 mg three times daily. The initial dose of enalapril is 2.5 mg and maintenance dose 10 or 20 mg twice daily. Trandolapril is long acting and is given once daily (initial dose 0.5 – 1.0 mg and maintenance dose 4 mg).

Hypertension

ACE inhibitors are recommended as *first-line treatment* for hypertension along with diuretics and β blockers. Except for captopril (given thrice daily), they require only once a day administration.

Adverse effects

The most common side effect of ACE inhibitors is a dry, non-productive cough (up to 20% of patients), bronchoconstriction, angioneurotic edema, which is probably due to inhibition of bradykinin breakdown. They may cause hypotension, but do not cause levels of lipids, glucose or uric acid to increase. ACE inhibitors that contain a sulfhydryl group (e.g., captopril) may cause taste disturbance, proteinuria and neutropenia.

Renal impairment may occur as a result of preferential vasodilation of the efferent arterioles in the kidney by ACE inhibitors, especially in patients with compromised renal functions.

ACE inhibitors can cause hyperkalemia and should be used with caution in patients with a decreased glomerular filtration rate and who are taking potassium supplements or who are receiving potassium-sparing diuretics.

ACE inhibitors are contraindicated in renovascular disease, aortic stenosis, pregnancy and patients who are hypersensitive to it.

ANGIOTENSIN-RECEPTOR BLOCKERS (ARBs)

Angiotensin II is an extremely powerful vasoconstrictor that acts on specific angiotensin II receptors on the blood vessel wall and on the renin-angiotensin system. Antagonist drugs bind to angiotensin II receptor and block the vasoconstrictor actions and the secretary effects on the zona glomerulosa of angiotensin II at the angiotensin II type 1 recptor. These actions result in decreased peripheral resistance.

Candesartan, irbesartan, losartan, telmisartan, valsartan and **olmesartan** are ARBs available for clinical use. All ARBs end with "sartan"

ARBs produce pharmacological actions similar to that of ACE inhibitors. In contrast to ACE inhibitors, they do not increase bradykinin levels, which may be responsible for adverse effects seen with ACE inhibitors, such as cough. ARBs are useful alternatives in patients who are unable to tolerate ACE inhibitors.

ARBs cause cough much less frequently than ACE inhibitors; the side effect profile is otherwise similar to that of the ACE inhibitors. Losartan specifically is uricosuric.

ALISKIREN

Aliskiren is a renin inhibitor, which binds the proteolytic site of renin, therapy preventing cleavage of angiotensinogen. As a consequence, levels of angiotensin I and II are reduced and renin concentration is increased. It has been approved for use as monotherapy or in combination therapy with diuretics, ACE inhibitors, and ARBs in lowering the blood pressure. As yet there are no clinical trial data with this new drug, so the effect of aliskinen on ontcome in hypertension, diatbetes, or cardiovascular disease remains unknown.

5.3 DIURETICS

Diuretics are drugs which cause a net loss of sodium ions and water from the body, resulting into an increase secretion of urine from the kidneys. Diuretics are not used in patients who can not empty their bladder (e.g. prostatic hyperplasia leading to urinary retention).

Classification

Diuretics are classified according to their site of action in the kidney tubule and their relative effects on sodium and potassium excretion. They belong to three main groups (Table 5.2):
- Thiazides and related drugs,
- "Loop" (high ceiling) diuretics, and
- Potassium sparing diuretics.

In addition, less often used diuretics are the carbonic anhydrase inhibitors and osmotically active drugs. Mercurial diuretics, because of their serious cardiac and renal toxicity are no longer used.

Site of action. Although an individual diuretic can act on several areas of the nephron, the major sites of action for the diuretics may be summarized as follows:

Table 5.2: Commonly used diuretics

Drug	Usual dose range (mg)	Drug	Usual dose range (mg)
Thiazide diuretic		**Loop diuretic**	
Bendroflumethiazide	2.5–15	Bumetanide	0.5–5
Benzthiazide	50–100	Ethacrynic acid	25–100
Chlorthalidone	12.5–50	Furosemide	20–320
Hydrochlorothiazide	12.5–50	Torsemide	5–10
Hydroflumethiazide	50–100	**Potassium-sparing diuretic**	
Methyclothiazide	2.5–5.0	Amiloride	5–10
Polythiazide	1–4	Triamterene	50–200
Quinethazone	25–100	**Aldosterone antagonist**	
Trichlormthiazide	1–4	Eplerenone	25–100
Thiazide related drugs		Spironolactone	25–100
Chlorothiazide	125–1,000		
Indapamide	2.5–5.0		
Metolazone	1.25–5		

- Those acting on the **proximal tubule:**
    - Osmotic diuretics
    - Carbonic anhydrase inhibitors
- Those acting on the **ascending limb of the loop of Henle:**
    - High-ceiling (loop) diuretics
    - Thiazide diuretics
    - Mercurial diuretics
- Those acting on the **distal tubule:** K^+ sparing diuretics

THIAZIDES

These are moderately potent diuretics, and with few exceptions are equally effective at equivalent doses

Bendroflumethiazide (bendrofluazide) is the most widely used thiazide in doses of 2.5–5 mg daily.

Other thiazide drugs do not offer any significant advantage over bendrofluazide.

Mechanism of action

Thiazides are medium potency natriuretic drugs. They inhibit NaCl reabsorption, particularly in the cortical portion of the ascending tubule of loop of Henle and at the beginning of the distal convoluted tubule, where less than 10% of the filtered sodium load is reabsorbed and cause excretion of only 5–10% of the total sodium load. Refractoriness to their action does not occur.

Thiazides enhance Ca^{2+} reabsorption both in the proximal and distal tubules. Thiazides are useful in the treatment of kidney stones caused by hypercalciurea.

Thiazides also increase excretion of potassium by the kidney.

Thiazides may produce mild vasodilation by inhibiting sodium entry into vascular smooth muscles. Indapamide in particular has pronounced vasodilating effect.

Pharmacokinetics

All thiazides are given orally and are well absorbed, except chlorothiazide which is not very lipid soluble and requires to be given in large doses. It is the only thiazide available for parental administration. They produce diuresis within 2 hours, but the duration varies between 12 hours or less (bendrofluazide) and 48 hours or longer (polythiazide). Long acting thiazides cause profound hypokalemia. All thiazides are secreted by the organic acid secretory system and compete with the secretion of uric acid. As a result, thiazide use may blunt uric acid secretion and elevate serum uric acid level.

Pharmacological actions

Thiazides increase the renal excretion of Na^+, Cl^-, HCO_3^- and K^+. Thiazides have a direct vasodilator effect.

Therapeutic uses

Congestive heart failure

Thiazides are used to treat mild to moderate edema of heart failure.

Hypertension

Thiazides are first-line drugs for the management of hypertension in patients with normal renal functions. Bendrofluazide in small doses (2.5 mg daily) lowers the blood pressure and rarely causes postural hypotension or biochemical disturbances. Addition of a β blocker or ACE inhibitor to thiazide treatment usually obviates the need for potassium supplements.

Cirrhosis of liver with ascites

Thiazides produce diuresis with reduction in the ascites and edema. Mental changes with disorientation may occur due to potassium deficiency produced by these drugs.

Nephrolithiasis

Thiazides increase calcium retention and may reduce stone formation and the frequency of renal colic.

Nephrogenic diabetes insipidus

Thiazide diuretics reduce polyuria and polydipsia in both types of (neurogenic and nephrogenic) disbetes insipidus. This paradoxic beneficial effect is mediated through plasma volume reduction, with an associated fall in GFR rate, enhanced proximal reabsorption of NaCl and water, and decreased delivery of fluid to the downstream diluting segments. Thus, the maximum volume of dilute urine that can be produced is lowered, and thiazides can significantly reduce urine flow in the polyuric patient.

Adverse effects

Thiazides, especially long acting (e.g. polythiazide, chlorthalidone), may result in biochemical disorders such as hypokalemia, hypomagnesemia, hyperuricemia, gout, hyperlipidemia (with increase in low density lipoproteins and triglyceride levels) and hyperglycemia. Serum potassium monitoring may be necessary when used with digitalis, in cirrhosis of liver and in acute myocardial infarction. Other side effects include weakness, muscle cramps and impotence. Thiazides are contraindicated in refractory hypokalemia and renal and hepatic impairment.

Thiazide related drugs

Chlorthalidone has a longer duration of action than thiazides and may be given on alternate days to control edema.

Indapamide produces minimal diuresis but lowers blood pressure as effectively as a thiazide. In contrast to thiazides, indapamide has little or no apparent influence on concentrations of serum potassium, urate, glucose or lipoproteins.

Xipamide has pronounced diuretic action but causes profound hypokalemia.

Metolazone, unlike other thiazides, exerts its action at the proximal as well as the distal tubule and may be useful in combination with a loop diuretic, even in patients with renal failure. Severe electrolyte disturbances have been reported and it should be reserved for resistant edema.

LOOP DIURETICS

The loop or "high ceiling" are powerful diuretics and act by inhibiting the reabsorption of sodium from the thick ascending limb (TAL) of the loop of Henle in the renal tubule, where normally about 25% of the filtered sodium load is reabsorbed. The loop diuretics have the advantage of inducing diuresis despite volume and electrolyte depletion.

Pharmacokinetics

Loop diuretics are rapidly absorbed after oral administration and have a characteristically rapid onset (30–60 minutes) and brief duration (4–6 hours) of action. Reduction in the secretion of loop diuretics may result from simultaneous administration of drugs, such as NSAIDs or probenecid.

Pharmacological actions

Loop diuretics inhibit $Na^+/K^+/2Cl^-$ transporter in the thick ascending loop (TAL) of Henle. The diuretic action of loop diuretics (inhibition $Na^+/K^+/2Cl^-$ transporter in TAL) is in part due to the production of prostaglandin (PGE_2). NSAIDs which inhibit prostaglandin synthesis can interfere with the action of loop diuretics.

Loop diuretics cause greater excretion of chloride than sodium and inhibit $Na^+/K^+/2Cl^-$ absorption from the thick ascending loop (TAL) of Henle, without absorbing water, as TAL is nearly impermeable to water. This positive potential normally drives divalent cation reabsortption in the loop and by reducing this potential loop diuretics cause an increase in Mg^{2+} and Ca^{2+} excretion.

Loop diuretics have direct effects on blood flow through several vascular beds. Furosemide increases renal blood flow. Furoseumide and ethacrynic acid reduce the pulmonary congestion and left ventricular filling pressures in heart failure. These effects in vascular tone may also be related to prostaglandins induced by furosemide.

Loop diuretics due to increased in Mg^{2+} and Ca^{2+} excretion may cause significant hypomagnesemia and hypocalcemia. Hypochloremic alkalosis can occur but it does not produce a refractory state. They increase renal blood flow without increasing glomerular filtration rate. Large doses promote uric acid excretion.

Therapeutic uses

The most important indication of the Loop diuretics is in acute pulmonary edema, edema associated with chronic heart failure, cirrhosis, and renal disease. However, cirrhotic patients are often resistant to loop diuretics because of decreased secretion of the drug in the tubular fluid and high aldosterone level. In contrast, cirrhotic edema is usually responsive to spirnolactone and eplerenone.

High dose intravenous furosemide has been used to treat elevated intracranial pressure and hypercalcemia of malignancy.

Furosemide (lasix) is the most widely used loop diuretic. Its bioavailability is poor, perhaps as low as 20%. It can be administered intramuscularly and more often intravenously. The dose is 20–40 mg.

Bumetanide is 40 times more potent on a weight basis than furoseminde and its bioavailability is much higher because of better oral absorption. It is more 'potassium sparing' than furosemide and is less likely to impair glucose tolerance or cause urate retention. It is preferred for those patients who fail to respond to oral furosemide.

Ethacrynic acid is a loop diuretic which possesses uricosuric action but is now little used because of high incidence of adverse reactions. However, it is used in sulfa-sensitive patients as an alternative to furosemide and bumetanide, which are sulfa derivatives.

Torsemide is 3 times more potent and longer acting than furosemide.

Adverse effects

Loop diuretics cause biochemical disturbances as seen with thiazides except on lipids. They may precipitate acute urinary retention in patients with prostatism and cause mild or asymptomatic thrombocytopenia and irreversible ototoxicity.

Loop diuretics can cause hyperuricemia and precipitate attacks of gout.

Loop diuretics are contraindicated in precomatose states associated with cirrhosis or renal failure with anuria or heart failure.

Drug interactions

Thiazide and loop diuretics can cause nephrotoxicity when combined with NSAIDs or aminoglycoside antibiotics. Thiazides increase lithium toxicity. Concurrent use of steroids increases potassium loss.

POTASSIUM SPARING DIURETICS

Potassium-sparing diuretics prevent K^+ secretion by antagonizing the effects of aldosterone in the late distal and cortical collecting tubules.

Spironolactone and **eplerenone** inhibit K^+ secretion by direct pharmacologic antagonism of mineralocorticoid receptors.

Spironolactone is a synthetic steroid that acts as a competitive antagonist to aldosterone.

Eplerenone is a spironolactone analog with much greater selectivity for the mineralocorticoid receptor. It is several hundred-folds less active on androgen and progesterone receptor than spironolactone, and therefore elperenone has considerably fewer effects.

Amiloride and **triamterene** do not block aldosterone, but instead directly interfere with Na^+ entry through the epithelial Na^+ channels (ENaC) in the apical membrane of the collecting tubule.

The actions of the aldosterone antagonists depend on renal prostaglandin production. The action of K^+ sparing diuretics can be inhibited by NSAIDs under certain conditions.

Therapeutics uses

Potassium sparing diuretics are most useful in states of mineralocorticoid excess or hyperaldosteronism. They are very weak diuretics but potentiate the action of thiazide and loop diuretics while causing retention of potassium.

Eplerenone has the least adverse actions and in low doses (25–50 mg/d) may interfere with some of the fibrotic and inflammatory effects of aldosterone. This action can reduce the progression of albuminuria in diabetic patients.

Eplerenone has been found to reduce myocardial perfusion defects after myocardial infarction. In one clinical study, eplerenone reduced mortality rate by 15% in patients with mild to moderate heart failure after myocardial infarction.

Adverse effects

Hyperkalemia

K^+ sparing diuretics reduce urinary excretion of K^+ and can cause even life-threatening hyperkalemia in renal disease or by the use of drugs which reduce or inhibit renin (β blockers, NSAIDs, aliskiren) or ACE inhibitors and angiotensin receptor inhibitors. Fixed-dosage combinations of K^+ sparing and thiazide diuretics should generally be avoided as thiazide associated adverse effects often predominate.

Hyperchloremic metabolic acidosis

In contrast to thiazide and loop diuretics which cause hypokalemic metabolic alkalosis, K^+ sparing diuretics cause hyperchloremic metabolic acidosis due to inhibition of H^+ secretion.

Gynecomastia

Synthetic steroids cause endocrine abnormalities by actions on other steroid receptors. Gynecomastia, impotence and benign prostatic hyperplasia occurring with spironolactone do not occur with eplerenone because of lack of action on androgen or progesterone receptors.

Acute renal failure

Triamterene with indomethacin can cause acute renal failure, which is not seen with other K^+ sparing agents.

Kidney stone

Triamterene, because of poor solubility, may precipitate in the urine causing kidney stone.

Contraindications

K^+ sparing diuretics in chronic renal inefficiency and along with other agents such as β blocker, ACE inhibitors can cause severe, even fatal hyperkalemia.

OTHER DIURETICS

CARBONIC ANHYDRASE INHIBITORS

Mechanism of action

Carbonic anhydrase inhibitors inhibit carbonic anhydrase enzyme, which reduces the number of H^+ ions available for Na^+–H^+ exchange and thus leads to decrease Na+ reabsorption. Carbon dioxide (CO_2) reabsorption from glomerular filtrate is suppressed and HCO_3^- excretion is increased.

Increase urinary excretion of Na^+, K^+ and HCO_3^- results in an alkaline urine leading to metabolic acidosis. The acidosis eventually induces a refractory state (i.e., decreased diuresis).

Carbonic anhydrase inhibitors also reduce the rate of aqueous humor and spinal fluid formation.

Therapeutic uses

Carbonic anhydrase inhibitors are no longer used as diuretics because of development of metabolic acidosis which limits their diuretic effect.

Acetazolamide (Diamox) is given orally (250 mg–1g daily in divided doses) for following conditions.

- Glaucoma to reduce rate of aqueous humour formation. Topically active carbonic antydrase inhibitors (dorzolamide, brinzolamide) are available and reduce intraocular pressure without producing detectable plasma levels. Thus diuretic and metabolic effects are eliminated with the topical agents.
- Petit mal epilepsy, in which they act as anticonvulsant and decrease the rate of spinal fluid formation.
- Mountain sickness to increase ventilation at altitude.
- Salicylate or barbiturate poisoning to alkalinize the urine and increase their excretion.

Adverse effects

Side effects are not common. Acetazolamide is an aromatic sulphonamide and rarely can cause blood dyscrasias and allergic skin reactions. Large doses may cause drowsiness and parasthesias.

OSMOTIC DIURETICS

Mechanism of action

Osmotic diuretics are filtered at the glomerulus but are poorly reabsorbed because of their molecular size. The presence of osmotic diuretics in the proximal tubule decreases reabsorption of Na^+ and water resulting in marked diuresis.

Therapeutic uses

Mannitol is used in cerebral edema by intravenous infusion in a dose of 50–200 g as a 20% solution over a period of 24 hours.

Adverse effects

Chills and fever may occur. Mannitol infusion is contraindicated in CHF and pulmonary edema.

5.4 DRUGS USED IN CHRONIC HEART FAILURE

The general principle of pharmacologic therapy of chronic heart failure (HF) involves the antagonism of neurohormones (renin-angiotensin system and adrenergic nervous system) that are increased in patients with HF and have deleterious effects on the myocardium and the peripheral vasculature. The following groups of drugs are used in the treatment of heart failure (Table 5.3).

Table 5.3: Commonly used drugs used for chronic heart failure

Drugs	Starting dose	Target dose
Thiazide diuretics		
Hydrochlorothiazide	12.5 mg daily	50 mg daily
Metolazone	2.5 mg daily	20 mg daily
ACE inhibitors		
Enalapril	2.5 mg 12 hourly	10 mg 12 hourly
Lisinopril	2.5 mg daily	20 mg daily
Ramipril	1.25 mg daily	10 mg daily
Angiotensin receptor blockers		
Losartan	25 mg daily	100 mg daily
Candesartan	4 mg daily	32 mg daily
Valsartan	40 mg daily	160 mg daily
β-blockers		
Bisoprolol	1.25 mg daily	10 mg daily
Carvedilol	3.125 mg 12 hourly	50 mg 12 hourly
Metoprolol	12.5 mg daily	200 mg daily

(Contd.)

(Contd.)

Drugs	Starting dose	Target dose
Aldosterone receptors antagonists		
Eplerenone	25 mg daily	50 mg daily
Spironolactone	12.5 mg daily	25 mg daily
Inotropic drugs		
Digoxin	0.125 mg daily	0.25 mg daily
Anti-arrhythmic drug		
Amiodarone	5 mg/kg I.V. over 20-120 mins then up to 15 mg/kg/24 hrs.	

- Diuretics
- ACE inhibitors and ARB
- β blockers
- Aldosterone receptors antagonists
- Digoxin
- Amiodarone

The treatment of heart failure requires a multidrug regimen to control symptoms, retard progression of the disease and prolong survival.

Diuretics

The diuretics drugs play a pivotal role in the treatment of heart failure since they are the only drugs that can adequately control the fluid retention; provide symptomatic relief more rapidly than any other drug; and modulate the responses to other drugs because the effects of neurohormonal antagonists (ACE inhibitors and β-blockers) are highly dependent on sodium balance.

Diuretics are generally given initially in low doses, which is gradually increased until signs and symptoms of fluid retention are alleviated. NSAIDs should not be given because they decrease the efficacy and increase the toxicity of diuretic therapy.

Thiazide diuretics (hydrochlorothiazide) can be used as initial agents in patients with normal renal functions in whom only a mild diuresis is desired. Loop diuretics (furosemide) should be used in patients who require significant diuresis and in those with markedly decreased renal function. Furosemide reduces preload acutely by causing direct venodilation when administered IV, making it a very useful drug for managing severe HF or acute pulmonary edema. Ethacrynic acid can be used in sulfa-sensitive patents, since furosemide is a sulfa derivative.

The principal adverse effects of diuretic are electrolyte depletion, neurohormonal activation and hypotension and azotemia.

Depletion of K^+ and Mg^+ can predispose patients to cardiac arrhythmias, particularly in presence of digitalis therapy. Concomitant treatment with ACE inhibitors, β blockers or aldosterone antagonist prevents the loss of electrolytes caused by diuretics.

ACE inhibitors or β blockers should always be combined with diuretics to counteract any activation of endogenous neurohormonal system that may be caused by diuretics.

Hypotension and azotemia are generally asymptomatic and require no specific treatment.

ACE inhibitors

ACE inhibitors attenuate vasoconstriction, vital organ hypoperfusion, hyponatremia, hypokalemia and fluid retention attributable to compensatory activation of renin-angiotensin system. The major advantage of ACE inhibitors over traditional (digitalis) treatment is their ability to inhibit the deleterious effects on the myocardium and the peripheral vasculature of the neurohormones.

The beneficial actions of ACE inhibitors are not only due to the interference with the formation of angiotensin II, but are also due to enhancement of the actions of kinins; kinin potentiation may add importantly to angiotensin suppression in mediating the effects of ACE inhibitors. The favorable effects of ACE inhibitors on the cardiac musculature are greater than those of angiotensin II receptor antagonists. The hemodynamic and prognostic benefits of ACE inhibitors may be attenuated by the co-administration of aspirin, which blocks kinin mediated prostaglandin synthesis.

ACE inhibitors decrease afterload, increase cardiac output and reduce the risk of death or hospitalization in patients with HF. ACE inhibitors have also been shown to reduce the mortality rate in patients with left ventricular systolic dysfunction or HF after an acute attack of myocardial infarction.

ACE inhibitors should not be used before (or instead of) diuretics in patients with a history of fluid retention, because diuretics are needed to maintain Na^+ balance and prevent the development of peripheral and pulmonary edema. ACE inhibitors reduce the need for large doses of diuretics and K^+ supplement and even attenuate many of the metabolic effects of diuretic therapy (e.g., hypokalemia and hyponatremia).

All the available ACE inhibitors can be used.

The adverse effects of ACE inhibitors are mainly due to the effects of kinin potentiation, which include angioneurotic edema and cough and their occurrence requires withdrawal of the drug and the use of alternate drugs i.e., angiotensin receptor blocker.

Angiotensin receptor blockers (ARBs)

These drugs act by blocking the action of angiotension II on the heart, peripheral vasculature and kidney. In heart failure, they produce beneficial hemodynamic changes that are similar to the effects of ACE inhibitors, but are generally better tolerated. They have comparable effects on mortality and are a useful alternative for patients who cannot tolerate ACE inhibitors. Unfortunately, they share all the more serious adverse effects of ACE inhibitors, including renal dysfunction and hypokalemia. They may be considered in combination with ACE inhibitors, especially in those with recurrent hospitalization for heart failure.

Aliskiren

Aliskiren a renin inhibitor used for hypertension, has been found to have similar efficacy as that of ACE inhibitors in heart failure.

β blockers

The use of β blockers was earlier avoided in the treatment of HF. Large clinical trials have shown the beneficial actions of β blockers which are now considered to be an important component of heart failure pharmacotherapy that block the cardiac effects of chronic adrenergic (endogenous neurohormonal system) stimulation, including myocyte toxicity. β blockers should be added to diuretic and ACE inhibitor therapy for patients with stable heart failure symptoms.

β blockers appear to reduce both the risk of death and risk of hospitalization for heart failure by 30 to 40% in patients already receiving ACE inhibitors. β blockers have been found to be highly effective particularly in reducing cardiac arrhythmias and sudden deaths in the first few weeks after diagnosis of HF.

The hemodynamic benefits of β blockers in HF include; an increase in ejection fraction, reduction in end-systolic volume, improvement in ventricular incoordination, improved ventricular filling time, and delaying the process of damage to cardiac muscle.

Individual β blockers have unique properties, and the beneficial effects of β blockers may not be a class effect. Therefore, β blockers with proven effects on patient survival in large clinical trials (bisoprolol, metoprolol, and carvedilol) should be used. Carvedilol seems to be significantly more efficacious than others in reducing mortality, presumably because it provides more comprehensive sympathetic antagonism.

β blockers, like ACE inhibitors, are given in very low doses initially, followed by gradual increments. Example of starting dose for β blocker includes carvedilol 3.125 mg twice daily with a target dose of 25 mg twice daily.

β blockers are not used in acutely severe HF or patients receiving digitalis or patients with advanced heart block or bronchospastic disease.

Aldosterone receptor antagonists

Spironolactone and eplerenone potassium sparing diuretics act by antagonizing an endogenous neuohormonal mechanism that may adversely affect the heart independent of its effects on Na+ balance. Low doses of spironolactone have been shown to reduce the risk of death by 25 to 30% due to HF in patients receiving ACE inhibitors. They improve long-term clinical outcome in patients with severe heart failure or heart failure following acute myocardial infarction.

Digitalis

Digoxin has little beneficial effect in preventing the progression of HF and there seems to be no justification for its use in early cases of HF, especially when the patient is asymptomatic.

Digoxin can be prescribed at any time, if symptoms persist after the use of diuretics and inhibitors of endogenous neurohormonal agents. Its main use in heart failure is to slow the pulse rate, particularly in atrial fibrillation.

Digoxin is not recommended for use in patients who have no symptoms or for the stabilization of patients with acutely decompensated heart failure.

Amiodarone

This is a potent anti-arrhythmic drug, but has little negative inotropic effect and may be valuable in patients with poor left ventricular function. It is only effective in the treatment of symptomatic arrhythmias, and should not be used as a preventive agent in asymptomatic patients.

5.5 CALCIUM CHANNEL BLOCKERS

In the myocardium and vascular smooth muscle, an essential step in the process of contraction is the entry of calcium ions in the cells

Calcium channel blocking (CCB) drugs or calcium antagonists act by selective blockade of the slow inward calcium channels into the myocardium and the vascular smooth muscles. Thus, myocardial contractility is reduced (negative inotropic effect), the formation and propagation of electrical impulses within the heart is depressed (decreased AV conduction) and coronary and systemic vascular tone is diminished (vasodilation).

On the basis of chemical structure and differential effects on the heart and blood vessels, calcium antagonist can be divided into three groups (Table 5.4).

Table 5.4: Calcium antagonist

Drugs	Effect on heart		Vasodilation	Uses
	negative inotropic	A-V depression		
Dihydropyridines	+	–	+++	Hypertension, angina
Diltiazem	++	+	+	Hypertension, angina
Verapamil	++	++	++	Hypertension, angina, cardiac arrhythmias

Dihydropyridines – all are ending with "dipine". They include **nifedipine, nicardipine, amlodipine, felodipine, isradipine lacidipine, nisoldipine, nitreridipine, benidipine, lercanidipine, nimodipine and clevidipine.**

Pharmacokinetics

Calcium antagonist is well absorbed after oral administration. Most of them undergo extensive first pass metabolism in the liver.

Dihydropyridines on the basis of their duration of action are classified into:

Short-acting	– nifedipine and nicardipine
Intermediate-acting	– isradipine and nitrendipine
Long-acting	– amlodipine, lacidipine, felodipine and nisoldipine

They are highly bound by serum proteins and are excreted as metabolites in the urine.

Pharmacological actions

Calcium antagonists mainly act on smooth and cardiac muscles because their physiological actions are dependent on calcium influx.

Skeletal muscle is not depressed because it uses intracellular pools of calcium to support excitation – contraction coupling and does not require as such transmembrane calcium influx.

Smooth muscle

Calcium antagonists relax bronchial, gastrointestinal, uterine smooth muscle but vascular smooth muscle appears to be the most sensitive. In the vascular system, arterioles appear to be more sensitive than veins: orthostatic hypotension is not common adverse effect. The reduction in peripheral vascular resistance and blood pressure is one mechanism by which these agents may benefit the patients with angina of effort. Reduction of coronary artery tone and prevention of focal coronary artery spasm involved in variant angina makes calcium antagonists the most effective prophylactic treatment for this form of angina pectoris.

Dihydropyridines, having a greater ratio of vascular smooth muscle effects, differ in their potency in different vascular beds. For example, nicardipine is claimed to be particularly selective for cerebral blood vessels and may also reduce cerebral damage after thromboembolic stroke.

Cardiac muscle

Cardiac muscle is highly dependent on calcium influx for normal function.

Calcium antagonists reduce cardiac contractility (negative inotropic effect) in a dose-dependant fashion. In some cases, cardiac output may also decrease. The reduction in cardiac mechanical function is another mechanism by which the oxygen requirement in patient with angina is reduced.

Impulse generation in the SA node, conduction in the AV node and action potential is reduced by verapamil, less with diltiazem and negligible with dihydropyriridines.

Other effects

Calcium antagonists may interfere platelet aggregation and prevent or attenuate the development of atheromatus lesions in animals, but these effects have not been established clinically.

Verapamil, in large doses, inhibits insulin release.

Calcium antagonists block P-glycoprotein responsible for efflux of many foreign drugs out of cancer cells and may partially reverse the resistance of cancer cells to many chemotherapeutic drugs.

Future clinical role of calcium antagonists in the treatment of osteoporosis, fertility disorders and male contraception, immune modulation, malaria and schistosomiasis, based on animal studies, require exploration.

Calcium antagonists have no significant effects on glucose tolerance, electrolytes or lipid profiles.

Therapeutic uses (Table 5.5)

Coronary heart disease

Dihydropyridine calcium antagonists often cause a reflex tachycardia, which may worsen angina and are best used in combination with a β-blocker. In contrast, verapamil and diltiazem cause bradycardia and are suitable for patients who are not receiving a β blocker (e.g. those with airways obstruction).

Table 5.5: Therapeutic uses of some commonly used CCB

Drugs	Indications	Dosage (Daily)
Dihydrophyridines		
Amlodipine	Angina, Hypertension	2.5–10 mg
Felodipine	Hypertension, Reynaud's phenomenon	5–10 mg
Nisoldipine	Hypertension	20–40 mg
Nitrendipine	Hypertension, angina, Reynaud's phenomenon	5–20 mg
Isradipine	Hypertension	2.5–10 mg twice
Nicardipine	Subarachnoid hemorrhage	20–40 mg three times
Nifedipine	Angina, hypertension, Reynaud's phenomenon	3–10 mcg/kg IV, 20–40 mg 8 hourly
Rate-limiting CCB		
Diltiazem	Angina, hypertension, Reynaud's phenomenon	75–150 mcg/kg; 30–80 mg 6 hourly
Verapamil	Angina, hypertension, arrhythmias, migraine	75–150 mcg/kg IV; 80–160 mg 6 hourly

a. Stable angina

Calcium antagonists lower the oxygen requirements of the ischemic myocardium by reducing BP and myocardial contractility.

b. Variant angina

Dihydropyridines cause dramatic relief in about 80% of patients who develop spontaneous episodes of chest pain at rest or at night that are associated with reversible ST segment elevation in the ECG and are thought to be associated with coronary artery spasm (vasospastic angina).

c. Acute coronary syndrome (unstable angina and MI)

Dihydropyridine calcium antagonist (e.g. nifedipine or amlodipine) can be added to the β blocker if there is persistent chest discomfort. Verapamil and diltiazem are the drugs of choice if a β blocker is contraindicated.

Verapamil has been reported to reduce mortality and the risk of reinfarction in post myocardial patients. Immediate release short-acting CCB increase the risk of adverse cardiac events and therefore are contraindicated in unstable angina.

Supraventricular tachycardia

Verapamil is used to slow the ventricular rate in many supraventricular arrhythmias and may sometimes prevent or abolish them. It is not useful in managing ventricular arrhythmias.

Hypertension

Dihydropyridines (e.g. amlodipine, nifedipine) are the first line antihypertensive drugs that are particularly useful in older people. Long acting or sustained release preparations are used since short acting dihydropyridines may increase mortality due to fluctuating response on blood pressure.

Dihydropyridines have been claimed to slow the progress of atherosclerosis.

Calcium antagonists relax arterial muscles and so reduce raised blood pressure. Their hypotensive effect is more striking when combined with other first-line antihypertensive drug.

Raynaud's syndrome

Nifedipine is useful for reducing the frequency and severity of vasospastic attacks, particularly the idiopathic variety than that secondary to collagen vascular disorders.

Subarachnoid hemorrhage

Nicardipine acts prefentially on cerebral arteries and is used for prevention and treatment of ischemic neurological defects following subarachnoid hemorrhage.

Noncardiac chest pain

Nicardipine decreases the pressure in the lower esophageal sphincter and is useful in patients with diffused oesophageal spasm and "nutcracker" esophagus, which is a common cause of non-cardiac chest pain.

Migraine

Nifedipine and verapamil have been reported to reduce the frequency of migraine headache.

Cardiomyopathy

Verapamil, particularly reduces cardiac symptoms and improves tolerance to exercise in hypertrophic cardiomyopathy, even in patients who have not responded to β blockers.

Calcium antagonists, unlike diuretics and β blockers, have not been found to be associated with particular problems in managing patients who have concomitant peripheral vascular disease, gout or asthma.

Adverse effects

Calcium antagonists reduce myocardial contractility and can aggravate or precipitate heart failure.

Ankle edema may result from the higher proximal capillary pressure consequent to dilation of the resistance vessels and does not usually respond to diuretics.

Relative short acting vasoselective (dihydropyridines) CCB have been found to enhance the risk of adverse cardiac events and should be avoided. Patients receiving β blocking drugs are more sensitive to the cardiodepressant effects of CCB.

Minor adverse effects include GIT disturbances (particularly constipation) with verapamil, headache and dizziness, and rashes, which may be transient.

Dihydropyridines should not be used in cardiogenic shock, unstable angina, advanced aortic stenosis and pregnancy.

Verapamil and diltiazem are cardiac depressants and are contraindicated in heart failure, or significantly impaired left ventricular function, second or third degree AV block and sick sinus syndrome.

Calcium antagonists enhance the action of digoxin, theophylline and carbamazepine by increasing their steady state blood concentrations.

Nimodipine has been withdrawn.

5.6 DRUGS USED IN ESSENTIAL HYPERTENSION

The cause of essential hypertension is still unknown. The elevation of blood pressure, unless severe, rarely produces symptoms, but over a period of time damages the heart, blood vessels and kidney, which may lead to coronary thrombosis, heart failure, strokes and less often to renal failure.

Appropriate lifestyle measures may obviate the need of drug therapy or reduce the dose and/or the number of drugs required in established hypertension.

Correcting obesity, reducing alcohol and salt intake, regular physical exercise and consumption of low saturated fat diet can lower BP and reductions in cardiovascular risk.

Drug therapy of essential hypertension is empiric and non-specific, and aims in lowering blood pressure, which is, achieved by drugs which:

- Lower peripheral resistance
- Lower cardiac output and
- Decrease blood volume.

A single antihypertensive drug is often not adequate and other antihypertensive drugs are usually added in a step-wise manner until a reduction in blood pressure to less than 140/90 mm Hg is achieved. Combination therapy may be desirable for other reasons, for example, low-dose therapy with two drugs may produce fewer unwanted effects than treatment with the maximum dose of a single drug. Some drug combinations have complementary or synergistic actions, for example, thiazides increase activity of the renin-angiotensin system while ACE inhibitors block it.

First line antihypertensive drugs (Tables 5.6 and 5.8)

- Diuretics
- ACE inhibitors
- Calcium channel blockers
- β blockers

Other drugs

- α_1 blockers
- Centrally acting sympatholytics
- Direct-acting vasodilator

Parenteral antihypertensive drugs

These are reserved drugs for refractory hypertension or specific circumstances such as hypertensive emergencies or hypertension in pregnancy.

Diuretics

Thiazide diuretics in low doses (e.g. 2.5 mg bendroflumethiazide) produce a maximal or near maximal blood pressure lowering effect, with very little metabolic disturbances and are considered to be the drugs of first choice because of their safety and benefit in reducing the incidence of stroke and cardiovascular events. Thiazides are particularly effective in patients with low renin hypertension, such as elderly, for whom they remain the drugs of choice.

Table 5.6: Commonly used drug for essential hypertension

Drugs by class	Initial dose	Usual dosage range
Thiazide diuretics		
Bendroflumethiazide	2.5 mg daily	2.5–15 mg
Indapamide	1.25 mg daily	2.5–5.0 mg
Loop diuretics		
Furosemide	40 mg daily	40–320 mg
Bumetamide	1.0 mg daily	1.0–5.0 mg
ACE inhibitors		
Enalapril	5 mg daily	5–40 mg
Ramipril	2.5 mg daily	2.5–20 mg
Lisinopril	10 mg daily	10–40 mg
Angiotensin receptor blockers		
Irbesartan	150 mg daily	150–300 mg
Valsartan	80 mg daily	80–320 mg
Calcium antagonists (dihydropyridines)		
Amlodipine	5 mg daily	5–10 mg
Nifedipine	30 mg daily	30–90 mg
Calcium antagonists (rate limiting)		
Diltiazem	200 mg daily	200–300 mg
Verapamil	240 mg daily	240-480 mg
β-blockers (cardioselective)		
Metoprolol	50 mg twice daily	100–200 mg
Atenolol	50 mg daily	50–100 mg
Acebutolol	400 mg daily	400–1200 mg
Bisoprolol	10 mg daily	10–40 mg

The fall in blood pressure is due to a reduction in blood volume, natriuresis and mild vasodilation by inhibiting sodium entry in the vascular smooth muscle cells. Indapamide in particular has a pronounced vasodilating effect.

Diuretics are more effective than α adrenergic antagonist (doxazoin) in the treatment of hypertension.

Loop diuretics are usually reserved for patients with renal in sufficiency or heart failure. Diuretics enhance the efficiency of many agents, particularly ACE inhibitors. Patients being treated with powerful vasodilators such as hydralazine or minoxidil usually require diuretics because these vasodilators cause significant salt and water retention.

The only compelling contraindication to thiazides is gout.

β blockers

These are no longer used as first line antihypertensive therapy, except in patients with another indication for the drug (e.g. angina). They decrease the incidence of myocardial infarction and heart failure. There mode of action is not clearly understood, but several factors probably play a role in their overall hypotensive effects which include, decrease in heart rate and cardiac output, alteration of baroreceptor reflex sensitivity, reduction in plasma renin and aldosterone activity, decrease in plasma volume, release of vasodilatory prostaglandins, and probably a CNS-mediated antihypertensive effect.

β blockers are very suitable antihypertensive drugs in myocardial infarction and angina. Cardioselective β blockers e.g., atenolol, metoprolol, bisoprolol and acebutolol are commonly used.

Labetalol and carvedilol are combined β and α adrenoreceptor antagonists which are sometimes more effective than pure β-blockers. Labetalol can be used as infusion in malignant phase-hypertension.

β blockers are contraindicated in bronchial asthma, chronic obstructive pulmonary disease and heart block.

ACE inhibitors

ACE inhibitors are considered to be the drugs of choice for hypertension when diuretics and β blockers are contraindicated or fail to control blood pressure.

Unlike, β blockers, ACE inhibitors improve the "quality of life" and do not interfere with the patient's lifestyle.

An ACE inhibitor can be used as a single drug to lower blood pressure or combined with other hypotensive drugs such as diuretics where it can reduce hypokalemia, hypercholesterolemia, hyperglycemia and hyperuricemia caused by diuretic therapy.

Long acting ACE inhibitors such as enalapril, fosinopril, ramipril are prodrugs and have the advantage of single dose administration.

As antihypertensives, the compelling indications of ACE inhibitors are heart failure, left ventricular dysfunction and diabetic nephropathy. They are absolutely contraindicated in renovascular disease and pregnancy.

Angiotensin-receptor blockers

Angiotensin-receptor blockers (ARBs) (losartan and valsartan) do not inhibit the breakdown of bradykinin and thus do not appear to cause the persistent dry cough which complicates ACE inhibitor therapy.

Angiotensin receptor blockers are only indicated in patients who are intolerant to ACE inhibitors.

Calcium channel blockers

Calcium channel blocking drugs are effective agents in the treatment of hypertension, particularly in patients with co-existent angina pectoris. or in isolated systolic hypertension in the elderly, when a low dose thiazide is contraindicated or not tolerated.

The dihydropyridine group of calcium antagonists is used for the treatment of hypertension and amongst them the choice lies with newer second generation drugs like amlodipine, felodipine, isradipine and lacidipine, which are more vasoselective and have longer half life requiring single dose administration. Side effects include flushing, palpitations and fluid retention. The rate limiting calcium antagonist can be useful when hypertension coexists with angina but they may cause bradycardia. The main side effect of verapamil is constipation.

Calcium antagonists should not be used in heart failure and heart block.

α_1 blockers

Prazosin, doxazosin and terazosin have a selective postsynaptic α_1 adrenergic receptor blocking property and cause vasodilation of both the arteries and veins. These drugs cause a fall of blood pressure with very little compensatory rise in pulse rate or cardiac output. Unlike β-blockers, these drugs do not adversely affect insulin sensitivity or blood lipids and can improve the negative effects on lipids induced by thiazides and β blockers.

α_1 blockers are less effective than first-line antihypertensive drugs, when used as monotherapy. They may be used with other antihypertensive drugs in the treatment of mild to moderate hypertension, but cause postural hypotension.

α_1 blockers also relax smooth muscle tone in the bladder neck, prostatic capsule and prostatic urethra and are used for benign prostatic hyperplasia, but may cause urinary incontinence, particularly in women.

Side effects of α_1 blockers include 'first dose effect' (increased fall in blood pressure), syncope, dizziness and headache, which are self limited and do not occur with continued therapy.

Centrally acting sympatholytics

These are potent antihypertensive agents that act by stimulating the presynaptic α_2 adrenergic receptors in the CNS. This simulation leads to a decrease in peripheral sympathetic tone, which reduces systemic vascular resistance. Also, it causes a modest decrease in cardiac output and heart rate.

Methyldopa: The only indication of methyldopa is in the treatment of pregnancy-related hypertension, where it serves as first-line therapy because of its proven safety. Other commonly used antihypertensive drugs in pregnancy carry the risk of fetal morbidity or mortality. Hydralazine, a direct-acting vasodilator, is an alternative agent, and both of these drugs can be given IV for treatment of eclampsia.

Side effects include drowsiness, dry mouth, postural hypotension and sexual dysfunction. Rarely, it may cause hemolytic anemia and hepatitis.

Clonidine is another centrally acting sympatholytic, which is mainly used to prevent the rise of noradrenalin in the brain that occurs during the withdrawal of opioids and accounts for the withdrawal symptoms during treatment of opioid addiction.

Direct-acting vasodilators

These are potent antihypertensive agents that act by causing dilation of the arterioles, but not of veins and are reserved for refractory hypertension. They cause salt and water retention and reflex sympathetic stimulation of heart. Therefore, treatment with direct-acting vasodilators is always combined with a diuretic and β blocker. These drugs should be used with caution or avoided in patients with ischemic heart disease because of the reflex sympathetic hyperactivity, which may precipitate angina or ischemic arrhythmias.

Hydralazine has been largely replaced by other safer hypotensive drugs, but is still used in serious hypertension during pregnancy. The disadvantages of hydralazine include:

- tachyphylaxis limits the sole use of the drug
- rapidly metabolized during first pass metabolism leading to considerable reduction of its bioavailability
- adverse effects, which include peripheral neuropathy, arthralgia, myalgia, and development of a lupus-like syndrome.

Minoxidil is a potent direct vasodilator, but rarely used because of potentially serious adverse effects, which include weight gain, hypertrichosis, hirsutism, ECG abnormalities, and pericardial effusion. Topical preparations of minoxidil have been used to stimulate scalp hair growth in baldness.

Nesiritide

Nesiritide, a recombinant form of human brain natriuretic peptide is a potent vasodilator that reduces ventricular filling pressure and improves cardiac output. Nesiritide may be used primarily in patient who continue to be symptomatic after initial treatment with diuretic and nitrates.

Choice of antihypertensive drug

Trials that have compared thiazides, calcium antagonists, ACE inhibitors and angiotension receptors blockers have not shown consistent differences in outcome, efficacy, side effects or quality of life. β-blockers, which previously featured as first-line therapy in guidelines (risk of cardiovascular disease), have a weaker evidence base.

The choice of antihypertensive therapy is usually dictated by the patient's age, response to initial therapy and drugs side effects. The usual approach is to start with ACE inhibitor in middle-aged and calcium antagonist or thiazide-type diuretic in elderly patients and then add up step-wise another antihypertensive drug till the optimum BP (139/83 mm/Hg) is achieved for reduction of major cardiovascular events.

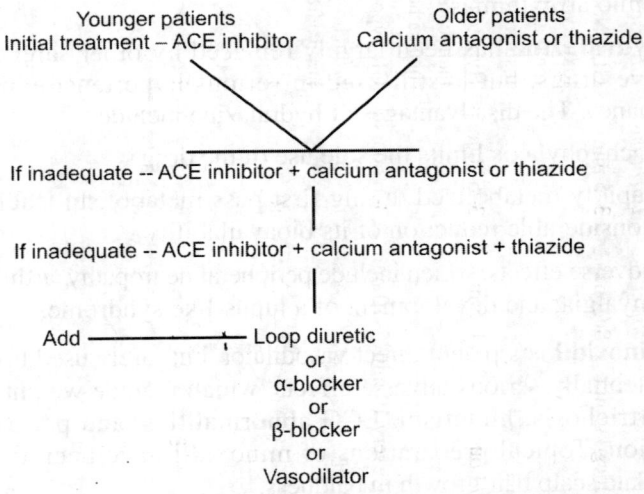

A stepwise approach to the management of hypertension

Parenteral antihypertensive agents

These are indicated for the immediate reduction of blood pressure in patients with hypertensive emergencies (Table 5.7). Great care must be taken when lowering a very high blood pressure, as a precipitate fall may cause renal failure or cerebral damage due to a

Table 5.7: Some intravenous antihypertensive agents

Drug	Dose	Onset	Duration	Adverse effects	Comments
Nitroprusside	0.25–10 mcg/kg/min	Seconds	3–5 min	GI, CNS, and cyanide, toxicity especially with renal and hepatic insufficiency, hypotension	Most effective and easily titrable. Used with β-blocker in aortic dissection
Nicardipine	5–15 mg/hour	1–5 min	3–6 hours	Hypotension, tachycardia, headache	May precipitate myocardial ischemia
Labetalol	20–40 mg every 10 min Max. 300 mg	5–10 min	3–6 hours	GI, hypotension, bronchospasm, bradycardia, heart block.	Avoid in congestive heart failure, asthma
Esomol	Loading dose 500 mg Maintenance 25–200 mg	1–2 min	10–30 min	Bradycardia, nausea	Avoid in congestive heart failure, asthma weak antihypertensive
Nitroglycerin	0.25–5 mcg/kg/min	2–5 min	3–5 min	Headache, nausea hypotension, bradycardia	Tolerance may develop. Useful primarily with myocardial ischemia
Hydralazine	5–20 mg	10–30 min	2–6 hours	Tachycardia, bradycardia, GI toxicity	Avoid in coronary artery disease, aortic dissection. Rarely used except in pregnancy.

(Contd...)

Table 5.7: Some intravenous antihypertensive agents (Contd.)

Drug	Dose	Onset	Duration	Adverse effects	Comments
Clevidipine	1–2 mg/hour Max. 32 mg/hour	2–4 min	5–15 min	Headache, nausea, vomiting	Lipid emulsion. Contraindicated in allergy
Trimethaphan	0.5–5 mg/Min	1–3 min	10 min	Hypotension, ileus, urinary retention, respiratory arrest, liberates histamine.	Useful in aortic dissection otherwiserarely used.

sudden reduction in the blood supply to the kidney and brain. The aim of treatment should be to reduce the diastolic blood pressure slowly to around 100 mm Hg. Patients should be monitored very closely to avoid an exaggerated hypotnsive response.

Sodium nitroprusside is the drug of choice for the most serious emergencies because of its rapid and easily controllable action. In the presence of myocardial ischemia nitroglycerine or a β blocker such as labetalol or esmolol is preferable.

Table 5.8: Therapeutic considerations of major oral antihypertensive drugs

Drug	Compelling indictions	Compelling contraindications	Major side effects
Diuretics	Most hpertensions Heart failure Elderly patients	Gout	Hypokalemia Dyslipidemia Hyperuricemia
β blockers	Angina After myocardial infarction Tachyarrhythmias Heart failure	Asthma Chronic obstructive pulmonary disease Heart block	Congestive heart failure Brochospasm Dyslipidemia
ACE inhibitors	Diabetic nephropathy Heart failure. After myocardial Infarction. Chronic renal insufficiency (early stages)	Pregnancy Hyperkalemia Bilateral renal artery stenosis	Cough Angioedema Hyperkalemia Fetal abnormalities
ARBs	As a substitute in patients intolerant to ACE inhibitors	Same as ACE inhibitors	
Calcium antagonists	Most hypertensions Angina Elderly patients	Heart block Congestive heart failure	Worsening of systolic function

5.7 NITRATES

Nitrates are the principal drugs for the treatment of acute attacks of angina pectoris and in anticipation of attacks, to prevent their occurrence.

Mechanism of action

The major mechanism of action include systemic venodilation with concomitant reduction in left ventricular end-diastolic volume and pressure, thereby reducing myocardial wall tension and oxygen requirements; dilation of epicardial coronary vessels; and increased blood flow in collateral vessels, particularly in ischemic regions. When metabolized organic nitrates release nitric oxide (NO) that binds to guanylyl cyclase in vascular smooth muscle cells, leading to an increase in cyclic guanosine monophosphate, which causes relaxation of vascular smooth muscle.

Nitrates also exert antithrombotic activity by NO-dependent activation of platelet guanylyl cyclase, impairment of intraplatelet calcium flux, and platelet activation.

The production of prostaglandin E or prostacyclin (PGI_2) and membrane hyperpolarization may also be involved.

Pharmacokinetics

Nitrates are readily absorbed from the buccal mucous membranes, the skin, the gastrointestinal tract, and the lungs. The nitrates undergo extensive first pass metabolism in the liver and need sufficiently large doses (to offset first pass metabolism) to be pharmacologically active. The oral bioavailability of the traditional organic nitrates (eg, nitroglycerin and isosorbide dinitrate is very low (typically <10-20%). The mononitrate metabolite of isosorbide dinitrate is an active metabolic and has an oral bioavailability of 100%.

Nitrates differ in their potency onset and duration of action (Table 5.9).

Table 5.9: The nitrates

Drug	Dose (mg)	Action Onset	Duration
Nitroglycerin			
Sublingual	0.3–0.6 mg	2 min	10–13 min
Spray	0.4 mg	1–2 min	10–13 min
Ointment	2% (7.5-40 mg)	10–20 min	7 hours
Transdermal	0.2–.08 mg	10–30 min	8–12 hours
Oral sustained release	2.5–13 mg	1–2 hours	4–8 hours
Intravenous	5–200 mcg/min	Tolerance may be seen in 7–8 hours	
Isosorbide dinitrate			
Sublingual	2.5–10 mg	2 min	up to 60 min
Oral	5–80 mg 2–3 times daily	10 min	up to 8 hours
Spray	1.25 mg daily	1–2 min	2-3 min
Chewable	5 mg	2 min	2 hours
Oral slow release	40 mg 1–2 daily	20 min	up to 8 hours
Intravenous	1.25–5.0 mg/hours	Tolerance in 7–8 hours	
Isosorbide mononitrate			
Oral	40 mg twice daily	20 min	12–24 hours

Pharmacological actions

The main action of nitrates is to relax all types of smooth muscle regardless of the cause of the pre-existing muscle tone. It has practically no direct effect on cardiac or skeletal muscle.

Vascular smooth muscle

The primary direct result is marked relaxation of veins with increased venous capacitance and decreased ventricular preload. Pulmonary vascular pressure and heart size are significantly reduced (decreased left ventricular diastolic pressure with decreased ejection time). In heart failure, preload is often abnormally high: the nitrates and other vasodilators, by reducing preload, may have a beneficial effect on cardiac output.

Dilation of large arteries results in lowering of after-load.

In patients with angina due to atherosclerotic obstructive coronary artery disease, redistribution of coronary flow from normal to ischemic regions (increased collateral flow) may play an important role in nitrate's therapeutic effects.

The beneficial effects of nitrates are due to a reduction in myocardial oxygen demand (lower preload and afterload) and an increase in myocardial oxygen supply (coronary vasodilation).

Other smooth muscle

Nitrates relax bronchial muscles and biliary tract smooth muscles with a reduction of biliary pressure. These actions are of no clinical valve, because of their brief duration of action.

Nitrates release nitric acid in erectile tissue causing relaxation of the nonvascular smooth muscle of the corpora cavernosa permitting inflow of blood into the sinuses of the cavernosa which causes erection. Adverse effects preclude its use in erectile dysfunction.

Therapeutic uses

The main use of nitrates is in the prophylaxis and treatment of an acute attack of angina. They can be used in several ways for the management of angina.

Sublingual nitroglycerin is the best drug for providing rapid symptomatic relief of an acute attack of angina. Nitroglycerin is also available as a metered dose aerosol, which is sprayed onto the oral mucosa. The aerosol spray has the advantage of chemically stable, may produce even more rapid relief from angina in some patients and may also be useful in patients affected by dry mouth, who find difficulty in dissolving sublingual tablet.

Isosorbide dinitrate (**sorbitrate**) is also active sublingually and is a more stable preparation for those who require nitrates infrequently.

Nitroglycerine and sorbitrate are also absorbed from skin, but more slowly than from the sublingual mucosa, bypassing the liver and are available as transdermal impregnated skin patches. These and other long acting nitrates can be given for prophylaxis, but development of tolerance limits their use on routine basis.

Nitroglycerine and sorbitrate can be used intravenously in patients with severe angina or myocardial infarction for the relief of pain and control of hypertension.

Sodium nitrate is used in cyanide poisoning because methemoglobin has a very high affinity for cyanide resulting in production of cyanmethemoglobin which can be further detoxified by the intravenous administration of Na thiosulfate. The thiocyanate ion, thus formed, is less toxic and readily excreted. Hydroxocobalmin, a form of vitamin B_{12} has a very high affinity for cyanide and is preferred over sodium nitrate.

Tolerance

Tolerance to the action of nitrates occurs when taken regularly for prophylaxis. Mechanisms involved for development of tolerance include the down regulation of receptors after continuous use of nitrates or increased liver metabolism. Tolerance is also due to depletion of reduced sulphydryl groups in vascular smooth muscle. Lower doses of nitrates combined with a calcium antagonist or beta blocker may obviate the nitrate tolerance.

Tolerance can be avoided by 6–8 hour nitrate free period, best achieved at night when the patient is inactive. If nocturnal angina is a predominant symptom, long-acting nitrates can be given at the end of the day.

Adverse effects

These are related to vasodilation and include:
- Throbbing headache, associated with meningeal artery pulsations.
- Severe orthostatic hypotension due to increased venous capacitance which may result in syncope.

- Palpitation (tachycardia) due to compensatory responses evoked by baroreceptors and hormonal mechanisms responding to decreased arterial pressure.
- Flushing due to dilation of skin vessels.
- Significant retention of salt and water due to venous capacitance.
- Dilation of cerebral vessels may result in an increase in cerebral pressure and, hence contraindicated if intracranial pressure is elevated.
- Nitrate ions in large amount can oxidize hemoglobin to methemoglobin to result in hypoxia, which can be treated by giving methylene blue intravenously. Hydroxocobalmin, a form of vitamin B_{12} has a very high affinity for cyanide and is preferred over methylene blue.

5.8 ANTICOAGULANTS

The anticoagulant drugs are used in the prophylaxis of venous thrombosis, where the thrombus consists of a fibrin web enmeshed with platelets and red cells.

Anticoagulants are generally ineffective in the treatment of arterial (white) thrombi which are composed mainly of platelets with little fibrin.

HEPARIN

Heparin is a complex mixture of acidic substances. It occurs naturally, and is stored in mast cells and basophils. It is a very potent anticoagulant.

It is derived from porcine intestinal mucosa or bovine lung tissue.

Mechanism of action

Heparin inhibits coagulation both in vivo and vitro.

Normally, factor Xa formed by the clotting cascade, when activated converts prothrombin to thrombin. Thrombin reacts with soluble fibrinogen to form fibrin strands, which enmeshes the platelets to form a clot.

Heparin inhibits coagulation by inactivation of factor Xa and thrombin by binding to antithrombin III. Therefore, heparin prolongs the activated partial thromboplastin time (aPTT) and the thrombin time (TT). Factor VIIa is unaffected. Because the anticoagulant effects of heparin administration normalize within hours of discontinuation and action of heparin is reversible by protamine sulphate, it is the drug of choice for patients with increased risk of bleeding.

Heparin suppresses the rate of aldosterone secretion and cell-mediated immunity and slows wound healing.

Pharmacokinetics

Heparin is not absorbed orally because of its highly negated charge and large molecular size. It is usually given by intravenous or sometimes by subcutaneous injection. It is not given by intramuscular injection because of formation of painful hematomas. Heparin is metabolized in liver by heparinase. The anticoagulant effect of heparin is seen with a minute or two of injection and passes off within a few hours. Heparin does not cross the placental barrier.

Therapeutic uses

Heparin is given as an intravenous loading dose (5000 units), followed by subcutaneous injection of 15000 units every 12 hours along with warfarin for 3 days (the period until oral anticoagulant becomes effective) for the treatment of deep vein thrombosis and pulmonary embolism, management of myocardial infarction, unstable angina and acute peripheral arterial occlusion

Low dose heparin by subcutaneous injection is used prophylactically in orthopedic surgery (particularly, if the pelvis or hip is involved) to prevent postoperative deep vein thrombosis and pulmonary embolism.

Heparin therapy is monitored by measurements of activated partial thrombosplastin time (aPTT) which should be kept between 1.5 and 2.5 times the control value.

Adverse effects

Hemorrhage is the most common side effect, which requires withdrawal of heparin. In emergency, protamine sulphate, a specific antidote, shall reverse the effects of heparin.

Other side effects of heparin include thrombobocytopenia, hyperkalemia (due to inhibition of aldosterone secretion), hypersensitivity reactions and osteoporosis after prolong use.

Heparin is contraindicated in hemophilia and other hemorrhagic disorders, peptic ulcer, recent cerebral hemorrhage, severe hypertension, severe liver disease and hypersensitivity to heparin.

Low molecular weight heparin (LMWH)

Heparin is a large molecule that can be broken down into a number of fragments, which also have anticoagulant properties and are known as low molecular weight heparins.

Dalteparin, enoxaparin, tinzaparin, certoparin reviparin, ardeparin, and **nadroparin** are low molecular weight heparin (LMWH) preparations. They offer certain advantages over unfractioned heparin;

- LMWH inactivates factor Xa to a greater extent than it does to thrombin; therefore, the aPTT is minimally prolonged and the patients may not need the same degree of monitoring.
- LMWH subcutaneously is as effective as intravenous unfractioned heparin.
- LMWH does not cross placental barrier and can be used during pregnancy.
- LMWH is long acting than unfractioned heparin and require less frequent dosings.
- LMWH can be used in lower doses for prevention of thrombosis.
- LMWH is less likely to cause thrombocytopenia and osteoporosis than unfractioned heparin.
- LMWH without laboratory monitoring of anticoagulant effect is safe and efficacious.

- LMWH is the first choice for long-term anticoagulation in pregnant women with thrombosis, and it is an alternative for patients who have clearly failed oral anticoagulation or have unacceptable INR liability.

Fondaparinux

It is a synthetic pentasaccharide, which is a selective inhibitor of factor Xa. It is structurally similar to the region of the heparin molecule that binds antithrombin and is used by SC route for deep vein thrombosis (DVT) prophylaxis. Unlike heparin and LMWH, it does not cause thrombocytopenia. Clinically, it has the best safety and efficacy profile, with LMWH being a reasonable alternative.

Rivaroxaban is the oral inhibitor of factor Xa. It seems to have efficiency and safety as that of LMWH.

Protamine sulphate

Protamine sulphate, a basic protein, reverses the action of heparin. It is a specific antidote for the acidic heparin and is given intravenously. It may cause a fall in blood pressure.

PARENTERAL DIRECT THROMBIN INHIBITORS (DTI)

The direct thrombin inhibitors exert their anticoagulant effect by directly binding to site of thrombin, thereby inhibiting thrombin's downstream effects. This is in contrast to indirect thrombin inhibitors such as heparin, LMWH and fondaparinux, which act through antithrombin.

Lepirudin, argatroban and **bivalirudin** are parenteral direct thrombin inhibitors, that differ mainly in their pharmacokinetic properties.

Lepirudin is cleared by the kidneys and accumulates in patients with renal insufficiency. The plasma half-life in 60 minutes.

Argatroban in metabolized by the liver. It is safer than lepirudin for heparian-induced thrombocytopenia (HIT) patients with renal insufficiency. The plasma half-life is 45 minutes.

Bivalirudin is degraded by peptidases and is partially excreted by kidneys. It has a plasma half-life of 25 minutes, the shortest half-life of all the parenteral DTI.

Bivalirudin causes less bleeding, which combined with is short durations of action makes it a useful alternative in patients undergoing percutaneous coronary intervention.

ORAL ANTICOAGULANTS

THE COUMARINS

Warfarin and phenindione are the oral anticoagulants. They act by inhibiting the reduction of vitamin K to its active form. Consequently, administration of coumarins leads to depletion of the vitamin-K dependent clotting factors II (prothrombin), VII, IX, and X and proteins C and S.

Warfarin is well absorbed orally, but requires 4–5 days before the full anticoagulant effect is achieved and for immediate effect, heparin is given concomitantly.

Phenindione is a short acting anticoagulant and is seldom used.

Therapeutic uses

Warfarin is used for prophylaxis of embolisation in rheumatic heart disease and atrial fibrillation and after insertion of prosthetic heart valve. It is used with heparin for the treatment of venous thrombosis and pulmonary embolism.

The prothrombin time should be measured before starting treatment, then daily in the early days of treatment, then up to every 12 weeks to maintain INR between 2 and 3.5 depending on the clinical situation. INR (International Normalised Ratio) is the patient's prothrombin time divided by normal prothrombin time. The prothrombin time (PT) is the time taken for clotting to occur in a sample of blood to which thromboplastin and calcium have been added. (Thromboplastin is formed naturally during the early stages of coagulation, and it converts the inactive prothrombin to thrombin).

Adverse effects

The main adverse effects are:
- hemorrhage
- skin rashes, fever and jaundice (phenindione)
- teratogenic effects (fetal abnormalities)

Coumarin-induced skin necrosis is a rare complication that can occur during initiation of warfarin therapy because of rapid depletion of the anticoagulant factor protein C.

Hemorrhage is the most important side-effect, which may result from over dosage. It is best treated by withdrawal of the drug. If necessary an infusion of fresh frozen plasma or **phytomenadione (vitamin K)** is given intravenously.

Warfarin is contraindicated in active peptic ulcer, severe liver disease, and renal failure and during pregnancy.

Drug interactions

The anticoagulant activity of warfarin is increased by antibiotics, NSAIDs, antiplatelet drugs, lipid lowering drugs, alcohol, cimetidine, anabolic hormones, antimalarials and phenytoin.

Barbiturates and oral contraceptives decrease the activity of warfarin.

NEW ORAL ANTICOAGULANT

New oral anticoagulants are direct thrombin inhibitors that target thrombus or factor Xa. They have a rapid onset of action and have half-lives that permits once or twice-daily administration.

Dabigatran etexilate is an oral thrombin inhibitor and **apixaban** is oral factor Xa inhibitor.

New oral anticoagulants have been designed to produce a practicable level of anticoagulation and are given in fixed doses without routine monitoring. Therefore, these drugs are more convenient to use than warfarin.

Dabigatran has been extensively compared with warfarin in various clinical studies and was found therapeutically more effective in stroke or systemic embolism. Its use was associated with significantly less intracerebral or life threatening bleeding as compared to warfarin. There was no evidence of hepatotoxicity with dabigatran.

Dabigatran is contraindicated in patients with a creatinine clearance of less than 15 m L/min.

The pharmacological properties of new oral anticoagulants may ultimately make them as drugs of choice and replace warfarin.

5.9 ANTIPLATELET DRUGS

Antiplatelet drugs reduce platelet "stickiness" (aggregation) and are helpful in inhibiting arterial thrombosis, where thrombi are formed partly by platelet aggregation and where anticoagulants have little effect. The main indications for the use of antiplatelet drugs are:
- hypertension
- angina pectoris
- myocardial infarction
- cardiovascular surgical procedures
- peripheral arterial disease
- transient ischemic stroke
- obliterative cardiomyopathy

Among the various antiplatelets, aspirin and clopidogrel are the most widely used drugs.

Antiplatelet therapy is a powerful means of reducing cardiovascular risk, but may cause bleeding, particularly intracerebral hemorrhage in a small number of patients. The benefits are thought to overweigh risk in hypertensive patients aged 50 or over, who have well controlled BP and either target organ damage, diabetes or coronary heart disease.

ASPIRIN

Aspirin is unique in that it causes irreversible inhibition of platelet cyclooxygenase leading to depletion of thromboxane for the life of the platelets. Thromboxane is responsible for platelet aggregation and its depletion by aspirin results in inhibition of platelet 'stickiness' to atheromatous plaques in arteries and thus prevents formation of arterial thrombus or its extension. Aspirin does not block all the pathways to platelets clumping.

Therapeutic uses

Aspirin within the dose range of 75–325 mg daily is taken regularly for the prophylaxis of vascular diseases and for the secondary prevention of thrombotic cerebrovascular episodes in cardiovascular diseases (myocardial infarction, stable angina, atrial fibrillation, and intermittent claudication) and following bypass surgery.

Aspirin may have a place in preventing eclampsia in pregnancy and in slowing the progress of diabetic retinopathy. The role of antiplatelet therapy is controversial in the management of pre-eclampsia, because hypertension is the consequence and not the cause and settles down with delivery.

The only contraindications to aspirin therapy are a history of documental drug allergy and active bleeding. Renal and hepatic toxicity are observed with aspirin overdose. Patients with aspirin allergy should receive clopidogrel.

ADENOSINE DIPHOSPHATE (ADP) ANTAGONISTS

Adenosine diphosphate is a powerful inducer of platelet aggregation secreted from platelet granules.

Clopidogrel, ticlopidine and **prasugrel** are ADP receptor antagonists that inhibit platelet activation and aggregation.

Clopidogrel is the preferred ADP antagonist and has replaced teclopidine because of lower risk of gastrointestinal bleeding, neutropenia and thrombotic thrombocytopenic purpura (TTP). It is absorbed and metabolized rapidly, and the onset of inhibition of platelet aggregation is more rapid than ticlopidine. Inhibition of platelet aggregation is detectable 90 minutes after an oral loading dose of 300 mg, which is maintained by administration of low doses (75 mg) daily.

Clopidogrel is more effective than aspirin in patients who have experienced a recent stroke or recent myocardial infarction and in patients presenting symptomatic peripheral arterial disease. The combination of clopidogrel and aspirin is more effective than aspirin alone in patients with unstable angina and non-ST segment elevation myocardial infarction.

Side effect is mainly hemorrhage. GIT, CNS, hepatic and biliary disorders have also been reported. It is contraindicated in active bleeding and breast-feeding.

Prasugrel has increased potency and results in greater and more uniform platelet inhibition compared to clopidogrel. It has a more rapid onset of action after an oral loading dose of 60 mg followed by a maintenance dose of 10 mg daily to achieve maximum platelet inhibition.

Prasugrel decreases adverse outcomes (cardiovascular death, MI and stroke) in acute coronary syndrome but increases fatal bleeding rates as compared to clopidogrel.

Prasugrel should be avoided in patients older than 75 years, less than 60 kg, and those with prior stroke or transient ischemic attacks.

ASPIRIN AND CLOPIDOGREL RESISTANCE

The reported incidence of resistance to these drugs varies greatly, from less than 5 to 75%.

Clopidogrel resistance is due to impaired cytochrome P450-mediated conversion of clopidogrel to its active metabolite. Prasugrel does not require cytochrome P450 – mediated conversion to an active metabolite and is useful in clopidogrel resistant cases.

GLYCOPROTEIN IIB/IIIA (GPIIB/IIIA) RECEPTOR ANTAGONISTS

The glycoprotein IIb/IIIa inhibitors block the interaction between platelets (GP IIb/IIIa receptors) and fibrinogen, thus targeting the final common pathway for platelet aggregation.

GP IIb/IIIa inhibitors (**abciximab, eptifibatide** and **tirofiban**) are given as IV infusion in high risk patients with refractory acute coronary syndrome, especially with significant ST-T changes or elevated cardiac enzymes.

The utility of GP IIb/IIIa inhibitors in conjunction with aspirin, clogidogrel and heparin therapy appears to be restricted in patients with elevated cardiac biomarkers (troponin, CK-MB and myoglobin) and those with diabetes.

Adverse effects include increased risk of bleeding especially when used in combination with clopidogrel and severe thrombocytopenia. Thrombocytopenia requires immediate discontinuation of the drug.

ADDITIONAL ANTIPLATELET DIRECTED DRUGS

Dipyridamole

Dipyridamole inhibits the uptake of adenosine into erythrocytes and other tissues. It allows metabolically released adenosine to accumulate in the plasma, which decreases coronary vascular resistance and increases coronary blood flow and coronary sinus oxygen saturation. Dipyridamole also prevents platelet aggregation. It is not very effective when given alone and is used as an adjunct to oral anticoagulation for prophylaxis of thromboembolism associated with prosthetic heart valves. It can also be used alone or with aspirin for secondary prevention of ischemic stroke and transient ischemic attacks.

Cilostazol is a newer phosphodosterase inhibitor that promotes vasodilation and inhibition of platelet aggregation. Cilostazol is used primarily to treat intermittent claudication.

NEW ANTIPLATELET DRUGS

Cangrelor and **ticagrelor** are direct acting reversible APD receptor antagonists.

Cangrelor is a short-acting antiplatelet and offers no significant advantage over clopidogrel.

Ticagrelor is an orally active reversible ADP antagonist, which has not only a more rapid onset and offset of action than clopidogrel, but also produces greater and more predictable inhibition of ADP-induced platelet aggregation. As compared to clopidogrel, it was found to be more effective in producing greater reduction in cardiovascular death, MI, and stroke. Although, not available yet for use, ticagrelor is the first new antiplatelet drug to demonstrate a greater reduction in cardiovascular death than clopidogrel in patients with acute coronary syndrome.

THROMBIN-MEDIATED PLATELET ACTIVATOR INHIBITOR

Vorapaxar and **atopaxar** are oral antagonists of protease activated receptor-1 (PAR-1), that causes activation of thrombin receptor on platelats. They are under investigation for use as an adjunct to aspirin or aspirin and clopidogrel.

5.10 LIPID LOWERING DRUGS

The hyperlipidemias are a group of disorders of metabolism in which there are increased amounts of various lipoproteins in the blood. The most important lipid in lipoproteins is cholesterol and there is strong evidence that a high level of blood cholesterol especially in the form of low-density lipoprotein (LDL), is associated with an increased risk of atherosclerotic vascular disease, particularly of coronary arteries. Lowering cholesterol concentration reduces the risk of cardiovascular events, including death, MI, stroke and coronary revascularization.

There is evidence that even in apparently healthy subjects with raised blood cholesterol, lowering the level reduces the risk of coronary disease.

Elevated serum triglyceride (TG) levels are an independent risk factor for atherosclerotic disease.

Patents with hypertriglyceridemia frequently have low levels of high-density lipoprotein (HDL) cholesterol.

In patients with baseline LDL cholesterol above 130 mg/dl (optimal LDL-C is less than 100 mg/dl), even though symptom free, there is a clear advantage in reducing the blood cholesterol, and this is achieved most effectively by using statins. In addition, other risk factors must be addressed: in particular, smoking, hypertension, diabetes mellitus, obesity and lack of exercise. Patients with elevated triglycerides need to restrict simple sugars and alcohol as well.

Drugs that lower LDL cholesterol and triglycerides include:
- Statins (the HMG-CoA reductase inhibitors)
- Bile acid binding resins
- Cholesterol absorption inhibitor
- Nicotinic acid (niacin)
- Fibrates
- Omega-3 fatty acids

STATINS (HMG-CoA reductase inhibitors)

Lovastatin, **pravastatin**, **simvastatin**, **fluvastatin**, **atrovastatin** and **rosuvastatin** are the statins having similar mechanism of action and side effects.

Statins inhibit cholesterol synthesis in the liver; reduce serum levels of total cholesterol, LDL-cholesterol and triglycerides. They elevate HDL-cholesterol.

The decrease in LDL-cholesterol results from an increase in hepatic LDL receptors (inhibition of cholesterol synthesis results in up-regulating activity of the LDL receptor). The increase in hepatic LDL receptors causes an increase in receptor mediated clearance of LDL from the blood.

Statins also cause decreased oxidative stress and vascular inflammation with increased stability of atherosclerotic lesions. This helps in limiting the atheromatous lesion and preventing its disruption which may result in thrombotic occlusion or distal embolisation of the vessel.

Statins reduce LDL-C by up to 60%, reduce TG by up to 40% and increase HDL-C by up to 10% (Table 5.10)

Pharmacokinetics

Absorption of statins varies from 40 to 75% when given orally except for fluvastatin which is almost completely absorbed. All

Table 5.10: Statins and lipoproteins

Statins	Dose range (mg PO/d)	Lipoproteins effects		
		TG%	LDL%	HDL%
Atrovastatin	10–80	13–32↓	38–54↓	4.8–5.5↑
Fluvastatin	20–80	5–35↓	17–36↓	0.9–12↑
Lovastatin	10–80	12–13↓	2.9–8↓	4.6–8↑
Pravastatin	10–80	3–15↓	19–34↓	3–9.9↑
Rosuvastatin	5–40	10–35↓	41–65↓	10–14↑
Simvastatin	10–80	12–36↓	28–46↓	5.2–10↑

TG: triglyceride; LDL: low density; HDL: high density; ↓: decreased; ↑: increased.

undergo extensive first pass metabolism in the liver. Most of the absorbed dose is excreted in bile; 5–20% is secreted in the urine. Plasma half-lives of these drugs range from 1 to 3 hours except for atrovastatin, which has a half-life of 14 hours and rosuvastatin, whose half-life is 19 hours.

Therapeutic uses

Statins are the treatment of choice for elevated LDL cholesterol. The lipid-lowering effect appears within the first week of use and becomes stable after approximately 4 weeks of use. Statins may be effective for patients with mild to moderate hypertriglyceridemia with concomitant LDL-C elevation.

Atrovastatin and rosuvastatin are most potent and longer acting and have good efficacy.

Adverse effects

Statins are generally well tolerated and serious side effects are rare (below 2%).

Common side effects (5% to 10% of patients) include GI upset (e.g. abdominal pain, diarrhea, bloating, constipation), myalgia, myositis and infrequently rhabdomyolysis especially in patients who are elderly, debilated and receiving other drugs that interfere with statin degradation, which usually involves cytochrome P450 or glucuronidation. Among the drugs, which increase the risk of rhabdomyolysis, are fibrates (greater risk with gemifibrozil), itraconazole, ketoconazole, erythromycin, clarithromycin, cyclosporine, mefazodone, and protease inhibitors.

Statins are contraindicated in active liver disease, pregnancy and breast-feeding.

CHOLESTEROL ABSORPTION INHIBITOR

Ezetimibe inhibits the specific intestinal membrane transporter (NPCILI) that absorbs dietary and biliary cholesterol at the brush border of the small intestine. Depletion of hepatic cholesterol up-regulates hepatic LDL-C receptor activity. This mechanism of action is synergistic with the effects of statins.

Ezetimibe is given in doses of 10mg orally once daily. No dosage adjustment is required for renal insufficiency, mild hepatic impairment, or in elderly patients. Monotherapy reduces LDL-C by 15–20%, and 17–25%, when combined with a statin.

Ezetimibe is well tolerated but its effect on cardiovascular disease end points is yet to be determined.

Ezetimibe is not recommended for use in patient with moderate to severe hepatic impairment.

BILE ACID SEQUESTRANT RESINS

Cholestyramine, colestipol and **colesevelam** are resins that bind bile acids in the intestine forming insoluble complexes, which are then excreted in the feces. The loss of bile acid leads to an increased bile acid synthesis from hepatic cholesterol. As with ezetimibe, the resultant depletion of hepatic cholesterol up-regulates LDL receptor activity and reduces LDL-C in a manner that is synergistic with the action of statins.

Bile acid sequestrants typically lower LDL-C and cause modest increase in HDL-C, but cannot be used as a monotherapy in patients with TG levels > 250 mg/dl, because they can raise TG levels.

Adverse effects include constipation, abdominal pain, bloating, nausea and flatulence.

Bile acid sequestrants may decrease oral absorption of many other drugs, including warfarin, digoxin, thyroid hormone, thiazide diuretics, amiodarone, glipizide and statins. Colesevelam causes fewer GI effects and interacts with fewer drugs.

NICOTINIC ACID (NIACIN, VITAMIN B_3)

Niacin in pharmacological oral doses (1 to 3 g daily) reduces peripheral fatty acid release and can lower LDL-C by > 15%, TG by 20 to 50%, and raise HDL-C up to 35%.

Niacin is very effective in combination with a statin to achieve target LDL levels in hypercholesterolemia in patients who do not reach LDL targets on the highest tolerated statin dose. It is also the most effective pharmacologic agent for increasing HDL levels.

Adverse effects

These can be minimized by taking the drug with meals and increasing the dosage gradually.
- Niacin produces prostaglandin-mediated intense flushing and itching.
- GI distress is common and peptic ulceration has occurred.
- Hepatic dysfunction can occur with high-dose regimens.
- Glucose intolerance and hyperuricemia can occur.

Niacin should be avoided in patients with a history of gout, active peptic ulcer and liver disease.

Acipimox is a synthetic analogue of nicotinic acid and is less liable to produce flushing and glucose intolerance, but is also less effective as a lipid lowering drug.

FIBRIC ACID DERIVATIVES (fibrates)

Gemfibrozil and **fenofibrate** primarily are triglyceride lowering drugs.

Mechanism of action and pharmacologic effects

Fibrates stimulates peroxisome proliferator activated receptor (PPAR) alpha (a nuclear receptor) which leads to:

a. Reduced synthesis of fatty acids, triglyceride and very-low-density lipoproteins (VLDL).
b. Increase synthesis of lipoprotein lipase which catabolises TG.

Fibrates also upregulate reverse cholesterol transport system via HDL. Consequently fibrates reduce TG up to 50% and increase HDL-C by up to 35% but LDL-C changes are variable. They can lower LDL-C up to 25% in patients with normal triglyceride levels, but may actually increase LDL levels in patients with elevated triglyceride levels.

Fibrates inhibit coagulation and promote thrombolysis which further contributes to their beneficial effects in cardiovascular disease.

Therapeutic uses

Fibrates are first choice drugs for hypertriglyceridemia, whether or not accompanied by hyperchotesterolemia. Since they do not control the cholesterol component combination therapy is often required which include: statin plus fish oil when TG is not too high: fibrate plus ezetimibe: statin plus niacin or statin plus fibrate.

Fenofibrate appears to be safer than gemfibrozil when used in combination with statins.

Adverse effects

- These agents are generally were tolerated. The most common untoward effects are mild gastrointestinal reactions.

- Side-effects profile is similar to statins, including myalgia, myopathy and abnormal liver function tests.

- Fibrates increase the incidence of cholelithiasis and cholecystitis.

- Fibrates displace warfarin from albumin, potentiating its anticoagulant effects.

- Fibrates should be avoided in patients with renal or hepatic dysfunction.

OMEGA-3 FATTY ACIDS

Eicosapentaenoic acid (EPA) and **docosahexaenoic acid** (DHA) comprise approximately 30% of the fatty acids in fish oil. EPA and DHA are potent inhibitors of VLDL, TG formation.

Omega-3 fatty acids are indicated in very high TG over 500 mg/dl (normal < 150 mg/dl), where a reduction up to 50% in TG may be achieved. They reduce the production of prostaglandins and have a mild antiplatelet action.

The combination of omega-3 fatty acids plus statin has the advantage of avoiding the risk of myopathy seen in the statin-fibrate combination.

Fish oil appears to be safe and well tolerated. Main side effects are burping, bloating and diarrhea.

5.11 DRUGS USED IN ANGINA PECTORIS

Angina pectoris (stable angina) is characterized by chest pain provoked by exertion and relieved by rest. It is due to narrowing of the coronary arteries, so that when myocardial work-load (oxygen demand) exceeds the capacity of myocardial blood supply (oxygen delivery), pain may ensue. The narrowing of the coronary arteries may be due to coronary spasm, but is generally due to advancing age coupled with risk factors such as hypertension, smoking and raised plasma cholesterol levels, which cause atherosclerotic lesions.

The aim of treatment of patients with stable angina is to reduce or relieve symptoms and to prevent the progression of the disease to angina at rest (unstable angina) and coronary thrombosis leading to myocardial infarction (MI) and death. Drugs do not reverse the underlying cause of angina, i.e. coronary artery atheromatous plaque.

Drugs used to reduce progression of stable angina to unstable angina (angina at rest), MI and death are lipid lowering drugs, antiplatelet/anticoagulant drugs, and ACE inhibitors, while to control symptoms are nitrates, β-blockers and calcium channel blockers.

Lipid lowering drugs

Statins in patients with elevated baseline total cholesterol levels reduce the risk of unstable angina, MI and even the need of revascularization. Simvastatin in fixed doses of 40 mg/day in patients with increased risk of coronary death because of prior MI, coronary artery disease or peripheral vascular disease, diabetes mellitus, treated hypertension or age 40 to 80 years with a total cholesterol greater than 135 mg/dl has been reported to reduce the risk of MI, stroke, and revascularization by one third regardless of cholesterol and LDL cholesterol levels at base line, age, sex or other treatments.

Antiplatelet drugs

Aspirin (325 mg every other day) in patients with stable angina has been shown to reduce cardiovascular events (MI) by 33% and is considered as a first-line agent in all patients with coronary artery and other vascular disease. Aspirin is also effective in primary prevention in patients without known coronary artery disease.

Clopidogrel (75 mg/day), though not so effective in primary prevention of risk factors, is at least as effective in secondary prevention in patients with an acute coronary syndrome and can be used as an alternative in patients who are allergic or intolerant to aspirin. Clopidogrel is associated with fewer gastrointestinal side effects, slightly more cutaneous reactions, and no excess total bleeding. There was no excess leucopenia or thrombocytopenia with clopidogrel compared with aspirin. The combination of aspirin and clopidogrel is used in selected patients at high risk.

Anticoagulant drugs

Warfarin is as effective as aspirin for secondary prevention but is associated with a higher risk of bleeding. Combination therapy with warfarin plus aspirin is superior to aspirin alone, provided INR is maintained greater than 2.0, though the risk of bleeding has to be kept in mind. Warfarin is indicated in patients with atrial fibrillation and in patients with left ventricular mural thrombosis.

ACE inhibitors

ACE inhibitors are widely used in the treatment of survivors of myocardial infarction, patients with hypertension or chronic ischemic heart disease (IHD) including angina pectoris, and those at high risk of vascular diseases such as diabetes. The benefit of ACE inhibitors are most evident in IHD patients at increased risk, especially if diabetes mellitus or left ventricular dysfunction is present, and those who have not achieved adequate control of blood pressure and LDL cholesterol with beta blockers and statins.

Anti-anginal drugs

Anti-anginal drugs represent an important component of the pharmacologic treatment of angina pectoris.

Nitrates

The choice of preparation depends on the acuity of patient's symptoms. Sublingual nitroglycerin (spray or tablets, 0.4 mg every 5 minutes for a total of 3 doses) is used at the first indication of angina attack or prophylactically before engaging in activities that are known to precipitate angina. Nitroglycerin reduces myocardial oxygen demand by reducing the preload (due to venous dilation) and afterload (due to arteriolar dilation) while enhancing myocardial oxygen delivery (due to epicardial artery dilation).

Long acting nitrates topically (transdermal nitroglycerine patches) or orally (isosorbide mononitrate SR) are used to prevent angina attacks and to improve exercise tolerance.

Nitroglycerine use is contraindicated in the presence of hypotension or if the patient has used sidenafil (Viagra) within the previous 24 hours.

Nitrates are generally are not used on a continuous basis because of the development of nitrate tolerance. 8 to 12 hours free of nitrate exposure daily avoids the development of tolerance which can be achieved by 6–8 hour nitrate-free period, best at night when the patient is inactive.

β blockers

β blockers are a key first choice of antianginal therapy. They reduce myocardial oxygen demand by inhibiting the increase in heart rate, arterial pressure, and myocardial contractility caused by adrenergic activation. Beta blockade reduces these variables most strikingly during exercise but causes only small reductions at rest. Long-acting beta-blocking drugs or sustained-release formulations offer the advantage of once-daily dosing. The therapeutic aims include relief of angina and ischemia. These drugs can reduce mortality and reinfarction rates in patients after myocardial infarction and are moderately effective antihypertensive agents.

Relative contraindications include asthma and reversible airway obstruction in patients with chronic lung disease, atrioventricular conduction disturbances, severe bradycardia, Raynaud's phenomenon, and a history of mental depression.

Side effects include fatigue, reduced exercise tolerance, nightmares, impotence, cold extremities, intermittent claudication, bradycardia (sometimes severe), impaired atrioventricular conduction, left ventricular failure, bronchial asthma, worsening claudication, and intensification of the hypoglycemia produced by oral hypoglycemic agents and insulin.

Beta blockers with relative β_1-receptor specificity such as metoprolol and atenolol may be preferable in patients with mild bronchial obstruction and insulin-requiring diabetes mellitus.

Calcium channel blockers

Calcium channel blockers are coronary vasodilators that produce variable and dose-dependent reduction in myocardium oxygen demand, contractility, and arterial pressure. These combined pharmacologic effects are advantageous and make these agents as effective as beta blockers in the treatment of angina pectoris. They are indicated when beta blockers are contraindicated, poorly tolerated, or ineffective. The indications for the use of calcium channel blockers are:

- Inadequate responsiveness to the combinations of beta blockers and nitrates; many of these patients do well with a combination of a beta blocker and a dihydropyridine calcium channel blocker.

- Adverse reactions to beta blockers such as depression, sexual disturbances, and fatigue.
- Angina with history of asthma or chronic obstructive pulmonary disease.
- Sick-sinus syndrome or significant atrioventricular conduction disturbances.
- Prinzmetal's (variant) angina.
- Symptomatic peripheral arterial disease.

Amlodipine and other second generation dihydropyridines are potent vasodilators and are useful in the simultaneous treatment of angina and hypertension. Short-acting dihydropyridines should be avoided because of the risk of precipitating infarction, particularly in the absence of concomitant beta blocker therapy.

Despite treatment with nitrates, beta blockers or calcium channel blockers, some patients with IHD continue to experience angina, and require additional medical therapy.

RANOLAZINE

Ranolazine, a piperazine derivative, may be useful for patients with chronic angina despite standard medical therapy. Its antianginal action is believed to occur via inhibition of the late inward sodium current (I_{Na}). The benefits of I_{Na} inhibition include limitation of the Na overload of ischemic myocytes and prevention of Ca^{2+} overload via $Na^+ - Ca^{2+}$ exchanger. A dose of 500–1000 mg orally twice is given.

Ranolazine is contraindicated in patients with hepatic impairment or drugs associated with QTc prolongation or when drugs that inhibit the CYP3A metabolic system (e.g. ketoconazole, diltiazem, verapamil, macrolide antibiotics, HIV protease inhibitors and large quantities of grape juice) are being used.

Potassium channel activators

Nicroandil, a potassium channel activator has actions like nitrates and calcium antagonists. It causes both arterial and venous dilatation and is reserved for the prevention and long term treatment of angina, in patients who remain symptomatic despite management with other drugs.

Side effects are like nitrates and include headache, flushing, nausea, and vomiting. Nicroandil is contraindicated in cardiogenic shock, left ventricular failure and hypotension.

5.12 FIBRINOLYTIC (THROMBOLYTICS) DRUGS

Fibrinolysis, normally, takes place to digest a blood clot. Plasminogen, a naturally occurring plasma globulin protein, is deposited on the fibrin strands. Plasminogen activators convert plasminogen into another protein called plasmin, which digests fibrin and fibrinogen amongst other proteins.

With the advent of plasminogen activators, it has become possible to use them as fibrinolytic drugs to dissolve the thrombi. They, therefore, complement the use of anticoagulants, which prevent the formation of clots in the first place.

The fibrinolytic drugs in use include:

Agents without fibrin specificity
- Streptokinase

Agents with fibrin specificity
- Alteplase (rt-PA)
- Reteplase (r-PA)
- Tenecteplse (TNK-tPA)

Streptokinase

Streptokinase is a non-selective plasinogen activator that induces a generalized fibrinolytic state characterized by extensive fibrinogen degradation. It is a streptococcal exotoxin and is isolated from β-hemolytic streptococci. It is antigenic in humans and leads to the development of antibodies, which restricts tits further use and requires the use of an alternate fibrinolytic drug if the treatment is warranted. Prior treatment with IV antihistamine (chlorpheniramine) and hydrocortisone is required to prevent anaphylactic reactions.

Alteplase

Alteplase is a recombinant tissue plasminogen activator (rt-PA). It is a more clot selective and does not cause adverse effects (allergy or hypotension) as compared to streptokinase.

Reteplase (r-PA)

Reteplase has reduced fibrin specificity but has a longer duration of action than alteplase. Its efficacy equals to streptokinase and alteplase.

Tenecteplase (TNK-tPA)

Tenecteplase is a genetically engineered variant of alteplase with slower plasma clearance, better fibrin specificity and high resistance to plasminogen-activator inhibitor – I.

FIBRINOLYTIC THERAPY

All plasminogen activators are given intravenously either as perfusion or bolus administration. Concomitant use of IV heparin reduces the risk of subsequent coronary occlusion.

Fibrinolytic therapy is most effective if given within 12 hours (particularly within 6 hours) of the onset of symptoms. Beyond 12 hours, fibronolysis yields little benefit. If angina symptoms or ischemic changes on the ECG persist at 60–90 minutes after the initiation of fibrinolytic therapy, patients should be considered for urgent invasive strategy–coronary angiography and subsequent revascularization, as warranted.

Bleeding complications are the most common adverse effects of fibrinolytic therapy, which may be of concern with intracranial hemorrhage. The risk of intracranial hemorrhage is increased two fold in patients older than 75 years, less than 70 kg, on anticoagulation therapy (Coumadin), or with severe hypertension (BP > 170/90). Fresh frozen plasma should be given to patients with intracerebral hemorrhage.

The contraindications of fibrinolytic therapy include active bleeding, defective homeostasis, recent major trauma, stroke/transient ischemic attacks, surgical procedures, acute pericarditis and GI/genitourinary bleeding and uncontrolled hypertension (BP > 180/110).

5.13 DRUGS USED FOR ACUTE CORONARY SYNDROME

Acute coronary syndrome (ACS) includes unstable angina (UA) and myocardial infarction (MI).

Unstable angina (UA) is closely related condition whose pathogenesis and clinical presentations are similar to MI but differ in severity. UA usually results from severe coronary artery narrowing, transient occlusion or microembolization of thrombus and/or atheromatous material.

The goal of pharmacologic management is to provide relief from chest pain and to limit thrombus formation. The drugs used include analgesics, antiplatelet, anticoagulant, antianginal and thrombolysis medication.

Analgesics

Intravenous opiates (initially morphine sulphate 5–10 mg or diamorphine 2.5–5 mg) and antiemetic (initially metoclopramide 10 mg) should be administered and repeated at intervals of 5–15 minutes until the pain is relieved or side effects (hypotension, respiratory depression) develop. In addition to relief of pain, opiates also lower sympathetic drive and thereby reduce vascular resistance, reduce myocardial oxygen demand, blood pressure, infarct size and susceptibility to ventricular arrhythmias.

Opiates should not be given by intramuscular route, because the clinical effects may be delayed by poor skeletal muscle perfusion, and a painful hematoma may form following thrombolytic or antithrombotic therapy.

Antiplatelet drugs

Aspirin (75–300 mg orally) daily improves survival, with a 25% relative risk reduction in mortality.

Aspirin (300 mg) should be given within the first 12 hours and therapy should be continued indefinitely if there are no side effects. In combination with aspirin (within 12 hours) the use of clopidogrel (300 mg loading dose, then 75 mg daily) confers a further reduction in the composite end point of cardiovascular death, MI or stroke without affecting overall major bleeding risk.

Anticoagulant drugs

Anticoagulation is a key component in the management of patients with UA and MI and should be routinely used in conjunction with aspirin.

Anticoagulation reduces the risk of thromboembolic complication, and prevents reinfarction after successful thrombolysis. Comparative clinical trials suggest that fondaparinux (2.5 mg SC daily) has the best safety and efficacy profile. Anticoagulation should be continued with warfarin if there in persistent atrial fibrillation or evidence of extensive anterior infarction or if echocardiography shows mobile mural thrombus, because these patients are at increased risk of systemic thromboembolism.

Antianginal drugs

Nitroglycerin (NTG) reduces myocardial oxygen demand and enhances myocardial oxygen delivery. Sublingual nitroglycerine (300–500 mg) is a valuable first-aid measure in UA or threatened infarction and intravenous nitrates (NTC 0.6–1.2 mg/hour or isosorbide dinitrate 1–2 mg/hour) are useful for the treatment of left ventricular failure and the relief of recurrent or persistent ischemic pain.

Beta-adrenergic blockers relieve pain by limiting cardiac ischemia and reducing myocardial oxygen demand, reduce arrhythmias and improve short-term mortality if given within 12 hours of onset symptoms. Intravenous (e.g. atenolol 5–10 mg or metoprolol 5–15 mg) followed by oral preparations can be used. Contraindication to β-blockers therapy include advanced AV block, active bronchospasm, decompensated CHF, cardiogenic shock, hypotension or bradycardia.

Calcium channel blockers can be used as third-line agent in patients continuing to have chest pain in the setting of adequate β-blockers and nitrate therapy. Verapamil and diltiazem, because of their rate-limiting action are the drugs of choice if β-blockers are contraindicated.

Other medical therapies

Blood transfusion improves oxygen-carrying capacity and myocardial oxygen supply. Patients presenting with UA/NSTEMI who are actively bleeding and /or significantly anemic should be transfused routinely. The recommended target hemoglobin and hematocrit is 10 mg/dl and 30%, respectively.

ACE inhibitors are useful in patients with LV dysfunction, hypertension, or diabetes. ARB_S are appropriate in patients who cannot tolerate ACE inhibitors.

Thrombolytic drugs

The appropriate use of thrombolytic therapy can reduce hospital mortality by 25–50% and this survival advantage is maintained for at least 10 years. The benefit is greatest for patients treated within the first 2 hours while beyond 12 hours thrombolytics yield little benefit. The major hazard of thrombolytic therapy is intracerebral bleeding. **Tenecteplase** (0.50 mg/kg bolus, total dose 30–50 mg) has a longer plasma half-life and whilst conferring similar intracerebral bleeding risk, has lower other major bleeding and transfusion risks.

HMG-COA reductase inhibitors *(statins)* are potent lipid-lowering agents that reduce the incidence of ischemia, MI and death. Statin therapy reduces adverse outcomes through lipid lowering, anti-inflammatory and atherosclerotic plaque-stabilizing effects.

NSAID$_S$ are associated with an increased risk of death, MI, myocardial rupture, hypertension and heart failure.. They should be discontinued in patients with ACS.

STROKES

Strokes are an important cause of death and disability. Most of them (80%) are due to interruption of vascular supply to a specific brain region, which can result from thrombi developing on atheroma, or emboli from atrial fibrillation blocking a branch of the cerebral circulation. Cerebral hemorrhage is another major cause of stroke.

Recombinant tissue plasma activator (**alteplase**) is the only proven therapy for non-hemorrhagic stroke, but the patient must be selected carefully, and administration of alteplase must commence within 3 hours of stroke onset. Fibrinolytic therapy is not indicated in conditions that include extensive infarction, recent surgery, head trauma, GI or urinary hemorrhage, seizure at stroke onset, bleeding disorder and severe uncontrolled hypotension.

Aspirin reduces atherosclerotic stroke morbidity and mortality and is used for acute and long-term treatment in doses of 160–325 mg/day. Other antiplatelet drugs are not recommended unless there are contraindications to the use of aspirin.

Anticoagulant therapy is indicated to prevent recurrent embolic strokes or in patients with mechanical heart valve implants.

The hallmark of strokes lies in preventive measures, which includes the management of risk factors such as hypertension, diabetes, smoking, elevated lipids and cholesterol. BP reduction even in normotensive stroke patients is beneficial. Oral contraceptives should be discontinued in women with strokes.

5.14 DRUGS FOR CARDIAC ARRHYTHMIA

Anti-arrhythmic drugs are potentially toxic and should only be used when drug therapy is required with the use of as few drugs as possible. Many arrhythmias are benign and do not require specific treatment. Precipitating or causal factors should be corrected e.g. excess alcohol or caffeine consumption, myocardial ischemia, hyperthyroidism, acidosis, hypokalemia and hypomagnesemia.

The antiarrhythmic drugs can be classified according to the effect on the intracellular action potential or by the site of action.

I. According to intracellular action potential

Class I: Membrane stabilizing agents (sodium channel blockers).

a. Block Na^+ channel and prolong action potential
- Quinidine and disopyramide

b. Block Na^+ channel and shorten action potential
- Lignocaine, mexiletine

c. Block Na^+ channel with no effect on action potential
- Flecainide, propafenone

Class II: β-adrenoceptor antagonists (β-blockers)
- Atenolol, bisoprolol, metoprolol, I-sotalol

Class III: Drugs whose main effect is to prolong the action potential
- Amiodarone, d-sotalol

Class IV: Calcium channel blockers
- Verapamil, diltiazem.

II. According to site of action

a. Sinoatrial node
- β-blockers, atropine, verapamil, diltiazem

b. AV node
- Adenosine, β-blockers, digoxin, verapamil, diltiazem

c. Atria, ventricles and accessory conducting tissue
- Disopyramide, flecainide, propafenone, amiodarone

d. Ventricles
- Lignocaine, (lidocaine), mexiletine, β-blockers

Class I drugs

Class I drugs act principally by suppressing excitability and slowing conduction in atrial or ventricular muscle. They act by blocking sodium channels, of which there are several types in cardiac tissue. These drugs should generally be avoided in patients with heart failure because they depress myocardial function, and class Ia and Ic drugs are often pro-arrhythmic.

Class 1a

These prolong cardiac action potential duration and increase the tissue refractory period. They are used to prevent both atrial and ventricular arrhythmias.

Disopyramide

Disopyramide is effective both for the prevention and treatment of atrial and ventricular tachycardia. It decreases excitability, slows conduction and has a potentially negative inotropic effect. It can be given either orally or intravenously in atrial or ventricular arrhythmias, including supraventricular tachycardia and ventricular extrasystoles.

Toxic effects include myocardial depression and hypotension, which may be clinically important and use of disopyramide is therefore contraindicated in heart failure and cardiogenic shock. It has anticholinergic activity, and urinary retention, dry mouth, and blurred vision often occur. Glaucoma may be precipitated.

Disopyramide is not used as a first-line antiarrhythmic drug.

Quinidine

Now rarely used as it increases mortality and causes GIT upset.

Class 1b

These shorten the action potential and tissue refractory period. They act on channels found predominantly in ventricular myocardium and are used to prevent ventricular tachycardia (VT) and ventricular fibrillation (VF).

Lignocaine (Lidocaine)

Lignocaine suppresses the excitability of the ventricular muscle with only moderate depression of the heart's action. In therapeutic doses it is not likely to cause cardiac arrest or a fall of blood pressure.

Lignocaine remains the **first- line drug** for treating ventricular arrhythmia after acute myocardial infarction, cardiac operations and digitalis intoxication. It is given by slow intravenous injection.

Adverse effects include nausea, vomiting, paraesthesia or drowsiness. High doses may cause CNS effects such as respiratory depression and convulsions and CVS effects such as hypotension and bradycardia which may lead to cardiac arrest. Beta-blockers, other antiarrhythmic drugs and cimetidine increase the risk of lignocaine toxicity. Diuretics (hypokalemia) antagonize the effects of lignocaine.

Mexiletine

Mexiletine has electrophysiological actions similar to those of lignocaine. It is used to treat ventricular arrhythmias by intravenous or oral route. Peak plasma concentrations are obtained 2–4 hours after oral administration with a half-life of 9–12 hours. Opioid analgesics reduce oral absorption. Adverse effects include neurological side effects such as drowsiness, confusion, convulsions, paresthesia, tremors and nystagmus. Cardiac side effects include hypotension, bradycardia and transient AV block.

Class 1c

These affect the slope of the action potential without altering its duration or refractory period. They are used mainly for prophylaxis of VF but are also effective in prophylaxis and treatment of supraventricular tachycardia or ventricular arrhythmias. They are successful for pre-excitation VT, because they block conduction in accessory pathways. They should not be used as oral prophylaxis in patients with previous MI because of pro-arrhythmia.

Flecainide

Flecainide is effective for prevention of atrial fibrillation (AF). Intravenous infusion may be used for pharmacological cardioversion of AF of less than 24 hours duration. It should be prescribed with an A-V node-blocking drug, such as a β-blocker to prevent pro-arrhythmia.

Flecainide is also useful for a wide range of arrhythmias including recurrent ventricular arrhythmias. It is as successful as amiodarone in converting AF to sinus rhythm. As with quinidine, it may induce dangerous arrhythmias, particularly following myocardial infarction.

Propafenone

Propafenone has beta blocking effects (class II) and minor calcium channel blocking activity. It also possesses anticholinengic activity. Propafenone has been shown to be effective in treating ventricular arrhythmias and atrial fibrillation.

Propafenone may induce conduction defects and may have arrhythmogenic (proarrhythmic) effects. It may cause atropine like side effects and rarely hypersensitivity reactions. Its use is contraindicated in conduction defects, uncontrolled congestive heart failure, marked hypotension and severe pulmonary obstructive disease.

Class II drugs

This group comprises the β-adrenoceptor antagonists (β-blockers). These agents reduce the rate of SA node depolarization and cause relative block in the AV node, making them useful for rate control in atrial flutter and AF. They can be used to prevent supraventricular andVT. They reduce myocardial excitability and reduce risk of arrhythmic death in patients with coronary heart disease and heart failure.

Non-selective β-blockers act on both $β_1$ and $β_2$ receptors. $β_2$ blockade causes side-effects such as bronchospasm and peripheral vasoconstriction. **Propranolol** is non-selective and is subject to extensive first-pass metabolism in the liver. The effective oral dose is therefore unpredictable and must be titrated after treatment is started with a small dose. Other non-selective drugs include **nadolol** and **carvedilol**.

Cardioselective β blockers act mainly on myocardial $β_1$ receptors and are relatively well tolerated. Atenolol, bisoprolol and metoprolol are all cardioselective β-blockers.

Sotalol is a racemic mixture of two isomers with non-selective β-blockers (mainly l-sotalol) and class III (mainly d-sotalol) activity. It may cause torsades de pointes (VT).

Sotalol is used for prophylaxis in paroxysmal supraventricular arrhythmias. It also suppresses ventricular ectopic beats and non-sustained ventricular tachycardia. It has been shown to be more effective than lignocaine in the termination of spontaneous sustained ventricular tachycardia due to coronary disease or cardiomyopathy.

Esmolol, a relatively cardioselective beta blockers with a very short duration of action, is used intravenously for the short-term treatment of supraventricular arrhythmias, sinus tachycardia or hypertension when induced during anesthesia.

Atenolol and **metoprolol** may be used as adjunctive treatment to digoxin to control the ventricular rate in atrial fibrillation, especially in-patients with thyrotoxicosis.

β-blockers may cause myocardial depression and hypotension or cardiac failure in patients with little cardiac reserve. They are contraindicated in asthma or history of obstructive airway disease, uncontrolled heart failure, cardiogenic shock and severe peripheral artery disease.

Class III drugs

Class III drugs act by prolonging the plateau phase of the action potential, thus lengthening the refractory period. These drugs are very effective at preventing atrial and VT. They cause QT interval prolongation and can predispose to torsades de points and VT, especially in patients with other predisposing risk factors.

Amiodarone

Amiodarone prolongs the refractory period in all cardiac tissue. It is also a non-competitive α and β adrenoreceptor antagonist, and may have some additional class I activity. It is effective in a wide range of supraventricular and ventricular arrhythmias particularly when other drugs are ineffective or contraindicated. It can be given by intravenous infusion as well as by mouth and has the advantage of causing little or no myocardial depression.

Non-cardiac side effects are common and are potentially serious. Cutaneous manifestations of photosensitivity are extremely common. Amiodarone contains a high concentration of iodine and may cause both hypothyroidism and thyrotoxicosis. More potential serious effects are hepatitis, pulmonary infiltration, neuropathy and corneal deposits of yellow brown granules.

Amiodarone potentiates the action of warfarin and digitalis.

Dronedarone a related drug that has a short tissue half-life with fewer side effects. It has recently been shown to be effective in preventing episodes of atrial flutter and fibrillation.

Class IV drugs

These blocks the 'slow calcium channel' which is important for impulse generation and conduction in atrial and nodal tissue, although it is also present in ventricular muscle. Their main indications are prevention of SVT (by blocking the AV node) and rate control in patients with AF.

Verapamil

Verapamil has main action on AV conduction. Ventricular rate in atrial fibrillation and flutter is controlled, and cardioversion of paroxysmal supraventricular tacchycardia (SVT) is often achieved. It can be given intravenously or orally. Intravenous verapamil may cause profound bradycardia or hypotension, and should not be used with beta blocker.

Myocardial depression may occur in patients with heart failure. Drug interaction may occur with digoxin and beta-blockers, which may result in increased digitalis intoxication and hypotension.

Verapamil is contraindicated in sick sinus syndrome, AV node disease and history of heart failure.

Diltiazem has similar properties.

OTHER ANTI-ARRHYTHMIC DRUGS

Atropine

Atropine sulphate (0.6 mg IV, repeated if necessary to a maximum of 3 mg) increases the sinus rate and SA and AV conduction, and is the treatment of choice for severe bradycardia or hypotension due to vagal overactivity. It is used for initial management of symptomatic bradyarrhythmias complicating inferior MI, and in cardiac arrest due to asystole. Side effects include dry mouth, thirst, blurred vision, atrial and ventricular extrasystole.

Adenosine

Adenosine has an inhibitory effect on the sinus and AV conduction. It is the drug of choice for terminating paroxysmal tachycardia (chemical cardioversion). Given intravenously, it has a very short duration of action, lasting for 20–30 seconds.

Dyspnoea, flushing and chest pain are common side effects, but are short lived. Bronchoconstriction may occur, which contraindicates the use of adenosine in asthma.

Digoxin

Digoxin is not an antiarrhythmic drug but is of great therapeutic value in slowing the ventricular rate, particularly in atrial fibrillation and flutter where the slower and more regular contractions allow the heart to function more efficiently and to raise cardiac output.

Digoxin tends to shorten refractory periods and enhance excitability and conduction in other parts of the heart (including accessory conduction pathways). It may therefore increase atrial and ventricular ectopic activity and can lead to more complex atrial and ventricular tachyarrhythmias.

5.15 HEMATINICS

Hematinics are the drugs, which are used for the treatment of anemia.

IRON DEFICIENCY ANEMIA

Iron is an essential constituent of hemoglobin. The normal diet supplies about 25 mg of iron a day, which meets the requirements of the body.

Iron deficiency occurs, when iron is lost from the body in the various forms of blood loss such as menstruation or parturition, chronic bleeding from GIT (ulcer, hookworm infestation) or when there is an increased requirement in conditions like pregnancy, lactation and malnutrition.

Iron, present in the diet, is converted into ferrous form in the stomach and is absorbed from the upper part of the small intestine. The absorption of iron is regulated by a carrier protein in the intestinal wall which limits its absorption to make good any deficiency and acts as a mucosal block to prevent entry of excess iron in the body. In the intestinal wall iron forms a loose compound with carrier protein which is known as ferroportin and is oxidized to ferric iron (Fe^{3+}) by a ferroxidase and actively transported into the blood across basolateral membrane. Iron in combination with plasma transferrin (transferrin-iron complex) is transported across the bloodstream to the bone marrow for the synthesis of hemoglobin and other storage sites like liver and spleen, where it is stored as ferritin and hemosiderin.

Iron is given to correct a deficiency and should be given by mouth unless there are good reasons to give it by parenteral route. The rise in blood haemoglobin concentration should be by about 100–200 mg per 100 ml per day. After the haemoglobin level has returned to normal treatment should be continued for 6 to 12 months to replace depleted iron stores of at least 0.5–1 g.

ORAL IRON

Ferrous sulphate is the drug of choice and is given in doses of 325 mg (65 mg elemental iron) three times daily.

Other iron preparations include **ferrous gluconate, ferrous fumarate** and compound preparations such as **ferrous glycine sulphate, polysaccharide iron complex** and **sodium iron edetate**. The incidence of side effects is related to the content of elemental iron. Ideally, oral iron should be taken on an empty stomach, since food may inhibit iron absorption.

Iron salts are astringent and may cause nausea, epigestric discomfort, abdominal cramps, constipation and diarrhea. Some patients have less severe gastrointestinal adverse effects with one iron salt than another and benefit from changing preparation.

Parenteral iron

The indications of intravenous iron are intolerance to oral iron, refractoriness to oral iron, gastrointestinal disease (usually inflammatory bowel disease) precluding the use of oral iron, and continuous blood loss that cannot be corrected, including dialysis.

Parenteral iron use has further increased because of the use of **recombinant erythropoietin** (EPO) therapy, which requires huge demand of iron, that cannot be met through the release of iron from body stores or oral iron absorption.

Recent improvements in the formulation of intravenous iron preparation have greatly reduced the risk of serious adverse reactions such as hypersensitivity reactions, inducting anaphylaxis that occurred with iron dextran.

Current preparations of **iron sucrose** and **sodium ferric gluconate** are safe and can be given in less than 5 minutes and usually require no test dose.

The dose may be calculated by estimating the decrease in volume of red blood cell mass. 1 mg of iron for each milliliter of volume of red blood cells blow normal is required to which approximately 1 g is added for storage iron. Thus, a woman whose hemoglobin is 9 g/dl should be treated with total of 1315 mg of parenteral iron, 315 mg for the increased red blood cell mass and 1000 mg to provide iron stores.

Anaphylaxis is much rarer than what used to be with old iron dextran preparation. Although a test dose (25 mg) of parenteral iron dextran is recommended, in reality a slow infusion of a larger dose of parenteral iron solution will afford the same kind of early warning as a separately injected test dose. Early in the infusion of iron, if chest pain, wheezing, a fall in blood pressure or other systemic symptoms occur, the infusion of iron should be immediately stopped. Generalized symptoms appearing several days after the infusion of a large dose of iron can include arthralgias, skin rash and low-grade fever. These may be dose related and do not preclude the further use of parenteral iron in the patient.

Iron overdose may be accidental in children or may occur in aplastic and other refractory anemias with hyperplastic bone marrow (especially thalassemia major) due to repeated blood transfusion and excessive iron absorption from the gut.

Desferoxamine, an iron chelating agent is given parenterally in iron poisoning. **Deferasirox is** an oral iron-chelating agent.

Other hypoproliferative anemias

Apart from iron-deficiency anemia, the hypoproliferative anemia is due to chronic inflammatory disease, renal disease and endocrine and nutritional deficiencies.

Appropriate treatment of underlying disease may lead to recovery of normal hemoglobin in anemia of endocrine and nutritional deficiencies.

Anemia of Chronic Disease (ACD) is a common type of anemia which occurs in the setting of chronic infection, chronic inflammation or neoplasia and is normally associated with a normal MCV (normocytic normochromic). The serum iron is low but iron stores are normal or increased.

ACD is due to high levels of production of hepcidin by liver due to inflammatory cytokines especially IL-6. Hepcidin is the principal iron regulatory hormone, which negatively regulates the function of ferroportin. Hepcidin binds to ferroportin on the membrane of iron exporting cells, such as small intestinal enterocytes and macrophages, internalizing the ferroportin and thereby inhibiting the export of iron from these cells into the blood and iron remains trapped inside the cells in the form of ferritin.

The treatment of ACD is not possible and requires blood transfusion as and when required.

Anemia of chronic kidney disease (CKD)

Progressive CKD is usually associated with a moderate to severe hypoproliferative anemia with a normal MCV and decreased reticulocytes. The anemia is primarily due to a failure of erythropoietin production by diseased kidney. Erythropoietin (EPO) stimulates erythroid proliferation and differentiation by interacting on red cell progenitors.

Epoetin alfa is a human recombinant erythropoietin and is used intravenously thrice weekly to treat anemia due to chronic renal failure, HIV-infected patients treated with zidovudine, cancer chemotherapy and in patients scheduled to undergo elective non-cardiac, non-vascular surgery.

Darbepoetin alfa, a modified EPO has three to four time's longer half-life than recombinant The most common adverse effects of EPO are hypertension and thrombotic complications.

MEGALOBLASTIC ANEMIA

Cyanocobalamin (vitamin B_{12}) is required for the maturation of the red blood cells. The deficiency of vitamins B_{12} leads to a failure in the production of erythrocytes and those, which do manage to mature, are abnormal, large and irregular in size and shape. Primitive red cells may also appear in the blood.

Vitamin B_{12} deficiency also leads to glossitis and degenerative changes in the nervous system. The syndrome produced by vitamin B_{12} deficiency is known as pernicious anemia or Addison's anemia. Vitamin B_{12} deficiency is due to failure of its absorption from the intestine due to lack of a factor (intrinsic factor) produced by the stomach.

Hydroxocobalamin has completely replaced cyanocobalamin as the form of vitamin B_{12} used for pernicious anemia. It is ineffective orally and is given is doses of 1 mg by intramuscular injection.

Folic acid is necessary for the maturation of red blood cells, and its deficiency will produce changes in the blood similar to those found in pernicious anemia. However, it has no effect on the degenerative changes in the nervous system of pernicious anemia.

Folic acid has few indications for long term therapy since most causes of folate deficiency yield to short course of treatment. It is contraindicated in pernicious anemia, because it will improve the anaemia but will worsen the neurological complications of pernicious anemia.

Therapeutic uses

Folic acid is given orally in doses of 5 to 15 mg. daily in folate deficiency megaloblastic anemia (e.g. due to poor nutrition, pregnancy or antiepileptics). Prophylactically, it is used in chronic hemolytic states in renal dialysis and during the first 3 months of pregnancy to minimize the risk of neural tube defects, which occur very early in pregnancy. The incidence of fotate deficiency is so high in the smallest premature babies that folic acid (e.g., 1 mg) should be given routinely during the first 6 weeks of life.

The World Health organization recommends routine supplementation with iron and folic acid in children to diminish infant mortality rate. However, studies indicate no survival benefit.

Folic acid is believed to reduce the incidence of cardiovascular disease.

Folinic acid

Folinic acid is also effective in the treatment of folate deficient megaloblastic anemias but it is generally used in association with cytotoxic drugs (methotrexate) to prevent methotrexate induced mucositis and myelosuppression.

DRUGS USED IN LEUCOPENIA

Depression of white blood cells occurs by cancer chemotherapy, immunosuppression or treatments associated with the AIDS virus. Drugs are available which stimulate the growth of white blood cells and can be used to decrease the risk of serious infections due to leucopenia.

Myeloid growth factors

Granulocyte-colony stinulating factor (G-CSF) and granulocyte macrophage colony stimulating factor (GM-CSF) the two myeloid growth factors were originally purified from cultured human cell lines.

Recombinant human G-CSF (rHuG-CSF, **filgrastim**) is produced in a bacterial expression system, while recombinant human GM-CSF (r Hu GM-CSF, **sargamostim**) is produced in a yeast expression system.

Pegfilgrastim, a variant of filgrastim has a much longer serum half-life and requires less frequent administration.

The functions of myeloid growth factors are:
- Stimulation of proliferation and differentiation of various myeloid progenitor cells.
- Activation of the phagocytic activity of mature neutrophils.
- Prolongation of the survival of neutrophils in the circulation.
- Mobilization of the hematopoietic stem cells in the peripheral blood – the use of peripheral blood stem cells (PBSCs) instead of bone marrow stem cells for autologous and allogeneic hematopoietic stem transplantation (G-CSF more potent).
- GM-CSF along with interleukin-2 stimulate T-cell proliferation at the site of inflammation.

Therapeutic uses

G-CSF and pegfilgrastim are better tolerated and are commonly used.

- Cancer chemotherapy—induced neutropenia, G-CSF reduces episodes of febrile neutropenia, requirements of broad-spectrum antibiotics, infections, and days of hospitalization after cytotoxic chemotherapy. Pegfilgrastim requires less frequent administration and shortens the period of severe neutropenia slightly more than G-CSF.
- Congenital neutropenia, cyclic neutropenia, myelodysplasia and aplastic anaemia.

  G-CSF and GM-CSF cause prompt and sometimes dramatic increase in neutrophil count with a decrease in the frequency of infections.

- Autologus stem cell transplantation to counter severe myelo-suppression by reinfusion of patient's own hematopoietic stem cells after high-dose chemotherapy.

  Replacement of bone marrow as the hematopoietic preparation used for autologous transplantation.

Adverse effects

G-CSF and pegfilgrastim can cause bone pain, which clears on the discontimation of the treatment.

GM-CSF can cause more severe side effects which include fever, malaise, arthralgias, myalgias, and a capillary leak syndrome characterized by peripheral edema and pleural or pericardial effusions.

Megakaryocyte growth factors

Platelets are released from the megakaryocyte. The major regulators of platelet production are the hormone thrombopoietin and interleukin 11 (IL-11).

Interleukin 11 and its recombinant form **opreleukin** are used for the treatment of thrombocytopenia in patients with nonmyeloid malignancies, who receive myelosuppressive cancer chemotherapy.

Romiplostin is nonimmunogenic peptide agonist of the thrombopoietin receptor, which is used for the treatment of patients with chronic idiopathic thrombocytopenia (ITP).

6

Gastrointestinal System

6.1 DRUGS FOR OROPHARYNX INFECTIONS

Salivation is not only important for normal physiological functions but also keeps the oral cavity free from infection. Several oral infections may supervene if salivary flow is markedly decreased

Xerostomia (dry mouth) may be caused by irradiation of the head and neck region, damage to or disease of salivary glands, or by drugs having atropine like side effects, notably those of the phenothiazine group and the tricyclic antidepressants. Several oral infections may supervene if salivary flow is markedly decreased. The incidence of oral infection is increased with drugs, which lower the resistance to infection (e.g., cytotoxic drugs, immunosuppressant) and some cytotoxic drugs cause ulceration of the mouth.

Glandosane and **Luborant** are the artificial saliva preparations, which act locally as salivary stimulants. They contain sodium carboxymethyl cellulose, properly balanced with electrolytes so that they have a neutral pH.

Pilocarpine tablets are restricted to use in xerostomia following irradiation for head and neck cancer.

Mouthwashes, gargles, and dentifrices

Mouthwash solutions prevent oral infections and are commonly used in patients undergoing dental treatment, for clearing mucus or cleaning the oral ulcers.

Thymol is a mild antiseptic and one tablet dissolved in warm water is adequate mouthwash solution for most of the patients.

Chlorhexidine gluconate is a more powerful antiseptic and used in a 0.2% solution (Corsodyl) for mouthwash and 1% dental gel for children and handicapped patients. It has a specific effect in inhibiting the formation of plaque on teeth.

Hydrogen peroxide is useful in the treatment of acute ulcerative gingivitis (Vincent's infection) since the organisms involved are anaerobes. It also has a mechanical cleansing effect due to frothing when it comes in contact with oral debris. **Sodium perborate** is similar in effect to hydrogen peroxide.

Povidone-iodine mouthwash is useful for mucosal infections but does not inhibit plaque accumulation.

There is no convincing evidence that gargles are effective.

Oral ulceration and inflammation

Simple mouthwashes (saline or thymol) and antiseptic mouthwashes (chlorhexidine or povidone-iodine) are often beneficial and accelerate healing of recurrent aphthae.

Local anaesthetic mouthwash (**Benzydamine**) or dental gel (**Choline salicylate**) may be effective in relieving the discomfort or oral ulceration.

Aphthous ulcers are small, painful, recurrent that are common in healthy people. The cause is not known, but may be related to stress, and the treatment is only partly effective. **Hydrocortisone** lozenges, **triamcinolone** dental paste or **tetracycline** mouthwashes are used.

Oropharyngeal anti-infective drugs

Infections of pharynx and tonsils are very common and are usually viral and do not require any specific treatment. Serious throat infections require the use of appropriate antibiotic given systemically and there is little indication for the local use of antibiotics in these circumstances.

Preparations administered in the dental surgery for the local treatment of periodontal disease include gels of metronidazole and of minocycline.

Fungal infections, caused by *Candida albicans*, give rise to thrush and other forms of stomatitis and are generally a sequel to the use of broad-spectrum antibiotics or of cytotoxics. Of the antifungal antibiotics used for mouth infection, **amphotericin** and **nystatin** are not absorbed from the intestine, and are used by local application in the mouth. **Miconazole** occupies an intermediate position, since it is used by local application in the mouth, but is also absorbed. **Fluconazole** and **itraconazole** are absorbed and are available for oral administration for oropharyngeal candidiasis.

Herpes simplex and herpes labialis are treated by **acyclovir** suspension and cream.

6.2 DRUGS FOR DYSPEPSIA AND GASTROESOPHAGEAL REFLUX DISEASE (GERD)

The predominant symptom of GERD is heartburn, due to the inflammation of the lower end of the esophagus and is usually due to reflux of the acid from the stomach, which may be associated with peptic ulcer.

ANTACIDS are useful in relieving symptoms of ulcer dyspepsia and of gastroesophageal reflex disease (reflex oesophagitis). With the advent of acid release inhibitors (H_2 blockers, proton pump inhibitors and selective antimuscarinics) antacids are no longer used in the treatment of peptic ulcers.

NON-SYSTEMIC ANTACIDS

Aluminium and magnesium containing antacids are relatively insoluble, very poorly absorbed, longer acting and most suitable for most antacid purpose. Liquid preparations are more effective than tablets.

Magnesium trisilicate or **magnesium carbonate** is the commonly used magnesium salts for dyspepsia. They may cause diarrhea.

Aluminium hydroxide in addition to reducing acidity also inactivates gastric pepsin. This antacid is slightly astringent and can cause constipation.

SYSTEMIC ANTACID

Sodium bicarbonate dissolved in water is used occasionally when a rapid relief of dyspepsia is intended. It should not be used for prolonged periods, as it causes alkalosis, which may lead to aggravation of hepatic, renal and cardiovascular disorders.

All antacids may affect the absorption of other medications by binding the drug or by increasing intragastric pH so that drug dissolution or solubility is altered. The antacids should not be given within 2 hours of administration of tetracycline, fluoroquinolones, itraconazole and iron.

Compound antacid preparations

Activated dimeticone (**simethicone**) is added to non-systemic antacid as an antifoaming agent to relieve flatulence. Such a combination may also be useful for the relief of hiccup in palliative care.

ALGINATES

Alginates float on the gastric contents and can also be added to an antacid, which protects the mucosa of the lower esophagus in case of a reflux and may be useful against gastroesophageal reflux disease.

SURFACE ANESTHETICS

Oxetacaine added to an antacid is of doubtful efficacy in gastroesophageal reflux disease.

ACID RELEASE INHIBITORS

Proton pump inhibitors (e.g. omeprazole) are the most potent inhibitors of gastric acid secretion and are indicated in severe gastroesophageal reflux disease, which do not respond to combined antacid preparation.

PROKINETIC DRUGS OR MOTILITY STIMULANTS

These are the drugs that improve gastroesophageal sphincter function and accelerate gastric emptying and small intestine transit. They include **metoclopramide, domperidone** (dopamine antagonists) and **cisapride** (cholinomimetic).

Metoclopramide and domperidone are mainly used in non-specific and cytotoxic induced nausea and vomiting due to their selective action on the CTZ, where their prokinetic action further acts as contributing factor for antiemesis. They may induce an acute dystonic action, particularly in young women and children.

CISAPRIDE, a prokinetic drug, is believed to promote release of acetylcholine in the gut wall. It does not have dopamine antagonist action as possessed by metoclopramide and domperidone. It is quite useful in gastroesophageal reflex, gastric stasis and dyspepsia. The most serious side effect of cisapride is serious cardiac arrhythmia, which may be even fatal. Others include abdominal cramps, diarrhea, hypersensitivity reaction and increased urinary frequency. Cisapride is contraindicated in heart diseases with a family history of QT interval prolongation or ventricular arrhythmia.

6.3 DRUGS FOR PEPTIC ULCER DISEASE

Multiple factors play a role in the pathogenesis of peptic ulcer disease (PUD). The two predominant causes are *H. pylori* infection and NSAID ingestion. Irrespective of etiologic agents, peptic ulcers develop as a result of an imbalance between mucosal protection/repair and aggressive factors. Gastric acid plays an essential role in mucosal injury.

Although acid secretion is important in the pathogenesis of PUD, eradication of *H. pylori* and therapy/prevention of NASID induced disease is the mainstay of the treatment.

The drugs used in the treatment of PUD include (Table 6.1)
  Acid inhibitory drugs
  Mucosal protective agents

H_2 receptor antagonists

Four H_2 receptor antagonists are available: **cimetidine, ranitidine, famotidine** and **nizatidine**. All four agents, at therapeutic doses, significantly inhibit basal and stimulated acid secretion to comparable levels. However, patients may develop tolerance to H_2 blockers, a rare event with PPIs.

Table 6.1: Drugs used in the treatment of peptic ulcer disease

Group	Drugs	Dose
Acid inhibitory drugs		
H_2 receptors antagonists*	Cimetidine	400 mg twice daily
	Ranitidine	300 mg once daily
	Famotidine	40 mg once daily
	Nizatidine	300 mg once daily
Proton pump inhibitors**	Omeprazole	20 mg once daily
	Lansoprazole	30 mg once daily
	Rabeprazole	20 mg once daily
	Pantoprazole	40 mg once daily
	Esomeprazole	20 mg once daily
	Dexlansoprazole	20 mg once daily
Mucosal protective agents		
Sucralfate	Sucralfate	1 g four times daily
Prostaglandin analogue	Misoprostal	200 µg four times daily
Bismuth-containing compounds	Bismuth subsalicylate (BSS)	524 mg four times daily

*at bedtime, **before breakfast

Comparable nighttime dosing regimens are cimetidine 800 mg, ranitidine 300 mg, famotidine 40mg, and nizatadine 300 mg. Duodenal and gastric ulcer healing rates of 85–90% are obtained within 6 weeks and 8 weeks respectively.

Cimetidine is rarely used because it inhibits hepatic cytochrome P 450 metabolism (raising the serum concentration of theophylline, warfarin, lidocaine and phenytoin) and may cause gynecomastia and impotence, due to of its weak antiandrogenic effects. Other rare reversible adverse effects reported with cimetidine include confusion and elevated levels of serum aminotransferses, creatinine and serum prolactin.

Systemic toxicities reported with H_2 receptor antagonists include pancytopenia, neutropenia, anemia and thrombocytopenia.

Ranitidine to a lesser extent can bind to hepatic cytochrome P450, famotidine and nizatidine do not.

The use of H_2 receptor antagonists has significantly declined with the advent of proton pump inhibitors. H_2 antagonists are especially effective in inhibiting nocturnal acid secretion (which largely depends on histamine), but have a modest impact on meal-stimulated acid secretion (which is stimulated by gastrin and acetylcholine as well as histamine).

Proton pump (H^+ - K^+ - ATPase) Inhibitors (PPIs)

Proton pump inhibitors covalently bind the acid-secreting enzyme H^+ - K^+ - ATPase or "proton pump" permanently inactivating it. Restoration of acid secretion requires synthesis of new pumps, which has a half-life of 18 hours. Thus, although these agents have a serum half-life of <60 minutes, their duration of action exceeds 24 hours.

There are six oral PPIs currently available: **omeprazole, rabeprazole, esomeprazole, lansoprazole pantoprazole** and **dexlansoprazole**. These are the most potent acid inhibitory agents available. They inhibit over 90% of 24-hour acid secretion, compared with fewer than 65% for H_2 receptor antagonists in standard doses. Another advantage is they do not cause tolerance and provide faster pain relief and more rapid ulcer healing as compared to H_2 receptor antagonists.

Omeprazole and lansoprazole are acid-labile and are administered as enteric coated granules in a sustained-release capsule that dissolves within the small intestine at pH of 6.

Pantoprazole is also available for intravenous use.

PPIs are lipophilic compounds; upon entering the parietal cell they are protonated and trapped within the acid environment of the tubulovascular and canalicular system. These agents potently inhibit all the phases of gastric acid secretion. Onset of action is rapid, with a maximum acid inhibitory action within 2–6 hours and duration of inhibitors lasting for 72–96 hours.

PPIs are best administered before a meal (e.g. in the morning before breakfast), because pumps need to be activated for these agents to be effective.

Rebound gastric hypersecretion has been described after discontinuation of PPIs. The clinical relevance of this lies in worsening symptoms of gastroesophageal reflux disease (GERD) or dyspepsia upon stopping of PPIs. Gradual tapering of the PPI and switching to H_2 receptor antagonists may prevent this from occurring.

PPIs are well tolerated and largely used drugs.

Omeprazole and lansoprazole inhibits hepatic cytochrome P450, which is not observed with other PPIs. However, caution should be taken when using theophylline, warafarin and phenytoin along with PPIs.

Adverse effects of PPIs are mainly related to their significant long-term acid suppression.

Long-term acid suppression, especially with PPIs has been associated with a higher incidence of community-acquired pneumonia and *C. difficile*-associated disease.

Long-term use of PPIs may result in reduction of intestinal absorption of calcium or inhibit osteoclast function leading to increased risk of hip fractures. Inhibition of intrinsic factor may lead to non-absorption of vitamin B_{12} but megaloblastic anemia is uncommon due to large stores of the vitamin in the body.

PPIs may exert a negative effect on the anti-platelet effect of clopidogrel and should be given with an interval of 12 hours (e.g. PPI before breakfast and clopidogrel at bedtime).

Therapeutic uses

- *Gastroesophageal Reflex Disease* (GERD)
  PPIs are the most effective agents for the treatment of non-erosive and erosive reflex disease, esophageal complications and extra esophageal manifestations of reflex disease.

- *Peptic ulcer disease*
  PPIs heal more than 90% of duodenal ulcers within 4 weeks and gastric ulcers within 6–8 weeks.

- *Non-ulcer Dyspepsia*
  PPIs like H_2 antagonists have modest efficacy (10–20%) for treatment of non-ulcer dyspepsia.
- *Mucosal Bleeding*
  Intravenous PPIs as well as H_2 antagonists are the preferred treatment for stress-related mucosal bleeding in critically ill patients.
- *Gastrinoma and other Hypersecretory Conditions*
  PPIs provide excellent acid suppression in metastatic or unresectable gastrinomos to prevent peptic ulceration, erosive esophagitis, and malabsorption.

Sucralfate

Sucralfate is a compound of aluminium and sucrose. It is insoluble in water and becomes a viscous paste within the stomach and duodenum, binding primarily to sites of active ulceration.

Sucralfate may act by several mechanisms; serving as a physiochemical barrier, promoting a trophic action by binding growth factors such as epithelial growth factor (EGF), enhancing prostaglandin synthesis, stimulating mucus and bicarbonate secretion and enhancing mucosal defense and repair. Toxicity is rare, with constipation being the most common. It should be avoided in patients with chronic renal insufficiency to prevent aluminium-induced neurotoxicity. Hypophosphatemia and gastric bezoar formation has been reported rarely.

Given the greater efficacy and safety of antisecretory agents and better compliance of patients, sucralfate is rarely used.

Bismuth containing preparations

Bismuth has direct antibacterial action against *H. pylori* and is used in combination with PPIs and antibiotics for its eradication.

Colloidal bismuth subcitrate (CBS) and **bismuth subsalicylate** (BSS) are the most widely used preparations.

Adverse effects with short-term usage include black stools, constipation and darkening of the tongue. Long-term usage with high doses, especially with the avidly absorbed CBS, may lead to neurotoxicity.

Prostaglandin analogues

Misoprostal, is a prostaglandin analogue that is used as a prophylactic agent in reducing the incidence of gastroduodenal ulcers in persons taking NSAIDs. The standard therapeutic dose is 200 mg four times daily.

Depletion of prostaglandin due to NSAIDs causes increased secretion of acid and reduced secretion of mucin, bicarbonate, surface active phosphilopid resulting in mucosal injury and preventing its repair by reducing epithelial cell proliferation.

The most common adverse effect is diarrhea. Major toxicities include uterine contractions and bleeding.

Instead of misoprostal, PPIs are more commonly used **alongwith NSAIDs to prevent mucosal damage. A lansoprazole naproxen combination preparation is ava**ilable to target at decreasing NSAID-related G1 injury.

Miscellaneous drugs

A number of drugs including anticholinergic agents and tricyclic antidepressants were used for treating PUD, but in light of their toxicity and availability of safer and potent antisecretory agents, they are no longer used.

H. pylori eradication

Helicobacter pylori, a spiral, gram-negative, urease-producing bacillus, is thought to be responsible for approximately 80% of ulcers that are not due to NSAIDs. Eradication of *H. pylori* promotes healing and markedly reduces recurrence of gastric and duodenal ulcers.

No single agent is effective in eradicating the organism and the treatment requires combination of two antimicrobial drugs with an antisecretory drug, usually a proton pump inhibitor.

The antimicrobial drugs used with the greatest frequency include amoxicillin, metronidazole, tetracycline and clarithromycin. One of the major problems for the failure of eradication of the infection is the development of resistance to one of the major antimicrobial drugs (e.g. clarithromycin or metronidazole). The other factor responsible for the treatment failure is the duration of treatment. The minimum duration of therapy should be at least 10 days, though 14 days of therapy provides better cure rates.

Antisecretory therapy provides rapid relief of pain, accelerates healing, and, with many drug (e.g. proton pump inhibitors, antibiotics and bismuth) combination improves the cure rate.

Many combination therapies are available for the treatment of *H. pylori* infections. However, failure of therapy to cure the infection is an increasing problem, which is due to the presence of antimicrobial-resistant *H. pylori* and poor compliance with therapy.

The available eradication regimens for *H. pylori* include dual, triple and quadruple therapies. Dual therapy is associated with a high failure rate and is no longer recommended. Triple therapy with a minimum duration of 10 days yields a cure rate as high as 91% among patients who comply with the full protocol. A good example of triple therapy is omeprazole 20 mg, clarithromycin 500 mg and amoxicillin 1 g taken twice a day for 10 days. Metronidazole is generally not included in he regimen because more than 90% of the *H. pylori* isolates are resistant to it.

Patients, who fail to respond to triple therapy for more than two attempts, require quadruple therapy consisting of omeprazole (20 mg once or twice daily), tetracycline (500 mg four times daily), metronidazole (500 mg three times daily) and bismuth (e.g., bismuth subsalicylate (2 tablets four times daily) for 14 days. Because this regimen generally has a higher cure rate than traditional triple therapies, it can also be initial therapy. An alternative salvage therapy uses high-dose omeprazole (40 mg three times daily) plus amoxicillin (1 g three times daily). Either approach has a high rate of success, even in the face of metronidazole resistance.

NSAID ASSOCIATED ULCERS

NSAID should be stopped as the first step in the therapy of an active NSAID-induced ulcer. If that is not possible, then treatment with one of the acid inhibitory agents (H_2 blockers or proton pump inhibitors) is indicated. For patients with rheumatoid arthritis who require active antiinflammatory therapy, prednisone (5–10 mg/day) can be given without apparently adversely affecting ulcer healing. Once the ulcer has healed, the patient can be given a selective COX-2 inhibitor or a traditional NSAID with concomitant misoprostol with or without one of the acid-inhibitory agents (H_2 blockers, proton pump inhibitors).

6.4 DRUGS FOR INFLAMMATORY BOWEL DISEASE (IBD)

Ulcerative colitis (UC) and Crohn's disease (CD) are chronic inflammatory bowel diseases which pursue a protracted relapsing and remitting course, usually extending over years.

It is thought that IBD develops because of an abnormal host response to an environmental trigger in genetically susceptible individuals. This causes inflammation of the intestine and release of inflammatory mediators such as TNF, IL-12 and IL-23 which cause tissue damage. In both the diseases the intestinal wall is infiltrated with acute and chronic inflammatory cells.

The treatment is based on the severity of disease, the location, and associated complications. The aim is to resolve the acute presentation and reduce further occurrences.

Drugs used in the treatment of IBD include:
- 5-Aminosalicylate (5-ASA)
- Corticosteroids
- Immunosuppressants
- Antitumor necroses factor alpha (anti-TNF-α) monoclonal antibodies
- Anti-integrin therapy
- Antibiotics
- Antidiarrheal agents

IBD can be categorized into three categories of severity for treatment namely mild to moderate, moderate to severe and severe or fulminant disease.

Mild to moderate disease

This includes patients whose vital signs and ESR are normal and have no disabling symptoms.

5-Aminosalicylate (5-ASA)

This is available in various formulations to act topically (not systemically), each targeting different parts of the gut. They modulate cytokine release from the mucosa by decreasing the production of arachidonic acid metabolites, particularly leukotrienes To prevent absorption of 5-ASA, a number of formulation have been designed to deliver 5-ASA to various distal segment of the intestine or the colon. These include azo compounds and various forms of mesalamine.

Azo compound

Sulfasalazine, balsalazide and **olsalazine** contain 5-ASA bound by an azo (N = N) bond to an inert compound or to another 5-ASA molecule from which active 5-ASA is released by bacterial breakdown by colonic bacteria.

Mesalamine compounds

Mesalamine is the term used for different proprietary formulations designed to deliver 5-ASA itself in various ways to deliver it to different segments of the bowel.

Pentasa is a mesalamine formulation that contains timeed-release microgranules that release 5-ASA throughout the small intestine.

Asacol has 5-ASA coated in a pH 7 sensitive resin that dissolves at the distal ileum and proximal colon.

Apriso also has a pH dependent release mechanism, and distributes mesalamine throughout the colon.

Lialda, a multimatrix delivery system mesalamine, uses a novel drug delivery system that allows sustained 5-ASA release throughout the colon while decreasing the frequency of administration.

Therapeutic uses

5-ASA drugs induce and maintain remission in UC and are the first-line agents for treatment of mild to moderate acute ulcerative colitis and CD.

5-ASA suppositories or enema may be better choice in lesions confined to rectum or distal colon, as they yield higher concentration of the 5-ASA which is more effective than oral therapy.

For lesions extending to proximal colon oral therapy is required. Mesalamine compounds which release 5-ASA in the small bowel are preferred for treatment of CD.

Adverse effect

Sulfasalazine has the highest incidence of adverse effects due to systemic absorption of sulfapyridine. Nausea, vomiting and abdominal pain may respond to dose reduction. Rare hypersensitivity reactions include skin rash, fever, agranulocylosis, hepatotoxicity, and paradoxical exacerbation of colitis. Folic acid supplementation is recommended as sulfasalazine can impair folate absorption.

In contrast to sulfasalazine, other 5-ASA formulations are well tolerated. Rarely, renal impairment has been reported, particularly in association with high doses of mesalamine formulation.

5-ASA is safe during pregnancy.

Antibiotics

Metronidazole and **ciprofloxacin** are commonly used in mild to moderate CD. They are not indicated in UC where the role of bacteria has not been established. Their role should be limited to colonic to ileocolonic CD, perianal disease, fistulas, and abscesses. Major concern is peripheral neuropathy with long-term metronidazole.

Glucocorticoids

Budesomide is a synthetic corticosteroid with first pass liver metabolism that limits systemic toxicity while retaining high local efficacy similar to oral corticosteroids. It is effective and safe for short-term use in mild to moderate ileocolonic CD and can replace mesalamine in inducing remission. Efficacy has not been reported in UC. Topical therapy is useful in IBD limited to distal left colon. Ulcerative proctitis or UC limited to rectosigmoid can be treated effectively with 5–ASA and/or glucocorticoids enemas or suppositories along with systemic therapy in severe cases.

Glucocorticoids have no role in maintenance therapy.

Moderate to severe disease

The aim of therapy is to induce remission rapidly with corticosteroids, and to maintain remission with immunosuppressive agents and/or biologic agents as appropriate.

Glucocorticoids are anti-inflammatory and effective in inducing remissions, especially with flare-ups of disease activity. Extracolonic manifestations of IBD (ocular lesion, skin disease, and peripheral arthritis) also respond to glucocorticoids. Bisphosphonates are co-prescribed to prevent osteopenia.

Prednisone is usually given orally (40 to 60 mg qd) and continued until symptom improvement. Higher doses have not been shown to be more efficacious but have significantly greater adverse effects. The dose is gradually reduced. Glucocordicoids are not recommended for maintenance therapy.

Immunosuppressive agents

6-Mercaptopurine, a purine analog and **azathioprine** cause preferential suppression of T-cell activation and antigen recognition. They are useful in maintaining glucocorticoid-induced remission in both UC and CD. They have more favorable side effect profiles than glucocorticoids and are used as steroid-sparing agents in severe or refractory IBD. Side effects include flu-like syndrome, with myalgia, leucopenia and pancreatitis.

Methotrexate is effective as a steroid-sparing agent in CD but not in UC. Drug intolerance is seen in 10–18%. Nausea, stomatitis, diarrhea, hepatotoxicity, bone narrow suppression, pneumonitits, teratogenicity are possible adverse effects. Folic acid reduces the risk of adverse effects without impairing anti-inflammatory effects.

Antitumor necrosis factor alpha (anti-TNF-α) **monoclonal antibodies** suppress inflammation and induce apoptosis of inflammatory cells. **Infliximab, adalimumab** and **certolizumab pegol** are the available anti-TNF-α agents beneficial in moderately to severely acute CD refractory to other approaches including immunosuppressants both for induction and maintenance of remission. They are also effective in severe acute UC.

Anti-TNF-α therapy has been associated with acute anaphylactic reaction, reactivation of tuberculosis, increased risk of infection, malignancy and worsening of heart failure. They are contraindicated in the presence of infections.

Anti-integrin therapy

Integrins are a family of adhesion molecules on the surface of leukocytes which may cause circulating leukocytes to adhere to vascular endothelium and subsequently move through the vessel wall into the tissue.

Natalizumab is a humanized IgG_4 monoclonal antibody, which blocks integrins and thus prevents migrating circulating inflammatory (leukocytes) cells into surrounding tissues.

Natalizumab is only indicated in patients of CD who have failed to respond to other therapies including anti-TNF-α antibodies.

Netalizumab may induce reactivation of humanpolyomavirus (JC virus) causing progressive multifocal leukoencephalopathy (PML). Risk for PML can be minimized by avoiding concomitant immunosuppressive agents and close monitoring.

Severe or fulminant disease

Severe or fulminating IBD requires intensive therapy with IV corticosteroids and broad-spectrum antibiotics. In absence of response **cyclosporine** serves as 'rescue' therapy to prevent surgery in UC. It has no value in CD. Minor complications include tremor, paraesthesia, abnormal liver function test and hirsutism. Major side effects are nephrotoxicity, infections and neurotoxicity (including fits).

Tacrolimus is a macrolide antibiotic with immunomodulatory properties (both on cellular and humoral immune systems) similar to cyclosporine. It is 100 times as potent as cyclosporine. It is well absorbed even in absence of bile and highly effective in steroid-dependent or refractory IBD as well as refractory fistulizing CD.

Antidiarrheal agents (codeine phosphate, loperamide, lomotil) may be useful as an adjunct to therapy to reduce gut motility and small bowel secretions. Loperamide improves anal function. Antidiarrheal agents are contraindicated in severe exacerbations and megacolon.

6.5 DRUGS FOR IRRITABLE BOWEL SYNDROME

Irritable bowel syndrome (IBS) is a functional disorder characterized by abdominal pain or discomfort, and altered bowel habits.

Treatment is mainly symptomatic with reassurance and dietary alterations.

Stool-bulking agents

High-fiber diets and bulking agents, such as bran or hydrophilic colloid, are frequently used in treating IBS. The water-holding action of fibers may contribute to increase stool bulk because of the ability of fiber to increase fecal output of bacteria. The dietary fibers may have beneficial effect on colonic physiology symptoms alternating diarrhea and constipation, pain and bloating.

However, most studies observe no responses in patient with diarrhea or pain-predominant IBS. It is possible that different fiber preparations may have dissimilar effects on selected symptoms in IBS.

A cross over comparison of different fiber preparations found that **psyllium** produced greater improvements in stool pattern and abdominal pain than bran. Furthermore, psyllium preparations tend to produce less bloating and distension and most gastroenterologists, consider stool-bulking agents worth trying in IBS-constipation predominant patients.

Antispasmodics

Anticholinergic drugs may provide temporary relief of symptoms such as painful cramps related to intestinal spasm. Physiologic studies demonstrate that anticholinergic drugs inhibit the gastrocolic reflex; hence, post prandial is best managed by giving antispasmodics 30 minutes before meals. Synthetic anticholinergics such as **dicyclomine** have less effect on mucous membrane secretions and produce fewer undesirable atropine like symptoms.

Antidiarrheal agents

Peripherally acting opiate-based agents are the initial therapy of choice for IBS-diarrhea predominant patients. Physiologic studies demonstrate increase in segmenting colonic contractions, delay in fecal transit, increase in anal pressures, and reductions in rectal perception with these drugs. Small doses of **loperamide** 2–4 mg every 4–6 h up to a maximum of 12 g/d can be prescribed. High dose of loperamide may cause cramping and may require another anti-diarrheal agent – bile acid binder cholestyramine resin.

Antidepressant drugs

Antidepressant medications have several physiologic effects that may be beneficial in IBS. In IBS-diarrhea predominant patients, the tricyclic antidepressant imipramine slows jejunal migrating motor complex transit propagation and delays orocecal and whole – gut transit, indicative of a motor inhibitory effect. Some studies also suggest that tricyclic agents may alter visceral afferent neural function.

The beneficial effects of tricyclic compounds appear to be independent of their effects on depression. The therapeutic benefits for the bowel symptoms occur faster and at a lower dosage. In contrast to tricyclic agents, **paroxetine** (SSRI) accelerates orocecal transit raising the possibility that this drug class may be useful in IBS-constipation predominant patients. The SSRI citalopram blunts perception of rectal distension and reduces the magnitude of the gastrocolic response. However, the efficacy of SSRIs in the treatment requires further studies for benefit confirmation.

Antiflatulence therapy

The management of excessive gas is seldom satisfactory, except when there is obvious aerophagia or disaccharidase deficiency. Avoiding flatogenic foods, exercising, losing excess weight, and taking activated charcoal are safe but unproven remedies. Pancreatic enzymes reduce bloating, gas, and fullness during and after high-caloric, high-fat meal ingestion.

Modulation of gut flora

Antibiotics have been found to benefit a subset of IBS patients. **Neomycin** 500 mg twice daily for 10 days is beneficial. Another non-absorbed oral antibiotic rifaximin at a dose of 400 mg three times daily was the only antibiotic that causes substantial, sustained benefit beyond therapy cessation in IBS patients. The drug has a favorable safety and tolerability profile compared with systemic antibiotic. However, currently there is still insufficient data to recommend routine use of this antibiotic in the treatment of IBS. Since altered colonic flora may contribute to the pathogenesis of IBS, use of **probiotics** is recommended to naturally alter the flora. **Bifidobactericum infantis** 35624 showed significant improvement in the composite score for abdominal pain, bloating/distension, and/ or bowel movement.

Serotonin receptor agonist and antagonists

Alosetron, a 5-HT_3 receptors antagonist reduces the perception of painful visceral stimulation in IBS. It also induces rectal relaxation, increases rectal compliance and delays colonic transit. Alosetron and or cilansetron (5-HT_3 antagonists) have been found more effective than placebo in achieving global improvement in IBS symptoms and relief of abdominal pain and discomfort.

A novel 5-HT_4 receptor agonist, such **tegaserod**, exhibit prokinetic activity by stimulating peristalsis. However, tegaserod has been withdrawn due to an increase in serious cardiovascular events.

Chloride channel activators

Lubiprostone is a bicyclic fatty acid which stimulates chloride channels in the apical membrane of intestinal epithelial cells. Chloride secretion induces passive movement of sodium and water into the bowel lumen and improves bowel function. Oral lubiprostone was effective in patients with constipation-predominant IBS in clinical trials. The major side effects are nausea and diarrhea.

Lubiprostone is a new class of compound for treatment of chronic constipation with or without IBS.

Irritable bowel symptoms require more of education, reassurance, and dietary/lifestyle changes. Drugs are only indicated for the treatment of moderate symptoms.

6.6 PURGATIVES

These are the drugs, which loosen the bowel and cause its evacuation. Purgatives, as a rule are not the treatment for constipation. The use of purgatives can only be justified in select conditions such as drug induced constipation, after anthelmintic treatment for the expulsion of parasites, hemorrhoids or severe life threatening condition, where straining increases the risk of rectal bleeding or exacerbation of the underlying illness (e.g. myocardial or cerebral ischemia), before surgery or radiological procedures to clear the bowel.

There are large numbers of purgatives, which may be classified as follows:

- Bulk purgatives : Bran, psyllium methylcellulose, ispaghula and sterculia
- Fecal softeners : Docusate sodium and liquid paraffin.
- Stimulant purgatives : Anthracenes and bisacodyl.
- Osmotic purgatives : Magnesium sulphate and lactulose.
- Chloride channel activator : Lubiprostone

- Opioid receptor antagonists : Alvimopan and methylnaltrexone
- 5-HT$_4$-receptor agonists : Cisapride

BULK PURGATIVES

These act by increasing fecal mass, which stimulates peristalsis. They are useful in the management of patients with colostomy, ileostomy, hemorrhoids, and fissures, chronic diarrhea associated with diverticular disease, irritable bowel syndrome and as adjuncts in ulcerative colitis.

Side effects of bulk purgatives include flatulence, distension, intestinal obstruction or fecal impaction and hypersensitivity reactions.

Bulk purgatives are contraindicated in intestinal obstruction, colonic atony and fecal impaction.

FECAL SOFTENERS

Docusate sodium acts both by softening the stools and stimulating the colon. It is indicated in painful conditions such as piles or anal fissures to relieve constipation and prior to radiological procedures.

Liquid paraffin is rarely used because it may cause anal seepage, lipoid pneumonia (if inhaled), and interference with the absorption of fat soluble vitamins.

STIMULANT PURGATIVES
Anthracenes

This group contains **cascara**, **senna**, **rhubarb** and **aloes**, which contain the anthraquinone glycoside, emodin. In the intestines, emodin is released, which gets absorbed into the blood-stream and acts on the large intestine, causing increased peristalsis. They take about 6–12 hours to act and are best given at bedtime. Senna is the only anthracene purgative used since other members of the anthraquinone group are powerful stimulants and may cause intestinal cramps. They should be avoided during pregnancy.

Bisacodyl (Dulcolax)

Bisacodyl stimulates the colon and takes about 10–12 hours to act. It can be taken orally in the form of tablets in the night or given as rectal suppositories in the morning for constipation and before radiological procedures and surgery. Side effects are minimal and include griping (tablets) or local irritation (suppositories).

Co-danthramer

It is a mixture of a fecal softener and a stimulant purgative (dantron). Because of its teratogenic effect in animals, it is only used in elderly patients with obstinate constipation or those whose constipation is due to opioid analsesics (e.g. terminally ill patients).

Colocynth, jalap and **castor oil** are other stimulant purgatives, which have a drastic purgative action. **Phenolphthalein** can cause rashes. They are no longer used.

OSMOTIC PURGATIVES

These act by retaining fluid in the bowel or by changing the pattern of water distribution in the feces. **Magnesium sulphate (Epson salt)** is the most commonly used saline purgative and is useful where rapid bowel evacuation is required. It is effective usually within 1–2 hours.

Lactulose is a semisynthetic disaccharide, which is not absorbed from the GIT. It is broken down in the large bowel with the production of various acids. It causes purgation by acting as osmotic purgative and as mild irritant. It prevents the proliferation of ammonia producing organisms and is useful in hepatic encephalopathy.

Polyethylene glycol (PEG) is an inert, unabsorbable, osmotically active sugar. Large balanced isotonic solution of PEG is commonly used as a bowel–cleansing agent before colonoscopy. The solution is designed with sodium sulfate, sodium chloride, sodium bicarbonate and potassium chloride so that no significant intravascular fluid or electrolyte shift occurs.

CHLORIDE CHANNEL ACTIVATOR

Lubiprostone acts by stimulating the type 2 chloride channel (CLC 2) in the small intestine and is used for chronic constipation and irritable bowel syndrome. It increases chloride-rich fluid into the intestine which stimulates intestinal motility.

Lubiprostone may cause nausea due to delayed gastric emptying and is generally avoided in pregnancy.

OPIOID RECEPTOR ANTAGONISTS

Alvimopan and **methylnaltrexone** block intestinal opioid receptors and are useful in preventing opioid – induced constipation in chronic opioid users (page 73).

SEROTONIN 5-HT$_4$ – RECEPTOR AGONISTS

Stimulation of 5-HT$_4$ receptors release neurotransmitters (acetylcholine, substance P, nitric acid and vasoactive intestinal peptide) which promote the peristaltic reflex.

Tegaserod, a 5-HT$_4$ partial agonist, has been withdrawn because of increased incidence of serious cardiovascular events.

Cisapride, another 5-HT$_4$ agonist causes QTc prolongation, which also leads to adverse cardiac toxicity.

Prucalopride, a highly potent 5-HT$_4$ agonist, does not appear to cause adverse cardiac effects and may prove to be a useful drug for treatment of chronic constipation.

Adverse effects of purgatives

The indiscriminate and chronic use of purgatives may be dangerous and can lead to:

- Loss of fluids and electrolytes
- Abdominal pain, rupture of an acutely inflamed appendix
- Damage to bowel
- Onset of labour pains
- Lipoid pneumonia with liquid paraffin
- Purgative habit

Purgatives should never be given to patients with undiagnosed abdominal pain.

6.7 INTESTINAL SEDATIVES

Several drugs may diminish the peristaltic activity of the intestine and are used in the spasm of colon and for symptomatic relief of diarrhea.

Anticholinergic drugs block the activity of parasympathetic system and are useful particularly in colon spasm.

Opioids reduce peristalsis and are use for symptomatic therapy in simple self-limiting GI infections in which diarrhea is frequent or troublesome inspite of the specific treatment or when a specific etiology is not identified. The most widely used is codeine phosphate.

Lomotil is a combination of atropine (anticholinrgic) and diphenoxylate (opioid) and **loperamide** (opioid) are the most effective non-specific antidiarrheal agents.

Pectin and **kaolin** preparations (bind toxins) and **bismuth subsalicylate** (antibacterial properties) is also useful in symptomatic treatment of acute diarrhea.

Bile acid - binding resins (e.g., **cholestyramine**) are useful in bile acid induced diarrhea.

Octreotide, a synthetic octapeptide with actions similar to somatostatin (a growth hormone antagonist) is useful in hormone-mediated secretory diarrhea, and can be of benefit in refractory diarrhea.

7

Respiratory System

7.1 COUGH PREPARATIONS

EXPECTORANTS

Expectorants are drugs that promote expulsion of bronchial secretions. The bronchial glands are supplied by vagus nerve and when nausea or vomiting occurs there is widespread vagal activity and a considerable increase in bronchial and salivary secretion. The assumption that mixtures containing sub-emetic doses of drugs like ammonium chloride, ipecacuanha, guaiphenesin and squill facilitate expectoration is incorrect, though they may serve a placebo effect.

Steam inhalation containing benzoin tincture, menthol or eucalyptus and mucolytic drugs by reducing sputum viscosity serves as very useful expectorants in chronic lung infections, though the antibiotics have declined their use.

MUCOLYTICS

Bromhexine, carbocisteine and **mecysteine** reduce sputum viscosity. They are taken orally 3 to 4 times daily and may be very effective expectorants in chronic asthma, bronchitis, and bronchiectasis in cleaning of the air passages. These drugs may cause occasional GIT irritation and rashes and are contraindicated in active peptic ulceration.

COUGH SUPPRESSANTS

Suppression of cough may be useful where there is no identifiable cause and the cough is unproductive, is tiring to the patient and disturbs the sleep. However, undue suppression of cough may cause sputum retention and this may be harmful in patients with chronic bronchitis and bronchiectasis.

DEMULCENTS

Cough arising from irritation of the upper respiratory tract are helped by demulcents. Demulcent cough preparations contain soothing substance such as glycerol, **diphenhydramine** (benadryl) or **brompheniramine** (antihistaminic) and menthol in the form of a syrup. The benefit from such preparations is from the sedative action of antihistamine and the soothing effect of the syrup.

ANTITUSSIVES

These are opioids that depress the cough center. **Codeine** depresses the cough centre. It can cause constipation and drug dependence. **Pholcodeine** has practically no analgesic or addicting property, and has fewer side effects and is as effective as codeine as an antitussive. Opioids are generally used in the form of linctus (oral solution 5–10 ml 3–4 times daily, 5 ml contain 15 mg of codeine phosphate or 5 mg of pholocodeine).

Dextromethorphan is a selective nonopioid antitussive with no narcotic, analgesic or addicting actions.

7.2 DRUGS FOR BRONCHIAL ASTHMA

Asthma is believed to be an autoimmune disease. The relationship between atopy (a propensity to produce IgE) and asthma is well established. Allergens cause synthesis of antibody IgE.

Bronchial asthma is a chronic disease, with episodic exacerbations that are interspersed with symptom free periods. The characteristic symptoms of an acute attack consist of dyspnoea, chest tightening and wheezing.

Possible factors for asthma development and its persistence include hypersensitive response of bronchial muscles to multiple environment factors, allergens, infection, and drugs.

Immunopathogenesis of asthma consist of synthesis of IgE antibody, due to exposure to allergen, which binds to mast cells in the airway mucosa. On re-exposure to allergens, antigen-antibody interaction on mast cell surfaces triggers release of mediators of anaphylaxis (histamine, tryptase, PGD_2, LTC_4 and PAF) which results in bronchoconstriction. Cytokines produced by T cells activate eosinophils and neutrophils which produce mediators that cause edema, mucus hypersecretion, and narrowing of the bronchial airways predisposing to episodes of acute attacks.

The treatment of bronchial asthma involves chronic management: use of an inflammatory disease modifying medication (long-term control medications) and as needed use of a short-acting bronchodilator (quick-relief medications).

Most of the antiasthmatic drugs can be given by a variety of inhaled devices and choice depends on patient preference and competence in using the device. The metered-dose inhaler (MDI) remains the most widely prescribed, because of the use of minimum doses and avoidance of systemic toxicity (Fig. 7.1). MDI reduces the deposition of the drug in oropharynx and increases the delivery of the drug to the lungs. The patients should be well versed in the use of MDI.

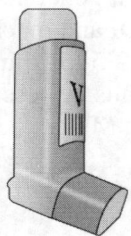

Fig. 7.1: How to use a metered-dose inhaler

- Remove the cap and shake the inhaler
- Breathe out gently and place the mouthpiece into the mouth
- Incline the head backwards to minimize oropharyngeal deposition
- Simultaneously, begin a slow deep inspiration, depress the inhaler plunger to release the drug and continue to inhale.
- Hold the breath for 10 seconds.

The main drugs for asthma can be divided into bronchodilators, which give rapid relief of symptoms mainly through relaxation of bronchial muscle, and controllers which inhibit the underlying inflammatory process.

Bronchodilators (relievers)—selective β_2 adrenoceptor stimulants, antimuscarinics and methylxanthines.

Drugs that prevent or suppress inflammation (controllers) – Corticosteroids, sodium cromoglicate, nedocromil and leukotriene receptor antagonist.

Antiasthmatic treatment essentially consists of regular prophylactic treatment with anti-inflammatory drugs, while bronchodilators (e.g. β_2 agonists) are used only to relieve an acute attack of bronchial asthma.

BRONCHODILATOR THERAPIES

Selective β_2 Agonists

Salbutamol (albuterol), terbutaline, pirbuterol and **metaproterenol** are short acting (peak action within 15–30 minutes which persists for 3–4 hours) available as MDI. They can also be given by hand-held nebulizer. The particles generated by a nebulizer are much larger than those from a MDI and much higher doses are required than those from a MDI (2.5–5.0 mg versus 100–400 mcg). Nebulizer therapy should thus be reserved for patients unable to coordinate inhalators form a MDI.

Mechanism of action

β_2-agonists stimulate β-adrenergic receptors in the bronchial muscle resulting in increased intracellular cyclic adenosine monophosphate (AMP), which relaxes smooth muscles cells of all airways and inhibits certain inflammatory cells, particularly mast cells.

The primary action of β_2-agonists is to relax bronchial smooth muscle, where they act as functional antagonists, reversing and preventing contraction of bronchial muscle by *all known bronchoconstrictors*.

β_2-agonists also have following nonbronchodilator effects that contribute to their efficacy in asthma.

- Inhibition of the release of bronchoconstricing mediators from the mast cells
- Inhibition of microvascular leakage and airway edema
- Increase mucocilliary transport by increasing ciliary activity
- Increased mucus secretion
- Decreased cough

β_2-agonists, in contrast to corticosteroids, have no effect on chronic inflammation.

Therapeutic uses

Short-acting β_2-agonists (SABAs) have a rapid onset of bronchodilation and are, therefore, used as needed for symptom relief. Increased use of SABAs indicates that asthma is not being controlled. They are also useful in preventing exercise induced asthma, if taken prior to exercise. SABAs are used in high doses by nebulizer or via a metered-dose inhaler with a spacer.

Terbutaline is the only β_2-agonists available for subcutaneous injection (0.25 mg) and has the same indication as that of adrenaline, i.e., severe asthma requiring emergency treatment when aerosolized therapy is not available or has been ineffective.

Long-acting β_2-agonists (LABAs) include **salmeterol** and **formoterol**, both of which have duration of action over 12 hours due to their high lipid solubility which dissolves in the smooth cell membrane and acts as a depot. They are given twice daily by inhalation. LABAs have replaced the regular use of SABAs, but LABAs should not be given in the absence of inhaled corticosteroids (ICS) therapy as they do not control the underlying inflammation. They do, however, improve asthma control and reduce exacerbations when added to ICS, which allows asthma to be controlled at lower doses of corticosteroids. This has led to the widespread use of fixed combination inhalers (Fig. 7.1) that contain a corticosteroid and a LABA, which have proved to be highly effective in the control of asthma.

Adverse effects

Adverse effects are not usually a problem with β_2-agonists when given by inhalation. The most common side effects are CNS and CVS symptoms like fine tremors, nervous tension, headache, and palpitations, which are seen more commonly in elderly patients. Adverse cardiac arrhythmic effect of B_2-agonists is unsubstantiated. Contrarily, irregularities in cardiac rhythm may improve with the improvements in gas exchange affected by bronchodilator action and oxygen administration,in patients presenting for emergency treatment of severe asthma.

β_2 stimulants can lead to hypokalemia particularly with concomitant treatment with theophylline, corticosteroids and diuretics or by hypoxia and requires monitoring of plasma potassium concentration in severe asthma.

Hypersensitivity reactions including paradoxical bronchospasm, urticaria and angioedema have been reported.

Tolerance

The chronic use of β_2-agonists does not reduce the bronchodilator response. Though there is down-regulation of β-receptors with chronic use, but this does not reduce the bronchodilator response as there is a large receptor reserve in bronchial muscle. By contrast, mast cells become rapidly tolerant, but their tolerance may be prevented by concomitant administration of ICS.

Safety

There is an association between asthma mortality and the amount of SABA used, but it is in fact poor asthma control, which is a risk factor for asthma death.

Mortality with use of LABA is related to the lack of use of concomitant ICS as the LABA therapy fails to suppress the underlying inflammation. This highlights the importance of always using an ICS when LABAs are given, which is most conveniently achieved by using a combination inhaler.

Antimuscarinics

Ipratropium is related to atropine and prevents cholinergic nerve-induced bronchoconstriction and mucus secretion. They are much less effective than β_2-agonists in asthma therapy as they inhibit only the cholinergic reflex component of bronchoconstriction, whereas β_2-agonists prevent all bronchoconstrictor mechanisms. Antimuscarinics are, therefore only used as an additional bronchodilator in patients with asthma that is not controlled by other inhaled medications.

Ipratropium may be given by nebulizer in treating acute severe asthma but should only be given following β_2-agonists, as it has a slower onset of bronchodilation.

Side effects are infrequent as there is little or no systemic absorption. The most common side effect is dry mouth and rarely urinary retention, constipation and glaucoma in elderly patients.

Methylxanthines

Theophylline, **theobromine** and **caffeine** are the naturally occurring methylated xanthine alkaloids. Caffeine is the constituent of coffee and tea and theobromine that of cocoa. Theophylline is only used in therapeutics as a bronchodilator in bronchial asthma.

Pharmacological actions

Theophylline inhibits the enzyme phosphodiesterase and blocks adenosine receptors in CNS, CVS, and smooth muscles that account for its bronchodilator and other (adverse) actions in asthma.

Theophylline stimulates the CNS (especially the higher centers), the heart-rate and force of contraction and secretions of acid and pepsin in the stomach. It relaxes the smooth muscles, which is most prominent on bronchi, especially in asthmatics. It has a mild diuretic action.

Theophylline in lower doses has anti-inflammatory effects, which is mediated by activating the key nuclear enzyme histone deacetylase-2, which is a critical mechanism for switching off activated inflammatory genes.

Pharmacokinetics

Theophylline has a narrow therapeutic index (small difference between the therapeutic and toxic dose) with substantial variation in metabolism, which makes it a difficult drug to use without monitoring its clinical response and blood concentration.

Theophylline is metabolized in the liver, which is dependent on a number of factors. The metabolism of theophylline is decreased with resultant high blood levels in heart failure, cirrhosis, viral infection, in the elderly, and by drugs such as cimetidine, ciprofloxacin, erythromycin, and oral contraceptives. The metabolism of theophylline is increased with resultant low blood levels in smokers and in chronic alcoholism, and by drugs such as phenytoin, carbamazepine, barbiturates and rifampicin.

The plasma clearance of theophylline varies widely. It is metabolized in the liver so the therapeutic dose in patients with liver disease may lead to toxic plasma concentration of the drug. Conversely, a number of factors may increase its clearance (Fig. 7.2).

Therapeutic uses

Sustained release **theophylline** preparations and ultrasustained release theophylline, **uniphyllin** once or twice daily gives stable plasma concentrations.

Theophylline may be used as an additional bronchodilator in patients with severe asthma when plasma concentrations of 10–20 mg/L are required, although these concentrations are often associated with side effects. Theophylline should be used only where methods to measure theophylline blood levels are available to exclude theophylline toxicity.

Low doses of theophylline, giving plasma concentrations of 5–10 mg/L, have additive effects to ICS and are particularly useful in patients with severe asthma. Indeed, withdrawal of theophylline from these patients may result in marked deterioration in asthma control. At low doses, the drug is well tolerated.

Aminophylline, a mixture of htheophylline with ethylenediamine, was used by very slow intravenous injection for the treatment of acute severe asthma but has been largely replaced by high doses of

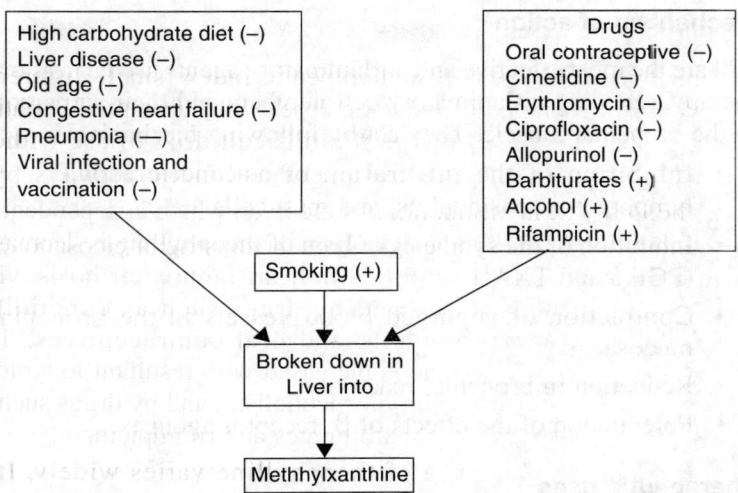

+ : (low blood levels) increased clearance; − : (high blood levels) decreased clearance

Fig. 7.2: Factors affecting the blood level and activity of methylxanthines.

inhaled SABAs, which are more effective and have fewer side effects. Aminophylline is occasionally used in patients with severe exacerbations that are refractory to SABAs.

Adverse effects

Side effects are related to plasma concentrations. The most common side effects are nausea, vomiting, and headaches and are due to phosphodiesterase inhibition. Diuresis and palpitations may also occur, and at high concentrations cardiac arrhythmias, epileptic seizures, and death may occur due to adenosine A_1-receptros antagonism. Theophylline side effects are related to plasma concentration and are rarely observed at plasma concentrations below 10 mg/L.

CONTROLLER THERAPIES

Corticosteroids

Inhaled Corticosteroids (ICS) are by far the most effective controllers for asthma, and their early use has revolutionized asthma therapy.

Mechanism of action

ICS are the most effective anti-inflammatory agents used in asthma therapy, reducing inflammatory cell numbers and their activation in the bronchial muscle. They act by following mechanisms:
- Inhibition of the infiltration of asthmatic airways by lymphocytes, eosinophils, and mast cells.
- Inhibition of the synthesis of bronchoconstrictor eicosanoids (PGF_2a and TXA_2)
- Contraction of engorged blood vessels in the bronchial mucosa.
- Reduction in bronchial reactivity.
- Potentiation of the effects of β_2 receptor agonists.

Therapeutic uses

ICS are by far the most effective controllers in the management of asthma (Table 7.1) and are beneficial in treating asthma of any severity and age. ICS rapidly improve the symptoms of asthma, and lung function improves over several days. They are effective in preventing asthma symptoms as well as severe exacerbations. Early treatment with ICS prevents irreversible changes in bronchial muscle that occur with chronic asthma, but do not cure the underlying condition. ICS are now given as first-line therapy with persistent asthma, but if they do not control symptoms at low doses, it is usual to add a LABA as the next step.

Adverse effects

Local side effects include hoarseness (dysphonia) and oral candidiasis. ICS have minimal systemic effects with moderate doses. At the highest recommended doses ICS may cause adrenal suppression, but there is no convincing evidence that long-term treatment leads to impaired growth in children or to osteoporosis in adults.

Systemic corticosteroids

Oral corticosteroids (OCS) are as effective as by intravenous route for the treatment of acute severe asthma. Prednisone (30–45 mg

Table 7.1: Comparative daily adult dosage for inhaled corticosteroids

Drug	Low dose	Medium dose	High dose
Triamcinolone 75 µg/puff	4–10 puffs	10–20 puffs	puffs >20 puffs
Beclomethasone 80 µg/puffs	2–6 puffs	6–8 puffs	>10 puffs
Budesonide aerosol powder (Turbuhaler) 160 µg/puff	1–2 puffs	2–3 puffs	>3 puffs
Inhalation suspension (Repules) 0.25, 0.5 mg/2 ml	1–2 repsules	2–4 repsules	>4 respsules
Flunisolide 80 µg, 250 µg/puffs	2–4 puffs	4–8 puffs	>8 puffs
Fluticasone 44, 110 and 220 µg/puff	2 puffs	3 puffs	>3 puffs
Mometasone 250 µg/puffs	1 puffs	2 puffs	3–4 puffs
Combination agent			
Budesonide/formeterol (MDI: 80/4.5, 160/4.5 µg/puff)	1–2 puffs bid: 80/4.5 µg/puff	2 puffs bid: 80/4.5 to 160/4.5 µg/puff	2 puff bid: 160/4.5 µg/puff
Fluticasone/salmeterol 100, 250, 500, mcg fluticasone + 50 mcg salmeterol	1 inhalation 100 mcg	1 inhalations 250 mcg	Inhalation 500 mcg

MID: metered-dose inhaler, bid, twice daily

once daily for 5–10 days) is used to treat acute exacerbations of asthma; no tapering of the dose is needed. About 1% of asthma patients may require maintenance treatment with the lowest OCS dose necessary to control the disease. Systemic side effects such as truncal obesity, bruising osteoporosis, diabetes, hypertension, gastric ulceration, proximal myopathy, depression, and cataracts are a possibility.

Cromolyn and nedocromil

Cromolyn and Nedocromil differ structurally but have same mechanism of action.

These drugs have no direct action on bronchial muscle. They inhibit both antigen and exercise-induced asthma and are of value when taken prophylactically. Their action appears to inhibit the activation of inflammatory cells (mast cells, eosinophils) by environmental allergens, and bronchoconstrictor eicosanoid synthesis.

Cromolyn and nedocromil are mainly indicated in seasonal or occupational related asthma, but they are much less effective than even a low dose of inhaled corticosteroids.

Cromolyn sodium (200 mcg/puff) for aerosol and 20 mg/2 ml for nebulization is used for the prophylaxis of asthma.

Cromolyn and nedocromil solutions are also useful in reducing symptoms of allergic rhinoconjunctivitis. Applying 2% solution by nasal spray for hay fever or eye drops several times a day is effective in about 75% of patients.

Adverse effects are usually minor and localized to site of application because of their poor solubility. Very rarely cares of pulmonary infiltration with eosinophils and anaphylaxis have been reported.

These drugs have relatively little benefit in the long-term control of asthma due to their short duration of action (at least four times daily by inhalation). They are safe and were popular in the treatment of childhood asthma; although now low doses of ICS are preferred as they are more effective and have a proven safety profile.

Leukotriene antagonists

Leukotrienes exert much effect that occur asthma like bronchoconstriction, bronchial hyperactivity, mucosal edema and mucus secretions.

Leukotrienes are formed by the action of 5-lipoxygenase on arachodonic acid and also synthesized by a variety of inflammatory cells in the airways including eosinophils, mast cells, macrophages and basophils.

Leukotriene D4 (LTD4) is a potent bonchoconstrictor and is recognized as the primary component of the slow-reacting substance of anaphylaxis (SRS-A) that is secreted in asthma and anaphylaxis.

Zileuton inhibits 5-lipoxygenase preventing synthesis of LTD4. Zafirlukast and montelukast are LTD4 receptor antagonist. They all improve asthma control and reduce the frequency of asthma exacerbation. Like cromolyn and nedocromil, they have only prophylactic valve, being much less effective than inhaled corticosteroids. Their main advantage lies in their oral administration, especially in children who comply poorly with inhaled therapy.

Montelukast, is most commonly used especially in children for the prophylaxis of asthma.

Leukotriene receptor antagonists are free from serious toxicities and montleukast (10 mg) is the most commonly used for the prophylaxis of asthma.

Montelukast should be strongly considered for patients with aspirin-induced asthma or for individuals who cannot master the use of an inhaler.

(Addition of omalizumab has been shown to reduce exacerbation rates and need for corticosteroids).

Anti-IgE monoclonal antibodies

IgE antibody plays a crucial role in the immunopathogenesis of asthma. It has been possible to raise antibodies against IgE antibody itself, which binds to IgE receptors (FC_E-RI and FC_E-R2 receptors) on mast cells and other inflammatory cells and thus prevents the binding of natural IgE produced by B lymphocytes.

Omalizumab is monoclonal antibody raised against IgE antibody itself that has been genetically humanized by replacing all but a small fraction of its amino acids with those found in human proteins.

Given by twice-weekly subcutaneous injections, omalizumab has been found to reduce the frequency and severity of asthma exacerbation, reduction in corticosteroid requirements. High costs restrict the treatment in selected individuals with severe disease characterized by frequent exacerbations.

Anaphylaxis occurs in 1 to 2 per 1000 usually within 2 hours of the first dose. Patients on omalizumab should be medically observed 2 hours after initial dose and then 30 minutes for subsequent dosing and should be equipped with a self-administered adrenalin.

8

Endocrine System

8.1 INSULIN AND ORAL ANTIDIABETIC DRUGS

Insulin is a protein hormone produced by the beta cells of the islets of Langerhans of the pancreas gland. It plays a key role in the regulation of carbohydrate, fat and protein metabolism. Lack of insulin or resistance to its action causes diabetes mellitus. There are two types of diabetes:

Type 1 Diabetes

This is known as **insulin-dependent diabetes mellitus (IDDM)** in which there is no circulating insulin in the plasma due to autoimmune destruction of pancreatic beta cells. Insulin deficiency leads to a rapid rise in the blood glucose concentration with subsequent loss of glucose with water and salt in the urine. Fats in the body are broken down releasing ketone bodies in blood, which cause acidosis. Protein breakdown releases amino acids in the blood, which are converted to pyruvate, glucose, and urea in the liver. The excess urea produced is excreted in urine resulting in negative nitrogen balance and weight loss may be marked. If not treated with insulin, patient will lapse into coma (hyperglycemic ketoacidosis).

Type 2 Diabetes

This is known as **non-insulin dependent diabetes mellitus (NIDDM)**, which is due to reduced secretion of insulin or due to peripheral resistance to the action of insulin. The blood glucose concentration is raised with glycosuria, but ketoacidosis is not common and the symptoms are often those of late complications of diabetes. These complications occur with both type of diabetes and are due to microvascular diseases including myocardial infarction, retinopathy, renal failure, and serious interference with the circulation to the legs sometimes requiring amputation and neuropathy.

Type 2 diabetes may be controlled on diet alone, but many require administration of oral antidiabetic drugs or insulin to maintain optimal glycaemic control.

INSULIN

Insulin lowers the concentration of glucose in the blood mainly by:
- Facilitating glucose transport across cell membrane resulting in increased uptake of glucose by the tissues.
- Facilitating glycogen synthesis from glucose in liver muscles and fat.
- Inhibiting gluconeogenesis (from protein) in liver and lipolysis in adipose tissue with increased production of fat and protein.

Sources of insulin

There are three sources of insulin, bovine, porcine and human. Bovine insulin extracted from beef pancreas is immunogenic and is rarely used.

Porcine insulin extracted from pork pancreas is very similar to human insulin.

Non-human insulin can stimulate the production of anti-insulin antibodies (AIA), which occasionally give rise to local and systemic allergic reactions, but immunological resistance to insulin action is uncommon

Human insulin is prepared semisynthetically by enzymatic modification of porcine insulin or biosynthetically by recombinant DNA technology using *Escherichia coli*. Virtually all insulin now used is human insulin.

Mechanism of action

Insulin interacts with a highly specific receptor located on the cell membrane of practically all cells, particularly liver and fat cells.

Glucose is transported from the blood into the cells across the cell membranes by so called glucose transporters, and insulin increases the activity of the glucose transporters.

Pharmacokinetics

Insulin is inactivated by GIT enzymes and must therefore be given by injection. The subcutaneous route is ideal for self-administration. A different site should be used each time to minimize fat hypertrophy. Liver and kidney are of primary importance in the degradation of insulin by a proteolytic enzyme.

Insulin administration

Insulin syringes

Most diabetic patients use disposable plastic insulin syringe available in 0.5 ml (up to 50 units) and 1 ml (up to 100 units) sizes for subcutaneous injection.

Pen devices

Insulin pen devices contain a cartridge of insulin that is automatically injected. Wide ranges of insulin are available in cartridges and are more convenient for the patient.

Jet injection

Jet Injection is high-pressure devices that eject insulin through a fine nozzle without a needle being used. Jet injections have not become popular because of delayed pain, greater bleeding and possibility of increased immunogenicity.

Syringe pumps

For intensive insulin requirements, soluble insulin can be given by subcutaneous infusion using a syringe pump. The rate of infusion can be modified to the patient's needs and produce an accurate control of the diabetes. However, this technique has a limited place since it requires regular monitoring of blood glucose by patients themselves with an access to expert advice at all times.

Insulin preparations

Insulin preparations are produced by recombinant DNA technology and are classified into short-acting and long-acting preparations (Table 8.1).

Table 8.1: Bioavailability characteristics of the insulin

Preparation	Onset of action	Peak action	Effective duration
Short-acting			
Aspart	5–10 minutes	1–1.5 hours	3–4 hours
Glulisine	5–10 minutes	1–1.5 hours	3–4 hours
Lispro	5–10 minutes	1–1.5 hours	3–4 hours
Regular	30–60 minutes	2 hours	6–8 hours
Long-acting			
Human NPH	2–4 hours	6–7 hours	10–20 hours
Insulin glargine	1.5 hours	Flat	24 hours
Insulin detemir	1 hour	Flat	17 hours
Insulin combination			
75% protamine lispro, 25% lispro	15 minutes	1.5 hours	10–16 hours
70% protamine aspart, 30% aspart	15 minutes	1.5 hours	10–16 hours
50% protamine lispro, 50% lispro	15 minutes	1.5 hours	10–16 hours
70% NPH, 30% regular	30–60 minutes	Dual*	10–16 hours

* Dual: two peaks—one at 2–3 hours and second one several hours later.

Short-acting insulin preparations

The short-acting preparations are regular insulin and rapidly acting insulin analogs. These are clear solutions at neutral pH and contain small amounts of zinc to improve their stability and shelf life.

The rapidly acting insulin has the advantage for allowing entrainment of insulin injection and action to rising plasma glucose levels following meals. The shorter duration of action also appears to be associated with a decreased number of hypoglycemic episodes, primarily because the decay of insulin action corresponds to the decline in plasma glucose after a meal.

Thus, insulin aspart, lispro, or glargine is preferred over regular insulin for prandial coverage.

The other advantages of rapidly acting insulin analogs are:

- Rapid onset of action permits the diabetic patient to take meals (within 20 minutes), without waiting as long as 60 minutes after regular insulin.
- The duration of action remains constant –4 hours irrespective of dosage, in contrast to regular insulin where duration of action is prolonged with larger doses.
- Commonly used in pumps because of improved post-prandial glucose control compared to regular insulin.

Regular insulin is soluble crystalline zinc insulin, which is particularly useful by intravenous infusion in the treatment of diabetic ketoacidosis and during the preoperative management of insulin-requiring diabetes. Regular insulin is indicated when the subcutaneous insulin requirement is changing rapidly, such as after surgery or during acute infections – although the rapidly acting insulin analogs may be preferable in these situations.

Long acting insulin preparations

NPH (neutral protamine Hagedorn or isophane) insulin – NPH is intermediate – acting insulin whose onset of action is delayed by combining 2 parts soluble crystalline zinc insulin with 1 part of protamine zinc insulin. This produces equivalent amounts of insulin and protamine so that neither is present in an uncomplexed form ("isophane"). Most patients require at least two injections daily to maintain a sustained insulin effect.

The disadvantage of NPH insulin is considerable loss of bioactivity if not refrigerated and/or not used within 1 month.

Insulin glargine

Insulin glargine is clear insulin which forms microprecipitates in the subcutaneous tissues, that slowly releases insulin into the circulation. It cannot be mixed with the other human insulin because of its acidic pH.

Insulin glargine has the advantage of single injection, whose action lasts for about 24 hours without any pronounced peaks to provide basal coverage. Moreover, as compared to NPH, it controls fasting hyperglycemia better, with less nocturnal hypoglycemia, if given as a single injection at bedtime.

The possible association between insulin glargine and increased cancer risk is being investigated and is controversial.

It is not recommended during pregnancy.

Insulin detemir

Insulin detemir has a fatty acid side chain (more lipophilic than native insulin) that prolongs its action by slowing absorption and catabolism. Twice daily injections are required to provide 24 hours coverage.

Mixing of short-acting insulin analogs with NPH is unstable as this combination may alter the insulin absorption profile. For example, lispro absorption is delayed by mixing with NPH.

In an attempt to remedy this, an intermediate insulin composed of isophane complexes of protamine with insulin lispro was developed called NPL (neutral protamine lispro). This insulin has same duration of action as NPH insulin. Premixed combinations of NPL and short acting insulin analog are available (Table 8.1). Combination of regular short acting insulin with NPH does not create any problem. While more convenient for the patient (only two injections/day), combination insulin formulations do not allow independent adjustment of short-acting and long-acting activity. Several insulin formulations are available as insulin "pen" which may be more convenient for some patients. Insulin delivery by inhalation is no longer available but remains under investigation.

Insulin regimens

In all insulin regimens, long-acting preparations (NPH, glargine or detemir) supply basal insulin, whereas regular, insulin aspart, glulisine or lispro insulin provides prandial insulin.

A shortcoming of current insulin regimen is that injected insulin immediately enters the systemic circulation, whereas endogenous insulin is secreted into the portal venous system. Thus, exogenous insulin administration exposes liver to subphysiologic insulin levels. No insulin regimen reproduces the precise insulin secretary pattern of the pancreatic islet. However, the more physiologic regimens entail more frequent insulin injections, greater reliance on short-acting insulin, and more frequent capillary plasma glucose measurements. Table 8.2 illustrates a regimen with a rapidly acting insulin analog and insulin detemir or insulin glargine that might be appropriate for a 70-kg person with type 1 diabetes eating meals providing standard carbohydrate intake and moderate to low fat content.

Table 8.2: Intensive insulin regimens for a 70-kg man with type 1 diabetes

	Breakfast	Lunch	Dinner	At bedtime
Carbodydrate intake	75 g	60 g	90 g	
Insulin regimens	Pre-breakfast	Pre-lunch	Pre-dinner	
Rapidly acting insulin analog*	5 units	4 units	6 units	
Insulin determir	6–7 units			8–9 units
or				
Rapidly acting insulin analog*	5 units	4 units	6 units	
Insulin glargine				15–16 units

*Insulin lispro, aspart, or glulisine

Rapidly acting insulin dose can be increased by 1 or 2 units if extra carbohydrate (15–30 g) is ingested or if the premeal blood glucose is > 170 mg/dl.

Factors altering insulin requirements

Insulin requirements may be in creased by infection, stress, accidental or surgical trauma, puberty, during second and third trimester of pregnancy, obesity and certain hormones (glucagon, adrenalin and growth hormone).

Insulin requirements may be decreased in patients with renal or hepatic impairment and with some endocrine disorders (e.g. addison's disease, hypopituitarism) or celiac disease.

Insulin-dependent diabetes mellitus (IDDM or type I diabetes)

In type I diabetes there is no circulating insulin due to autoimmune destruction of pancreatic beta cells. The insulin regimen used is a combination of short and intermediate acting insulin injected twice a day before breakfast and before the evening meal to mimic the normal insulin blood concentration. Alternatively soluble insulin three times a day may provide a good glycemic control.

Adverse effects

- *Hypoglycemia* is a potential problem and is more likely to occur with human insulin. Alcohol and beta blockers may aggravate it. Warning signs of hypoglycemia such as faintness, dizziness, tremors, sweating and abnormal behavior are thought to be brought about by he compensatory secretion of adrenalin. It can be relieved by giving sugar or parenteral glucagon, if required. Failure of treatment may lead to convulsions, coma and death.

    β blockers mask the symptoms of hypoglycemia in patients of diabetes receiving insulin.

- *Local reaction:* Irritation at the site of injection can lead to fat hypertrophy, which can be minimised by rotating the injection sites. Local allergic reaction and infection may occur due to impurities.

- *Immunogenic response:* Non-human insulin can stimulate the production of anti-insulin antibodies (AIA), which may lead to hypersensitivity reaction and to insulin resistance.

- *Growth promoting properties* of insulin may be a factor in the microvascular complications of diabetes including microangiopathy, nephropathy, neuropathy, retinopathy and atherosclerosis.

- *Weight gain* is an undesirable effect of intensive insulin therapy.

Diabetic ketoacidosis (diabetic coma)

Patients with type I diabetes who are not treated or who develop infection during treatment, may rapidly pass into a diabetic coma, which is a potentially fatal complication. It is less likely to occur in type 2 diabetes.

Diabetic coma gives rise to prominent GI symptoms, dehydration respiratory distress, shock, and coma and is due to very high blood and urinary glucose levels, production of large quantities of ketone bodies leading to acidosis (ketoacidosis), and severe diuresis resulting in depletion of sodium, potassium and water.

The aim of the treatment is fluid replacement, adequate insulin administration, and maintenance of normal plasma potassium levels, which constitutes a first-line management of diabetic ketoacidosis. Bicarbonate, phosphate, magnesium, antimicrobials or anticoagulants therapies may be required as part of specific therapy, once the patient has been stabilised.

Fluid replacement would restore the circulating blood volume, replenish total body water deficits and ensure its maintenance. This is achieved by giving infusion of normal saline at a speed depending on degree of dehydration and cardiac and renal status.

Insulin therapy: Sufficient insulin requires to be administered to turn off ketoacidosis and correct hyperglycemia. Soluble human insulin is given intravenously by an infusion pump and the dose is adjusted to produce a decrease in blood glucose of 50–75 mg/dl/hour. Once oral intake resumes, insulin can be administered by subcutaneous injection.

Potassium supplements: Potassium should be added routinely to IV fluids, regardless of plasma levels on admission, because insulin therapy causes a rapid shift of potassium into the intracellular compartment. The goal is to maintain plasma potassium in the normal range and thereby prevent the potentially fatal cardiac effects of hypokalemia.

Potassium supplements are contraindicated in patients with hyperkalemia (ECG evidence), renal failure or oliguria confirmed by bladder catheterisation.

Bicarbonate therapy is not necessary routinely, but is indicated in patients who develop shock or coma, severe acidosis; acidosis-induced cardiac or respiratory dysfunction and severe hyperkalemia.

Restoration of electrolyte and water balance is usually sufficient to correct the acidosis by excreting acid urine.

Frequent examination of the urine for sugar and ketones, the blood sugar hourly and of the electrolytes is important in monitoring the treatment.

IV antimicrobial therapy for any possible bacterial or fungal infections and prophylactic subcutaneous heparin to prevent common deep vein thrombosis is indicated.

ORAL ANTIDIABETIC DRUGS

Oral antidiabetic drugs are used to supplement dietary control and exercise in the treatment of non-insulin dependent (type 2) diabetes.

Type 2 diabetes is characterized by three major pathophysiologic abnormalities, namely impaired insulin secretion leading to relative insulin deficiency, insulin resistance and increased hepatic glucose output (due to hepatic insulin resistance).

Several oral glucose lowering drugs target pathophysiologic processes in type 2 diabetes with different mechanism of actions (Fig. 8.1), but their action mainly depends upon a supply of endogenous insulin. These antidiabetic drugs mainly fall into the following three categories:

Insulin secretagogues	Sulphonylureas, meglitinides, incretin-based therapies
Lower glucose output	Biguanides, thiazolidinediones
Delay glucose absorption	α-glucosidase inhibitors

In addition other drugs whose role is uncertain in type 2 diabetes are pramlintide, bile acid binding resins, and bromocriptine.

INSULIN SECRETAGOGUES

Sulphonylureas

Sulphonylureas have been in use for the treatment of type 2 diabetes for many years and have the strongest evidence of

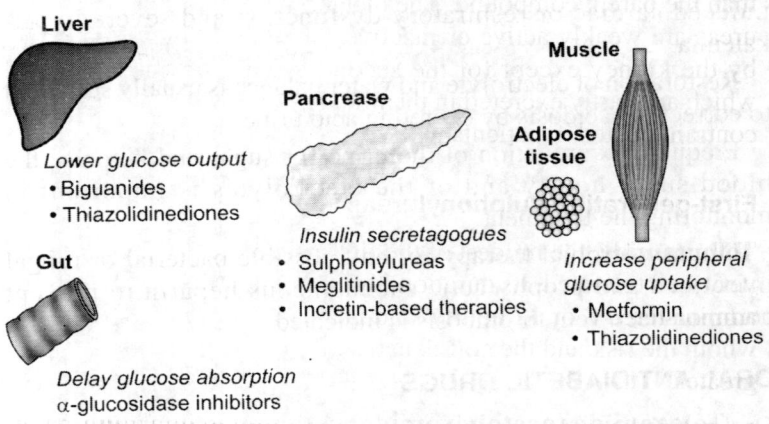

Fig.8.1: Mechanism of action of oral type 2 antidiabetic drugs.

preventing complications of diabetes. They are conventionally divided into first-generation and second-generation agents, which differ primarily in their potency and adverse effects.

Mechanism of action

The main action of sulphonylureas is to increase insulin release from the pancreas.

Sulphonylureas act by binding to specific receptors on the surface of pancreatic beta cells, which is linked to a K^+ channel. Activation of insulinotropic receptors closes K^+ channels, resulting in depolarization of the beta cell. This depolarized state permits calcium to enter the cell and actively promote insulin release.

Long-term administration of sulphonylureas reduces serum glucagon levels, which may contribute to the hypoglycemic effects. The suppressive effect on glucagon may be as a result of enhanced release of both insulin and somatostatin, which inhibit alpha-cell secretion.

Pharmacokinetics

Sulphonylureas are well-absorbed orally. They are metabolized by the liver, except acetohexamide whose metabolite is more active than the parent compound. The metabolites of all other sulphonylureas are weakly active or inactive. The metabolites are excreted by the kidney except for the second generation sulphonylureas which are partly excreted in the bile. Sulphonylureas are generally contraindicated in patients with severe liver or kidney impairment.

First-generation sulphonylureas

Tolbutamide, the mildest of the first-generation sulphonylureas is very well tolerated. Its duration of action is relative short, is usually administered 8 or 12 hourly, and is a useful drug in the elderly in whom the risk and the consequence of inducing hypoglycemia are greater.

Tolazamide, acetohexamide and **chlorpropamide** have a longer half-life, a greater incidence of hypoglycemia, more frequent drug interactions, and now are rarely used (almost obsolete).

Second-generation sulphonylureas

These have a more rapid onset of action and provide better coverage of the postprandial glucose rise. They reduce both fasting and postprandial glucose. They are 100–200 times more potent than tolbutamide. They should be used with caution in patients with cardiovascular disease or in elderly patients, in whom prolonged hypoglycemia would be especially dangerous.

Glyburide (1.5–20 mg) is unique among sulphonylureas in that it not only binds to the pancreatic beta cell membrane sulfonylurea receptor but also becomes sequestered within the beta cell, which contributes to its prolonged biologic effect despite of its relatively short half-life.

Glyburide has a few adverse effects other than its potential for causing hypoglycemia, which at times can be prolonged. Flushing has been reported after alcohol ingestion. Elderly patients are particularly at risk for hypoglycemia even with relatively small daily doses.

Glipizide (5–40 mg) is metabolized at least 90% in the liver to inactive metabolites and 10% is excreted unchanged in the urine.

Glipizide therapy should therefore not be used in patients with liver failure. Because of its lower potency and shorter duration of action, it is preferable to glyburide in elderly patients.

Glicalzide (40–320 mg) is another intermediate acting sulfonylurea with duration of action of about 12 hours. It is metabolized in liver and the metabolites have no hypoglycemic action. It is also a preferred preparation for elderly patients.

Glimepiride (1 – 8 mg) is a potent long-acting hypoglycemic drug, which is completely metabolized by the liver to relatively inactive metabolites. It should be avoided in the elderly.

Specific disadvantages

Hypoglyecmia is the most common adverse effect, especially with potent longer acting agents, which may be of great concern in elderly patients.

Weight gain, a common side effect, results from the increased insulin levels and improvement in glycemic control.

Increased cardiovascular risk. However, glyburide has not been associated with increased cardiac mortality.

Drug interaction

Some sulphonylureas have significant drug interaction with alcohol and some drugs including, warfarin, aspirin, ketoconazole, alpha glucosidase inhibitors, and flucinazolin.

MEGLITINIDES

These insulin secretagogues are called prandial glucose regulators. **Repaglinide** and **nateglinide** are not sulphonylures but also interact with the ATP - sensitive potassium channel. There is no sulfur in their structure and may be used in type 2 diabetes with sulfur or sulfonylurea allergy.

Meglitinides have short half-life and are given with each or immediately before meal to reduce meal-related glucose excursions. These drugs can be used as monotherapy or in combination with biguanides.

Hypoglycemia is the main side effect, though it may be less marked than sulfonylurea. The incidence of hypoglycemia with meglitinides is lowest of all the secretagogues and does not require dose titration. Like sulphonylureas, they also cause weight gain.

Meglitinides have the advantage of being safe in patients with kidney impairment or in the elderly.

INCRETIN-BASED THERAPIES

The secretion of insulin in response to glucose by mouth is greater than by intravenous infusion. In part, this is caused by secretion of gut hormones, or incretins, which potentiate glucose-induced insulin secretion. Glucagon like peptide (GLP-1) is an incretin hormone which stimulates insulin secretion in a glucose-dependent manner, thus hypoglycemia does not occur. In addition GLP-1 is rapidly proteolyzed by dipeptidyl peptidase 4 (DPP-4) and is cleared rapidly by the kidney. As a result, GLP-1's half-life is only 1–2 minutes and cannot be used therapeutically. Two GLP-1 receptor agonists **exenatide** and **liraglutide** are available for clinical use. Specific disadvantages of GLP-1 receptors agonists are:

- Require to be given by subcutaneous injection
- Nausea occurs in over 40% of the patients
- Increased risk of hypoglycemia when used with other insulin secretagogues
- Acute pancreatitis
- Renal failure

Liraglutide has been found to cause medullary thyroid carcinoma in rats and is contraindicated in individuals with medullary carcinoma of the thyroid and multiple endocrine neoplasia.

DPP-4 Inhibitors

As GLP-1 is rapidly degraded by the enzyme dipeptidyl peptidase 4, inhibitors of this enzyme can be used to prolong its biological effect.

Sitagliptin, **saxagliptin** and **vildagliptin** are DPP-4 inhibitors, which are given orally. They prolong endogenous GLP-1 action. These drugs do not cause weight gain or loss. The main adverse effects appear to be a predisposition to nasopharyngitis or upper respiratory tract infection.

Sitagliptin may cause serious allergic reactions including anaphylaxis, angioedema and exfoliative skin conditions including Stevens-Johnson syndrome. Pancreatitis has also been reported.

DRUGS THAT LOWER GLUCOSE OUTPUT

Biguanides

Metformin is the only biguanide available for use. Phenformin was discontinued because of its association with lactic acidosis and lack of any documentation of any long-term benefit from its use.

Mechanism of action

The mechanism of action of metformin has not been precisely defined. It has no hypoglycemic effect in non-diabetic individuals, but in diabetes, insulin sensitivity and peripheral glucose uptake are increased. Metformin's therapeutic effects primarily derive from activation of AMP-regulated kinase (AMPK) in liver and muscle, which reduces hepatic gluconeogenesis and lipogenesis and increases glucose uptake by muscles and adipose tissue. There is some evidence that it impairs glucose absorption from the gut and reduces plasma glucogan levels.

Metformin requires some endogenous insulin for its glucose-lowering action. It does not increase insulin secretion and hypoglycemia with therapeutic doses is essentially unknown. Metformin is therefore more appropriately termed as a *euglcemic* or *antihypergycemic* medication rather than an oral hypoglycemic agent.

Pharmacokinetics

Metformin is well absorbed from the gut, has a half-life of 1.5–3 hours, is not bound to plasma proteins and is not metabolized, being excreted unchanged by the kidneys.

Therapeutic use

Metformin is the *first-line therapy* for patients with type 2 diabetes. Its use is not associated with a rise in body weight and it may be beneficial for the overweight or obese patient as it improves both fasting and postprandial hyperglycemia and hypertriglyceridemia without weight gain. In addition, as the glucose-lowering effect of metformin is synergistic with that of sulphonylureas, the two can be combined when either alone has proved inadequate. It can also be given in combination with most other anti-diabetic medications. Metformin is given with food, usually starting with 500 mg 12-hourly gradually increased, as required, to a maximum of 1 g 8-hourly.

Metformin is ineffective in patients with type 1 diabetes.

Adverse effects

The most frequent side effects of metformin are gastrointestinal symptoms (anorexia, nausea, vomiting, abdominal discomfort, diarrhea, metallic taste).

Metformin can increase susceptibility to lactic acidosis. Therapeutic doses of metformin reduce lactate uptake by the liver, but serum lactate rise minimally if at all, since other organs such as the kidney can remove the slight excess. Its use is contraindicated in patients with impaired renal or hepatic function, cardiorespiratory insufficiency or alcoholism in whom the risk of lactic acidosis is significantly increased.

Absorption of vitamin B_{12} appears to be reduced during long-term metformin therapy but the serum vitamin B_{12} levels usually remain in the normal range. However, periodic serum vitamin B_{12} levels should be checked in patients with symptoms of peripheral neuropathy or if a macrocytic anemia develops.

THIAZOLIDINEDIONES

These drugs (also called TZD drugs, glitazones or PPARγ agonists) bind and activate peroxisome proliferator-activated receptor-γ, a nuclear receptor present mainly in adipose tissue that regulates the expression of several genes involved in metabolism.

TDZ enhance the actions of endogenous insulin, partly directly (in the adipose cells) and partly indirectly (by increased adiponectin and decreased release of resistin which alter insulin sensitivity in the liver). Observed effects of TDZ include decreased circulating insulin levels, decreased free fatty acid levels and deceased hepatic glucose output. Like biguanides TDZ do not cause hypoglycemia.

TDZ have significant effects on vascular endothelium, the immune system, the ovaries, lipid metabolism and tumor cells.

Piogliatazone and **rosiglitazone** are the available TZDS for clinical use. TDZ are usually prescribed as second-line therapy with metformin or as third-line therapy in combination with sulfonylurea and metformin (known as triple therapy).

TDZ are most likely to be effective in patients with pronounced insulin resistance (e.g., abdominal obesity) and redistribute fat away from the abdominal stores into subcutaneous depots. TDZ, though highly efficacious in the prevention of type 2 diabetes, are not very popular because of the adverse effects of weight gain, peripheral edema, CHF, fractures, macular edema. Rosiglitazone may increase cardiovascular risk. These drugs are contraindicated in pregnancy, breast-feeding, liver and cardiovascular disease.

DRUGS THAT DELAY GLUCOSE ABSORPTION

Alpha-glucosidase inhibitors competitively inhibit the α-glucosidase enzymes in the gut that digest starch and sucrose. **Acarbse**, **miglitol** and **vaglibose** are available and taken with meals. They lower post-prandial blood glucose and modestly improve overall glycemic control.

The main side-effects are flatulence, abdominal bloating and diarrhea. Miglitol should not be used in end-stage chronic kidney disease, where its clearance is impaired.

OTHER DRUGS

Pramlintide
Amylin is secreted with insulin from pancreatic beta cells; its role in normal glucose homeostasis is uncertain. However, based on the rationale that patients who are insulin deficient are also amylin

deficient, an analogue of amylin – pramlintide was found to reduce postprandial glycemic excursions in type 1 and type 2 diabetic patients taking insulin.

Pramlintide injected just before a meal slows gastric emptying and suppresses glucagon but does not alter insulin levels. Pramlintide is approved for insulin – treated patients with type1 and type 2 diabetes. Pramlintide is well tolerated.

BILE ACID – BINDING RESINS

Bile acid metabolism is abnormal in type 2 diabetes. The mechanism by which bile acid-binding resins lower blood glucose is not known. **Colesevelam** is prescribed prior to meals in type 2 diabetes. The most common side effects are gastrointestinal (constipation, abdominal pain and nausea). Bile acid-binding resins can increase plasma triglycerides.

BROMOCRIPTINE

Dopamine receptor agonist bromocriptine has been approved for that treatment of type 2 diabetes, though its role in the treatment of type 2 diabetes is uncertain.

INSULIN

Insulin, as initial therapy in type 2 diabetes may be required under following circumstances:

- In patients with severe weight loss
- In renal or hepatic disease which precludes the use of oral glucose lowering drugs
- In acutely ill hospitalized patients
- Progressive nature of the disease leading to relative insulin deficiency in long-standing diabetic patients.

Combination insulin therapy may be required in patients with type 2 diabetes when oral antidiabetic drugs fail to reach the glycemic target. Long-acting insulin (glargine) at bedtime is more effective, since fasting hyperglycemia and increased hepatic glucose production are prominent features of type 2 diabetics.

Choice of initial glucose-lowering Agent

The choice of therapy depends on the levels of hyperglycemia. Patients with mild to moderate hyperglycemia (200-250 mg/dl) generally respond to a single oral glucose-lowering agent. Metformin is usually the choice because of its efficacy, known side-effect profile and relatively low cost. Patients with more severe hyperglycemia (> 250 mg/dl) may require a second agent (combination therapy) to achieve the glycemic target and with severe hyperglycemia (250–300 mg/dl) triple therapy. Several medication combinations are available in different dose sizes; all have in common one which lowers glucose output e.g., metformin or thiazolidinedione combined either with sulfonylurea or DPP-4 inhibitor.

Insulin can be used as initial therapy in severe hyperglycemia or in patients who are symptomatic from the hyperglycemia. This approach is based on the rationale that more rapid glycemic control will reduce "glucose toxicity" to the islet cells, improve endogenous insulin secretion and possibly allow oral glucose-lowering agents to be more effective, which may permit withdrawal of insulin.

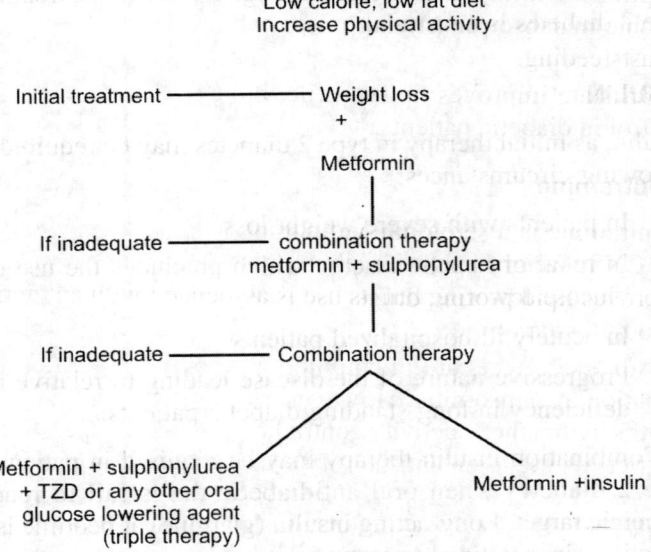

A step-wise approach to the management of type 2 diabetes

ANTIOBESITY DRUGS

Obesity is a serious health hazard, associated with many health problems including CVS diseases, diabetes mellitus, gallstones and osteoarthritis. Antiobesity drugs should be avoided and the treatment should consist of a balanced diet, exercise and changes in lifestyle. Appetite suppressants such as amphetamines, tobacco and thyroid hormones should not be used in the treatment of obesity.

Orlistat and sibutramine are the only drugs that are currently approved for use in patients with high risk of complications from obesity.

Orlistat

Oslistat inhibits pancreatic and gastric lipases and therapy decreases the hydrolysis of ingested triglycerides, reducing dietary fat absorption by 30%. The drug is not absorbed and adverse side-effects relate to the resultant fat malabsorption on the gut: namely, loose stools, oily spotting, fecal urgency, flatus and the malabsorption of fat-soluble vitamins. Orlistat is contraindicated in chronic malabsorption syndrome, cholestasis, and pregnancy and breast-feeding.

Orlistate improves lipid profile, blood pressure and glycemic control in diabetic patients.

Sibutramine

Sibutramine is a serotonin and noradrenalin reuptake inhibitor in the CNS. Weight loss with sibutramine is greater than orlistat. It improves lipid profile, but its use is associated with an increase in blood pressure.

Adverse effects are uncommon and include dry month, constipation and insomnia. However, risk in blood pressure due to central sympathetic activity contradicts its use in hypertension and restricts its use as an anti-obesity drug.

Rimonabant

Rimonabant is a cannabinoid receptor antagonist that acts in the hypothalamus to reduce appetite. It improves lipid profile, blood pressure, and glycemic control in diabetic patients. The major adverse effects of rimonabant are mood disorders with even risk of suicide, which restricts its use.

8.2 THYROID AND ANTITHYROID DRUGS

THYROID DRUGS

Thyroxine (T_4) and triiodothyronine (T_3) are the two hormones stored in the thyroid gland as thyroglobulin.

Thyroid hormones are important for normal growth and development and for energy metabolism. T_4 in the tissues is converted to T_3, which is the active hormone and T_4 is generally regarded as a prohormone.

Thyroid hormone increases the metabolism of lipids, carbohydrates and proteins and this calorigenic effect is manifested as an increase in basal metabolic rate. It has a very important action on normal growth, partly by a direct action on cells and partly indirectly by stimulating the normal secretion of growth hormone. It is essential for the maturation of the CNS.

Therapeutic uses

Thyroid hormone is used in hypothyroidism and the treatment is usually continued for the rest of patient's life.

In infants, congenital absence or incomplete development of the thyroid results in **cretinism**, which is characterized by stunted development of the baby, causing dwarfism, mental retardation, and coarsened facial features and skin. It is also called **congenital hypothyroidism**.

In adults thyroid deficiency may be due to different causes which include:

- Primary hypothyroidism (due to disease of the thyroid itself) accounts for more than 90% of cases.
- Insufficient iodine in the diet; this is called simple or nontoxic goiter.

- Chronic lymphocytic thyroiditis (Hashimoto's disease), which is the most common and is an immunological disorder, when the body reacts against the protein thyroglobulin, which is the mechanism for storing T_3 and T_4 in the thyroid gland.
- Iatrogenic hypothyroidism due to thyroidectomy or radioactive iodine (^{131}I) therapy.
- Secondary hypothyroidism due to TSH is uncommon but may occur in disorders of the pituitary or hypothalamus.
- Drugs that may cause hypothyroidism include lithium, interferon-alpha, interleukin-2, thalidomide, NSAIDs, glucocorticoids, X-ray contrast agents, sympatholytics, sulphonylureas and tranquillisers.

When thyroid deficiency is severe it causes a condition called **myxedema,** which is mainly characterised by symptoms like, mental impairment, slow or slurred speech and hoarseness, bradycardia, fatigue, myalgias, constipation, cold intolerance, facial and periorbital edema, dry skin and non-pitting edema.

Thyroxine sodium (**T_4, levothyroxine sodium**) is the drug of choice for maintenance therapy. The treatment is started with small doses, which are increased until the desired effects are produced. It is desirable to monitor the therapy with occasional T_4 and TSH estimations to ensure the correct dose.

Liothyronine (T_3, Triiodothyronine) has actions similar to thyroxine but are much more rapid in onset. It is not so useful in the treatment of myxedema but is the treatment of choice in myxedema coma, when given intravenously.

Adverse effects

Excessive doses of thyroid hormones lead to cardiovascular disorders (anginal pain, arrhythmia, and tachycardia), muscle cramps, GIT disorders (especially constipation), muscle weakness and loss of weight. Hypnotics should be avoided for insomnia.

ANTITHYROID DRUGS

Antithyroid drugs are used for hyperthyroidism, either to prepare patients for surgical excision of the thyroid gland, or for its regular treatment. The common types of hyperthyroidism are diffuse toxic goiter (also called thyrotoxicosis or Grave's disease) and toxic nodular goiter. The treatment of choice for diffuse toxic goiter is by drugs whereas for toxic nodular goiter is surgery. Antithyroid drugs used for the treatment of thyrotoxicosis are aqueous iodine solution (Lugol's solution), radioiodine (radioactive iodine; ^{131}I) and thionamides.

Aqueous iodine solution

It is also called **Lugol's solution** and is only indicated (1–2 drops orally given 12 hourly) to inhibit thyroid hormone secretion release as part of the treatment of thyroid crisis and also as premedication before thyroid surgery to make the thyroid gland less vascular. Its actions are temporary and after 10 days or so, the beneficial actions start wearing off. It is likely to give rise to allergic reactions.

Radio-iodine

Radio-iodine (radioactive iodine; ^{131}I) is the treatment of choice for almost all patients of Grave's disease except during pregnancy.

It is a radioactive isotope of iodine that is taken selectively by thyroid gland, where it emits powerful rays that kill cells. It is a rare example of a "magic bullet": i.e. a drug that targets the thyroid gland, because of its selective property of trapping the circulating iodine in the blood. A single dose permanently controls hyperthyroidism in 90% of patients. Radioiodine emits both β-particles and γ-rays and has a short half-life of about 8 days.

Radio-iodine does not increase the risk of malignancy, since its cytotoxic effects are mainly confined to thyroid gland because of relative short path of β-particles, which destroys quickly the thyroid tissue and the radioactivity decays away completely because of its short half-life. The common side effect is hypothyroidism, which occurs in more than half of patients within the first year and continues to develop at a rate of approximately 3% / year. Hypothyroidism is easily treated by administration of thyroxine.

THIONAMIDES

Carbimazole, methimazole and **propylthiouracil** are thiourea derivatives that act primarily by interfering with the synthesis of thyroid hormone.

Mechanism of action

These drugs inhibit thyroid hormone synthesis, possibly by preventing the oxidation of iodide to iodine. Propylthiouracil also blocks the conversion of T_4 to T_3 in target tissues. They do not have any permanent action on thyroid function and the symptoms recur, if the therapy is stopped.

Pharmacokinetics

Thionamides are well absorbed orally. Carbimazole is a prodrug and is rapidly metabolized in the blood to methimazole. They are distributed throughout the extracellular water and have a short half life. Though, not concentrated in thyroid, they have a prolonged effect on the thyroid and need only to be given once daily. These drugs are metabolized in the liver.

Carbimazole should be used with care during pregnancy, as excessive doses may suppress the fetal thyroid. It is also excreted in maternal milk and may cause goiter and hypothyroidism in the newborn.

Therapeutic uses

Methimazole and propylthiouracil are commonly used. They act quickly to block the oxidation of iodide, but the beneficial effects are delayed because the circulating T_3 and T_4 have a long half-life and the thyroid has large stores of the hormones in the colloid. Propylthiouracil has a more rapid onset of action because of its extrathyroidal (conversion of T_4 to T_3) inhibiting action.

In the majority of patients with Graves' disease, hypothyroidism recurs within 6 months after therapy is stopped. Spontaneous remission is likely to occur in mild, recent-onset hyperthyroidism and if the goiter is small.

Adverse effects

Minor side effects include rashes, joint pains, enlarged lymph nodes and transient depression of the white cell counts. Life-threatening side effects include agranulocytosis, hepatitis, vasculitis and drug-induced lupus erythematosus. Drug should be discontinued if jaundice or symptoms of agranulocytosis (e.g. fever, chills, and sore throat) develop.

Symptomatic therapy

β blockers reduce those symptoms of thyrotoxicosis that are due to over activity of the sympathetic system, such as palpitation, tremor, sweating and anxiety until hyperthyroidism is controlled by specific therapy. Verapamil can be used to control tachycardia in lieu of β blockers, if the latter is contraindicated.

8.3 CORTICOSTEROIDS

The adrenal cortex produces a number of hormones which belong to three main groups:

MINERALOCORTICOID HORMONE

Aldosterone is the principal mineralocorticoid that causes retention of Na^+, phosphate, Ca^+ and bicarbonate and reduction of serum K^+. It acts on Na^+ and K^+ transport in the distal tubule of the kidney to enhance Na^+ reabsorption. Its secretion is governed by the renin mechanism and its main function is to ensure maintenance of constant body fluid volume. It is not used as a drug.

SEX CORTICOID HORMONES

These are secreted in small amounts and are of no pharmacological importance.

GLUCOCORTICOID HORMONES

Cortisol or **hydrocortisone** is the main glucocorticoid hormone released from the adrenal cortex. Its main physiological role is concerned with metabolism of carbohydrate, fat and protein, maintenance of cardiovascular and skeletal muscle functions, a feeling of well being and modification of the responses of body in conditions of stress.

In addition to cortisol, there are a number of synthetic hormones with similar actions and the whole group is called the corticosteroid or steroid hormones.

The pharmacological actions of glucocorticoids generally fall under three main groups: a) general metabolic and systemic effects, b) negative feedback effects on the anterior pituitary and hypothalamus and c) suppression of disease process.

General metabolic and systemic effects

Carbohydrate and protein metabolism

Glucocorticoids tend to cause hyperglycemia due to a decrease utilization of glucose by peripheral tissues, an increase in gluconeogenesis, an increase production of glucose from protein and decrease sensitivity to insulin. Prolonged treatment may rarely give rise to diabetes mellitus. Glucocorticoids decrease protein synthesis and increase protein breakdown, particularly in muscles. This catabolic action may result in muscle wasting (proximal myopathy) and thinning of the skin, which becomes susceptible to bruising. They increase uric acid secretion.

Fat metabolism

Glucocorticoids promote lipolysis. The peripheral tissues loose fat which is deposited over face, neck and shoulders giving rise to round "moon-like" face with a picture similar to that of Cushing's disease.

Bone

Glucocorticoids inhibit osteoblast formation as well as intestinal absorption of calcium. They stimulate the secretion of parathyroid hormone that mobilizes calcium from bone. The bone production is thus reduced resulting in osteoporosis, which may cause osteoporotic fractures of the hip or vertebrae in the elderly. High doses are associated with a vascular necrosis of the femoral head.

Stomach

Glucocorticoids increase secretion of gastric acid and pepsin and may exacerbate peptic ulcer. Their anti-inflammatory action may mask the symptoms of perforation of peptic ulcer.

Central nervous system

Glucocorticoids usually produce a feeling of well being (euphoria). In patients with mental disorders, they may cause serious mental disease, a serious paranoid state or depression with risk of suicidal tendency. Large doses of glucocorticoids may increase intracranial pressure.

Miscellaneous effects

In children, administration of glucocorticoids results in suppression of growth.

Negative feedback effects

Glucocorticoid administration depresses the secretion of corticotropin releasing hormone from the hypothalamus and adrenocorticotropin hormone from the anterior pituitary with a resultant decrease in secretion of endogenous glucocorticoids and atrophy of adrenal cortex.

Adrenal atrophy can persist for years after stopping prolonged corticosteroid therapy and any illness or surgical emergency may require corticosteroid therapy to compensate for lack of sufficient adrenocortical response.

Suppression of disease processes

Glucocorticoids have potent anti-inflammatory and immunosuppresive effects. The anti-inflammatory action may be due to the synthesis of a new protein, lipocortin, which inhibits the production of prostaglandins, leukotrienes and platelet activating factor by inflammatory cells.

In certain disease antibody producing system may become deranged and produce antibodies against various body tissues. Diseases, which arise in this way, are called "autoimmune" and steroids, by suppressing the antibody system, can be useful in the management of such autoimmune disorders.

Anti-inflammatory and immunosuppressive effect constitutes the main uses of glucocorticoids and their other pharmacological actions are responsible for the adverse effects seen in therapy.

Glucocorticoids have marked antitumor effects in acute leukemias and lymphomas. They have anti-lymphocytic action. They enhance appetite and produce a sense of well being in the management of symptomatic end-stage malignant disease. In cerebral tumors, they help in reducing edema.

Pharmacokinetics

Glucocorticoids are readily absorbed from GIT. Almost 90% of the drug is bound to plasma proteins. They are metabolized in the liver. Inhaled corticosteroids using spacer devices have high topical potency due to increased airway deposition and a low systemic bioavailability due to reduced oropharyngeal deposition.

Preparations

Hydrocortisone and cortisone, the natural hormones exhibit some mineralocorticoid activity. Large number of semisynthetic analogues of the natural hormones do not possess mineralocorticoid activity and can be given in anti-inflammatory (pharmacological) doses without the adverse effect of sodium retention (Table 8.3).

Hydrocortisone: The relative high mineralocorticoid activity makes it unsuitable for disease suppression on a long-term basis. It is used on a short-term basis by intravenous injection for emergency conditions.

Prednisolone: It has predominant glucocorticoid activity and is the steroid most commonly used for long-term disease suppression.

Deflazacort: It is derived from prednisolone and has a high glucocorticoid activity.

Triamcinolone: It causes marked muscle wasting which may result in proximal myopathy. It is not indicated for chronic therapy.

Table 8.3: Comparison of the main corticosteroid agents (using hydrocortisone as a standard)

Drug	Relative affinity for glucocorticoid receptor	Approximate relative potency in clinical use			Equivalent oral dose (mg)	Preparations	Comments
		Anti-inflammatory	Topical	Na retaining			
Short-acting (8–12 hours)							
Hydrocortisone (cortisol)	1	1	1	1	20	Oral, injectable, topical	Drug of choice for replacement and emergencies.
Cortisone	0.01	0.8	0	0.8	25	Oral	Cheap, inactive until converted to hydrocortisone. Not used as anti-inflammatory because of mineralocorticoid effects.
Intermediate-acting (12–24 hours)							
Prednisone	0.05	4	0	0.3	5	Oral	Inactive until converted to prednisolone. Anti-inflammatory and immunosuppressive.

(Contd.)

Table 8.3: Comparison of the main corticosteroid agents (using hydrocortisone as a standard) *(Contd.)*

Drug	Relative affinity for glucocorticoid receptor	Approximate relative potency in clinical use			Equivalent oral dose (mg)	Preparations	Comments
		Anti-inflammatory	Topical	Na retaining			
Prednisolone	2.2	5	4	0.3	5	Oral, injectable	Drug of choice for anti-inflammatory and immunosuppressive effects.
Methyl prednisolone	11.9	5	5	0.25	4	Oral, injectable	Anti-inflammatory and immunosuppressive.
Triamcinolone	1.9	5	5	0	4	Oral, injectable, topical	Relatively toxic, mainly used topically.
Long-acting (over 24 hours)							
Dexamethasone	7.1	30	10	0	0.75	Oral, injectable, topical	Anti-inflammatory, immunosuppressive used especially when water retention is

(Contd.)

Table 8.3: Comparsion of the main corticosteroid agents (using hydrocortisone as a standard) (Contd.)

Drug	Relative affinity for glucocorticoid receptor	Approximate relative potency in clinical use		Equivalent oral dose (mg)	Preparations	Comments
		Anti-inflammatory	Topical	Na retaining		
Betamethasone	5.4	25–40	10	0	0.6	Oral, injectable, topical	underdesirable, e.g cerebral edema, drugs of choice for suppression of ACTH production.

Methylprednisolone, betamethasone and **dexamethasone** lack significant mineralocorticoid activity, which make them particularly suitable for high dose therapy in cerebral edema, where water retention would be a disadvantage.

Topical corticosteroids (*see* page 539)

Corticosteroid inhalations. Inhaled corticosteroids are useful adjunct to β_2 receptor agonists in the management of asthma. Beclomethasone, budesonide and flutucasone are highly lipophilic and employed.

Therapeutic uses

The therapeutic uses of corticosteroids may be considered under two headings:
- Suppression of some disease process (nonadrenal disorders)
- Replacement of steroid hormones which for some reasons are deficient.

Nonadrenal disorder

Glucocortocoids affect almost all cells of the body and are useful in the treatment of a diverse group of diseases unrelated to any known disorder of adrenal function (Table 8.4).

Since corticosteroids are not usually curative, pathologic process may progress while clinical manifestations are suppressed. Therefore chronic therapy with these drugs should be undertaken with great care and only when absolutely indicated or more conservative measures have failed. The doses and duration of administration should be kept to the minimum required for the treatment.

When prolonged therapy is anticipated, it is advisable to screen the patient for tuberculosis, since glucocorticoid therapy can reactivate dormant tuberculosis. The presence of diabetes, peptic ulcer, osteoporosis, glaucoma, hypokalemia, infections, psychological disorders, cardiovascular function and weight and height should be assessed.

Corticocoid therapy should not be decreased or stopped abruptly to prevent faring up of the disease process.

Table 8.4: Use in nonadrenal disorders

Disorder	Examples
Allergic reactions	Angioneurotic edema, asthma, bee stings, contact dermatitis, drug reactions, allergic rhinitis, serum sickness, urticaria
Collagen-vascular disorders	Giant cell arteritis, lupus erythematosus, mixed connective tissue syndromes, polymyositis, polymyalgia rheumatica and giant cell arteritis, rheumatoid arthritis, psoriatic arthritis, reactive arthritis, temporal arteritis
Eye diseases	Acute uveitis, allergic conjunctivitis, choroiditis, optic neuritis
Gastrointestinal diseases	Inflammatory bowel disease, nontropical sprue, subacute hepatic necrosis, autoimmune pancreatitis
Hematologic disorders	Acquired hemolytic anemia, acute allergic purpura, leukemia, autoimmune hemolytic anemia, idiopathic thrombocytopenic purpura, multiple myeloma
Systemic inflammation	Acute respiratory distress syndrome (sustained therapy with moderate dosage accelerates recovery and decrease mortality)
Inflammatory conditions of bones and joints	Arthritis, bursitis, tenosynovitis
Neurologic disorders	Cerebral edema (large doses of dexamethasone are given to patients following brain surgery to minimize cerebral edema in the postoperative period), multiple sclerosis
Organ transplants	Prevention and treatment of rejection (immunosuppression)
Pulmonary diseases	Aspiration pneumonia, bronchial asthma, prevention of infant respiratory distress syndrome, sarcoidosis, cystic fibrosis, tuberculosis with antituberculous drugs for meningitis
Renal disorders	Nephrotic syndrome
Skin diseases	Atopic dermatitis, dermatoses, lichen simplex chronicus (localized neurodermatitis), mycosis

(Contd.)

Table 8.4: Use in nonadrenal disorders *(Contd.)*

Disorder	Examples
	fungoides, pemphigus, seborrheic dermatitis, xerosis
Thyroid diseases	Malignant exophthalmos, subacute thyroiditis
Miscellaneous	Hypercalcemia, mountain sickness, lymphomas, primary or secondary cerebral tumours, necrotizing vasculitis, myasthenia gravis, inflammatory myopathies

Certain prophylactic measures should be undertaken such as calcium administration, avoidance of elective surgery, large doses of antacids, containing aluminum hydroxide, because it binds phosphate and may be a cause of hypophosphatemic osteomalacia. Hypogonadism, infections and edema should be treated.

Replacement therapy

Small (physiological) doses of steroids are needed in adrenal insufficiency, which may arise in Addison's disease, hypopituitarism, or adrenalectomy. A combination of hydrocortisone and fludrocortisone is indicated since hydrocortisone alone does not provide sufficient mineralocorticoid activity for complete requirements.

Adverse effects

The benefits obtained from glucocorticoids vary considerably. Use of these drugs must be carefully weighed in each patient against their widespread effects on every part of the organism. The major undesirable effects of glucocorticoids are the result of their hormonal actions, which lead to the clinical picture of iatrogenic Cushing's syndrome (Fig. 8.2).

Prolonged treatment with systemic high-dose corticosteroids causes a variety of adverse effects that can be life threatening (Table 8.5).

Steroids are contraindicated in systemic infections unless specific antibacterial therapy is given and with live virus vaccines.

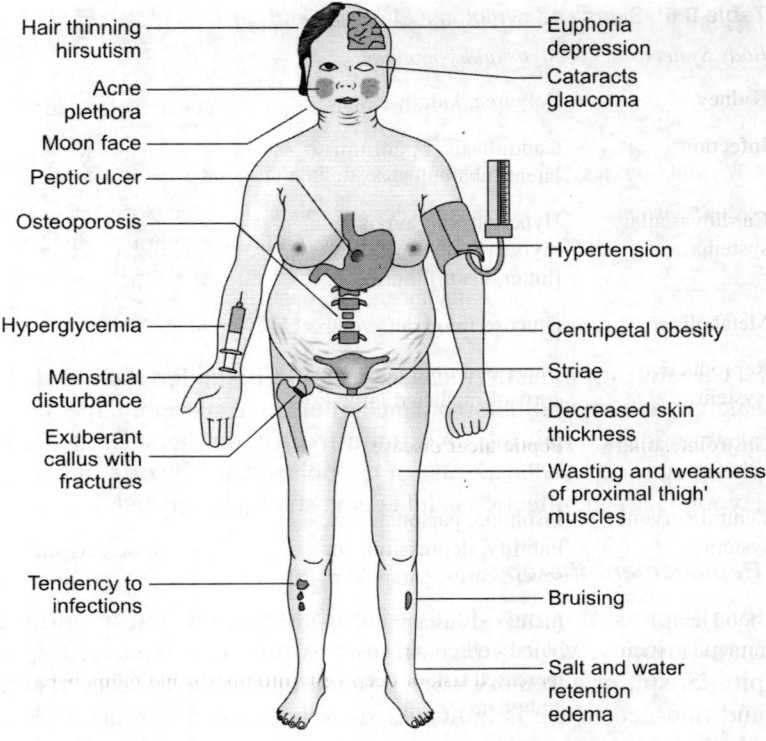

Fig. 8.2: Cushing syndrome showing adverse effects of glucocorticoids.

Table 8.5:	Signs and symptoms of corticoids toxicity
Body system	*Signs and symptoms*
Body fat	Weight gain, central obesity, rounded face, fat pad on back of neck ("buffalo hump")
Skin	Facial plethora, thin and brittle skin, easy bruising, broad and purple stretch marks, acne, hisutism
Bone	Osteopenia, osteoporosis (hip, vertebral fractures), avascular necrosis of femoral head, decreased linear growth in children, growth suppression
Muscle	Weakness, proximal myopathy (prominent atrophy of gluteal and upper leg muscles)

(Contd.)

Table 8.5: Signs and symptoms of corticoids toxicity

Body System	Signs and symptoms
Kidney	Polyurea, kidney stones
Infection	Candidiasis, opportunistic infections, reactivation of latent tubarculosis
Cardiovascular system	Hypertension, hypokalemia, edema, atherosclerosis, myocardial infarction, stroke, atrial fibrillation or flutter, heart failure
Metabolism	Glucose intolerance/diabetes, dyslipidemia
Reproductive system	Decreased libido, in women amenorrhea (due to cortisol-mediated inhibition of gonadotropin release)
Gastrointestinal system	Peptic ulcer disease
Central nervous system	Insomnia, parsonality change, irritability, emotional liability, depression, sometimes cognitive defects, in severe cases, paranoid psychosis
Blood and immune system	Increased susceptibility to infections, increased white blood cell count, eosinopenia, hypercoagulation with increased risk of deep vein thrombosis and pulmonary embolism
Eye	Glaucoma, cataract
Mineralocorticoid	Salt retention, potassium loss, edema
Glucocorticoid	Adrenal atrophy

8.4 FEMALE SEX HORMONES

GONADOTROPHINS

Follicular stimulating hormone and luteinizing hormone are the gonadotrophins secreted by anterior pituitary, which act in concert to release female sex hormones responsible for the fertility and maintenance of pregnancy or menstruation.

In women, the principal function of FSH is to direct ovarian follicle development. Both FSH and LH are needed for ovarian steroidogenesis. In the ovary both LH and FSH in the follicular stage of the menstrual cycle lead to the production of estrogens. In the luteal phase of the menstrual cycle, estrogen and progesterone production is primarily under the control first of LH and then, if pregnancy occurs, under the control of human chorionic gonadotropin (hCG). Human chorionic gonadotropin is a placental protein nearly identical with LH; its actions are mediated through LH receptors.

FSH (**urofollitropin** or **follitropin alfa** and **follitropin beta**), LH (**lutropin alfa**) and hCG (**choriogonadotrophin alfa** [rhCG]) are mainly used for the controlled ovulation hyperstimulation that is the cornerstone of assisted reproductive technologies such as in vitro fertilization (IVF).

The most serious complications of gonadotropins are ovarian hyperstimulation syndrome and multiple pregnancies.

The ovarian hyperstimulation syndrome is a more serious complication that occurs in 0.5-4% of patients and is characterized by ovarian enlargement, ascities, hydrothorax, sometimes resulting in shock.

GONADOTROPIN-RELEASING HORMONE AND ITS ANALOGS

Gonadotropin-releasing hormone (GnRH) is secreted by neurons in the hypothalamus, which regulate the release of anterior pituitary FSH and LH.

Pulsatile GnRH secretion releases FSH and LH, while nonpulsatile administration of GnRH or GnRH analogs inhibit the release of FSH and LH by the pituitary.

GnRH analogs are used to produce gonadal suppression in men with prostate cancer. They are also used in women, who are undergoing assisted reproductive technology procedure or who have a gynecologic problem that is benefited by ovarian suppression.

Gonadorelin is a synthetic human GnRH. **Goserelin**, **histrelin**, **leuprolide**, **nafarelin** and **triptorelin** are synthetic GnRH analogs. The GnRh agonists are occasionally used for stimulation of gonadotropin production. They are used more commonly for the suppression of gonadotropin release.

Female infertility

Drugs used for ovulation include clomiphene citrate, gonadotropins and pulsatile GnRH.

Clomiphene is a non-steroidal estrogen antagonist that increases FSH and LH levels by blocking estrogen negative feedback at the hypothalamus. It induces ovulation in about 60% of women with polycystic ovary syndrome (PCOS) and is the initial treatment of choice.

Aromatase inhibitors have also been found useful in the treatment of infertility. Gonadotropins are highly effective for ovulation induction and are used to induce the development of multiple follicles in unexplained infertility and in older reproduction–age women. Disadvantages include a significant risk of multiple gestations and the risk of ovarian hyperstimulation.

Pulsatile GnRH administration to treat infertility is not common because of technical problems in their use. Other uses of pulsatile GnRH include male infertility (not popular) and diagnosis of delayed puberty due to hypogonadotropic hypogonadism.

Suppression of gonadotropin production

- *Controlled ovarian hyperstimulation*
  Synthetic GnRH analogs (leuprolide or nafarelin) are used to suppress endogenous LH surge that may trigger premature ovulation during controlled ovulation hyperstimulation in assisted reproductive technology procedure.
- *Endometriosis*
  Endometriosis is a syndrome of cyclical abdominal pain in premenopausal women due to aberrant growth of endometrium outside the uterus particularly in the dependent parts of the pelvis and ovary. The GnRH analog greatly reduce estrogen and progesterone concentrations and prevents cyclical changes which reduces the pain of endometriosis.

- *Uterine fibroids*
  Uterine fibroids are benign, estrogen sensitive, fibrous growths in the uterus that can cause menorrhagia with associated anemia and pelvic pain. GnRH analogs reduce fibroid size and reduce pain.
- *Prostate cancer*
  Antiandrogen therapy is the primary medical therapy for prostate cancer. Combined antiandrogen therapy with continuous GnRH analogs and an androgen receptors antagonist such as **flutamide** is as effective as surgical castration in reducing serum testosterone concentrations and effects.
- *Other uses*
  Other clinical uses for gonadal suppression by continuous use of GnRH analogs include advanced breast and ovarian cancer and dysfunctional uterine bleeding. The major adverse effects with continuous use of GnRh analogs include symptoms of menopause, osteoporosis and ovarian cysts.

ESTROGENS

Estrogens are necessary for the development of female secondary characteristics. The important actions of estrogens are myometrial hypertrophy and endometrial hyperplasia, sensitization of uterine muscle to certain stimulating agents, increase in the duct tissue in the breast and inhibition of production of prolactin by pituitary.

Estrogen used therapeutically belongs to three groups:
- Natural estrogens : **Estradiol, estrone** and **estriol**
- Synthetic estrogens : **Ethinyl estradiol, mestranol and quinestrol**
- Nonstroidal synthetic estrogens : **Diethylstilbestrol, chlorotrianisene** and **methallenestril**

Therapeutic uses

Estrogens are mainly used for hormone replacement therapy (HRT), in neoplastic diseases and for oral contraception.

Hormone replacement therapy

Natural and nonsteroidal synthetic estrogens have a more appropriate profile for HRT than synthetic estrogens. They are used during and after menopause to relieve vasomotor symptoms, hot flushes and atrophic vaginitis. They are very effective in preventing osteoporosis, which is a serious problem in postmenopausal women. Progestogen is combined with estrogen to prevent the risk of carcinoma of the uterus.

Estrogen can be given by different routes. Topical estrogen can be used in atrophic vaginitis. Oral preparations of estrogens are subject to first pass metabolism, therefore, subcutaneous or transdermal administration is more akin to endogenous hormone activity.

Tibolone is a synthetic hormone that combines estrogenic and progestogenic activity with weak androgenic activity. It is used to control postmenopausal symptoms.

Side effects of HRT are nausea, weight gain, headache, fluid retention and risk of breast cancer and venous thrombosis.

HRT is contraindicated in thromboembolic disorders, breast or endometrial cancer, undiagnosed uterine bleeding and liver diseases.

Adverse effects

Adverse effects of variable severity have been reported with the therapeutic use of estrognes.

Uterine bleeding

Estrogen therapy is a major cause of postmenopausal uterine bleeding.

Cancer

Prolonged estrogen therapy increases the incidence of breast cancer. Endometrial carcinoma is another risk factor in patients who take large doses of estrogens alone for 5 or more years. However, the concomitant use of a progestin prevents this increased risk, and may in fact reduce the incidence of endometrial cancer to less than that in general population. Diethylstilbestrol should not be given during pregnancy as there have been reports of adenocarcinoma of the vagina in their children. Moreover the risk for infertility, ectopic pregnancy, and premature delivery are also increased. It is now recognized that there is no indication for the use of diethylstilbestrol in pregnancy and it should be avoided.

Other effects

Estrogen therapy is associated with an increased in frequency of migraine headaches as well as cholestasis, gall bladder disease and hypertension.

Contraindications

Estrogens should not be used in patients with estrogen – dependent neoplasm such as carcinoma of the endometrium or at high risk for carcinoma of the breast.

THE PROGESTOGENS

Progesterone is the natural progestin and is mainly produced by the ovary. It is concerned in the maintenance of the pregnancy by thickening and development of the secretary phase in the endometrium and by damping down the excitability of the uterine muscle.

Progestogens used therapeutically belong to two groups:
- **Progesterone and its analogue:** Progesterone, hydroxyprogesterone, medroxyprogesterone and megestrol.
- **Testosterone analogues:** Norethisterone, norgestrel, levonorgestrel, norgestimate, desogestrel and gestodene.

Progesterone and its analogues are less androgenic and do not cause virilisation,. However, they have adverse effects on plasma lipids and increase the possibility of vascular diseases.

Testosterone analogues have no adverse effects on lipids and are commonly used.

Therapeutic uses

The major uses of progestational hormones are for hormone replacement therapy and hormonal contraception, where its combination with estrogen reduces the risk of uterine cancer. In addition, they are useful in producing long-term ovarian suppression, which has been employed in the treatment of dysmenorrhea, endometriosis and bleeding disorders when estrogens are contraindicated, and for contraception.

Progestins do not appear to have any place in the therapy of threatened or habitual abortion, but have been found to delay premature labor.

Adverse effects

Progestational compounds may have adverse effects on cardiovascular system; increase in blood pressure and reduction in plasma HDL levels. There has been reports that progestin plus estrogen replacement therapy in postmenopausal women may increase breast cancer risk significantly compared with the risk in women taking estrogen alone.

ORAL CONTRACEPTIVES

The combined oral contraceptive pill containing estrogen and progestogen is the most effective method of fertility control. It prevents conception by inhibition of ovulation by reducing the output of pituitary gonadotrophins, prevention of penetration of sperm by changing the character of the mucus of the cervix and by prevention of implantation of the ovum by making the endometrium hyperproliferative or hypersecretory or atrophic.

The oral contraceptive pill usually contains ethinylestradiol (30–50 microgram) and progestogens (norethisterone or levonorestrel or desogestrel or gestodene). The combined pill preparations are available in low strength (ethinylestradiol 20 microgram), standard strength (ethinylestradiol 30 microgram) and high strength (ethinylestradiol 50 microgram). The choice depends on the age and presence of risk factors for venous and arterial thrombosis such as obesity, diabetes, hypertension, migraine, varicose veins etc.

Use of preparations which only contain progestogens may be made in patients with venous thrombosis where estrogens are contraindicated, though progestogen contraceptives have a higher failure rate than combined pills. They are suitable for older women and those with cardiovascular diseases, diabetes and migraine. Progestogen preparations are available as oral pills, intramuscular injections and intrauterine devices.

Oral contraceptive pills, progestogen alone or combined pill, if taken within 72 hours of unprotected intercourse are effective in reducing the risk of pregnancy (**postcoital contraception**). Nongestrel twice daily for 1 day is being available as emergency post-coital contraceptive kits.

Side effects of progestogen only pill are amenorrhea (most common), nausea, vomiting, breast discomfort, depression and weight changes.

The major side effects of the combined pill are due to estrogen and for this reason the estrogen content of these preparations is kept as low as possible. Venous and cerebral thrombosis, thromboembolic complications, vascular diseases (e.g. coronary thrombosis and strokes) are due to estrogen. Increased risk of breast cancer and the cancer of cervix is another serious side effect of the combined pill.

The associated arterial disease (e.g. hypertension) is due to progestogen fraction of the pill, which alters the blood lipids. Oral contraceptives reduce the risk of endometrium and ovarian cancer.

The use of combined pill is contraindicated in pregnancy, cardiovascular diseases, carcinoma of breast or genital tract, undiagnosed vaginal bleeding, liver diseases, migraine, chorea or deteoriation of otosclerosis and porphyria.

Drugs, which induce hepatic enzyme activity, decrease the efficacy of the contraceptive pills. The most important drug in this respect is rifampicin but antiepileptics (carbamazepine, phenytoin, phenobarbital), isoniazid, griseofulvin and broad spectrum antibiotics also reduce the efficacy of the pill.

Beneficial effects of oral contraceptives

It has become apparent that reduction in the dose of the constituents of oral contraceptives reduces the adverse effects and provides many benefits unrelated to contraception. These include a reduced risk of ovarian cysts, ovarian and endometrial cancer, benign breast disease and a lower incidence of ectopic pregnancy. Iron deficiency and rheumatoid are less common and premenstrual symptoms, dysmenorrhea, endometriosis, acne and hirsutism may be ameliorated with their use.

Centchroman (saheli) is a nonsteroidal estrogen antagonist developed by CDRI, India and is used as oral contraceptive. Its exact mode of action is not known. It is claimed to prevent implantation of the ovum and to be free of the side effects of contraceptive pill.

ESTROGEN AND PROGESTERONE INHIBITORS / ANTAGONISTS

Tamoxifen a partial estrogen agonist – antagonist (selective estrogen receptor modulator [SERM]) is extensively used in the palliative treatment of breast cancer in postmenopausal women and chemoprevention of breast cancer in high-risk women. It also prevents the loss of lumbar spine bone density and plasma lipid changes with a reduction in the risk of atherosclerosis following spontaneous or surgical menopause. The agonist activity of tamoxifen may increase the risk of endometrial cancer.

Raloxifene is another estrogen agonist – antagonist (SERM) at some but not all target tissues. It has similar effects like tamoxifen on bone and lipids, but not on the endometrium or breast.

Raloxifene is used for the prevention of postmenopausal osteoporosis and prophylaxis of breast cancer in women with risk factor.

Mifepristone

Mifepristone binds strongly to the progesterone receptors and inhibits the activity of progesterone. It has luteolytic properties when given in midluteal period, which provides the basis for using mifepristone as a contraceptive. *A single dose of 600 mg is an effective emergency postcoital contraceptive.* Mifepristone along with a vaginal pessary containing prostaglandin E_1 or oral misoprostol is highly effective in terminating pregnancy during the first 7 weeks after conception.

Mifepristone may be useful in the treatment of endometirosis, cushing's syndrome, breast cancer, meningiomas that contain glucocorticoid or progesterone receptors.

Danazol

Danazol has weak progestational, androgenic and glucocorticoid activities. It also suppresses pituitary gonadotropin production. Danazol has been used in the treatment of endometriosis and fibrocystic disease of the breast, but its androgenic effects (acne, edema, hirsutism) usually make this treatment intolerable; in practice, it is rarely used.

8.5 MALE SEX HORMONES, ANTI-ANDROGENS, ANABOLIC STEROIDS AND DRUGS FOR IMPOTENCE

MALE SEX HORMONES

Testosterone, the natural androgen, is produced by the interstitial cells of testis. It is responsible for the secondary male sex characteristics including distribution of hair, deepening of the voice and the growth of genitals. The leuteinizing hormone (LH) of the pituitary controls its release from the testis. Testosterone also has an anabolic action.

Therapeutic uses

Testicular hormone deficiency

Testosterone is used in testicular hormone deficiency due to hypopituitarism. It is given orally, as an implant or skin patches. Esters of testosterone (Sustanon) can be given intramuscularly every 3 weeks and released slowly from the injection site.

Mesterolone is similar to testosterone and is given orally. Unlike testosterone, spermatogenesis is not impaired with mesterolone.

Carcinoma of the breast

Testoterone is effective in about 39% of postmenopausal patients with adanced carcinoma of the breast for relieving symptoms and causing temporary regression of secondary deposits. It does, however, have virilizing effects and causes the growth of facial hair, deepening of the voice and acne, when given to women.

Adverse effects

Testosterone may lead to prostate abnormalities, prostate cancer and cholestatic jaundice. It may also cause electrolyte disturbances including sodium retention with edema and hypercalcemia, increased bone growth and virilism in women.

Testosterone is contraindicated in breast cancer in men, prostate cancer, liver tumors, hypercalcemia and pregnancy.

ANTI-ANDROGENS

Cyproterone acetate and **flutamide** block the action of testosterone at the cell receptors. They inhibit spermatogenesis and produce reversible infertility.

Anti-androgens are used in various endocrine disorders, where there is overproduction of male hormone causing hirsutism in the female (when it is combined with estrogen) and severe hypersexuality and sexual deviations in the male. They are also used in patients with metastatic prostate cancer refractory to gonadorelin analogue therapy. Anti-androgens are hepatotoxic and are mainly indicated to palliate symptoms of advanced prostate cancer.

Finasteride is a specific inhibitor of testosterone metabolism and interferes with its action on the prostate gland. The size of the prostate gland is reduced and the obstructive symptoms of enlarged prostate are relieved. Its use is limited to benign prostatic hyperplasia, where it improves the urinary flow rate.

The other drugs used for benign prostatic hyperplasia are selective alpha-blockers such as prazosin.

ANABOLIC STEROIDS

These are the derivatives of male sex hormones that have less virilisation effects in women, but have significant anabolic action (protein building property). Their protein building property was thought to be useful to hasten convalescence and in senile osteoporosis (a condition due to lack of protein in bone), but clinically their effectiveness is not proven. Their use as body builders or tonics is quite unjustified. They are abused by athletes. The use of anabolic steroids is only limited in the treatment of some aplastic anaemias.

DRUGS FOR IMPOTENCE

Male erectile dysfunction is commonly due to psychological factors, but endocrine abnormalities and certain drugs (e.g. alcohol, tricyclic antidepressants, neuroleptics, antihypertensives, cimetidine) may also result in a failure to produce a satisfactory erection. Erection depends on the relaxation of the penile smooth muscle, with subsequent engorgement with blood following necessary stimulus.

Prostaglandin E_1 (alprostadil) or **papaverine** given by intra-cavernosal injection relaxes smooth muscle and produces a satisfactory erection. The procedure is not only cumbersome, but leads to multiple penile problems. Erection lasting for longer than 4 hours (priapism) is an emergency requiring penile aspiration, intra-carvernosal injection of sympathomimetic vasoconstrictors or even surgical intervention.

Sildenafil (viagra) inhibits the phosphodiesterase 5 in the blood vessels of penis leading to vasodilatation and enhanced erection, when taken an hour or two before intercourse. It has the advantage of oral administration and being highly effective.

Common side effects of sildenafil are dyspepsia, headache, flushing, dizziness, visual disturbances and increased intraocular pressure.

Sildenafil is contraindicated in recent stroke or myocardial infarction, hypotension (it should not be used in patients receiving nitrates) and hereditary degenerative retinal disorders.

Antibiotics (erythromycin), antifungal, antiviral and ulcer healing (cimetidine) drugs increase the plasma sildenafil concentration and may cause priapism.

9

Prostaglandins and Drugs Acting on Uterus

Prostaglandins (PG) are the only autacoids that are used in therapy because of their cytoprotective activity in the GIT mucosa, antiplatelet activity, uterine stimulant and vasodilator actions.

Natural prostaglandins are not used in clinical practice because of their limited availability, unstability, shorter half-life and cost, but their analogues are popular drugs mainly for their oxytoxic effects.

ABORTION

PGE_2 and PGF_{2a} have potent oxytocic actions. There analogues are used for first and second-trimester abortion and for priming or ripening the cervix before the abortion. These prostaglandins appear to soften the cervix by increasing proteoglycan content and changing the biophysical properties of collagen.

Dinoprostone, a synthetic preparation of PGE_2 is administered vaginally to induce abortion in the second trimester of pregnancy, for missed abortion for benign hydatidiform mole, and for ripening of the cervix for induction of labor in patients at or near term.

Misoprostol (PGE_1) combined with antiprogestins (e.g., mifepristone) is used to produce early abortion.

Carboprost (PGF_{2a}) tromethamine is used to induce second-trimester abortions and to control postpartum hemorrhage that is not responding to conventional methods of management.

UTERINE STIMULANTS

Apart from prostaglandins, the other drugs which stimulate uterine contractions are oxytocin and ergometrine. They are also termed as oxytocics or ecbolics.

OXYTOCIN

Oxytocin and antidiuretic hormone (vasopressin) are the two hormones secreted by the posterior lobe of the pituitary gland. Oxytocin causes contraction of the uterine muscle. This effect is not marked until the later stages of pregnancy. At parturition, extremely small amounts of oxytocin cause powerful uterine contractions. Estrogens sensitize the uterus to the action of oxytocin and release of prostaglandin may be a contributing factor to its oxytocic action.

Oxytocin, in therapeutic doses, induces contractions in the fundus and body of the uterus only without affecting the lower segment and full relaxation occurs in between the contractions.

Oxytocin also causes contraction of cells surrounding mammary alveoli which leads to milk ejection.

Oxytocin is used to induce labor for conditions requiring early vaginal delivery such as Rh problems, maternal diabetes, pre-eclampsia, or ruptured membranes. It is also used to induce or augment labor when uterine contractions are inadequate.

Oxytocin can be used in the immediate postpartum period for the control of uterine hemorrhage after vaginal or cesarean delivery. It is sometimes used during second-trimester abortions.

Oxytocin for induction of labor is given at an initial infusion rate of 0.5–2 mU/min, which is increased every 30–60 minutes until a physiologic contraction pattern is established.

Syntocinon (synthetic oxytocin) is used, since the natural oxytocin contains small amounts of vasopressin. It is given by intravenous infusion, total dose not exceeding 5 units for induction of labour for medical reasons (hypotonic uterine inertia) and in incomplete, inevitable or missed abortion.

Oxytocin may cause uterine over stimulation leading to fetal distress, asphyxia, death and uterine rupture. Anaphylactic reactions are rare and large doses may cause placental abruption and amniotic fluid embolism. It should not usually be combined with prostaglandin to induce labor.

Oxytocin is contraindicated in conditions where vaginal delivery is inadvisable including the presence of uterine scar from major surgery, fetal distress, and severe CVS disease.

ERGOT ALKALOIDS

Ergot, a fungus that grows on rye, contains a large number of bioactive substances, of which alkaloids are of clinical importance. Ergot alkaloids are divided into:

Amine alkaloids : Ergometrine (ergonovine)
Peptide alkaloids : Ergotamine and ergotoxine

Bromocriptine, dihydroergotimine and methysergide are semi synthetic ergot alkaloids.

Peptide alkaloids have vasoconstrictor properties and are used in migraine (*see* page 106).

Ergometrine and methylergometrine are oxytocic. Small doses cause rhythmic contractions of uterus, but with larger doses they become more or less continuous. They have little effect on other smooth muscles.

Ergometrine and methylergometrine (methergine) in a dose of 500 (orally) or 250 (intramuscularly) microgram are used in the routine management of the third stage of labour after child birth to cause the uterus to contract and thus prevent postpartum hemorrhage and to stop bleeding due to incomplete abortion.

Common side effects of ergometrine are GIT disorders, chest pain, vasoconstriction and transient hypertension.

Ergometrine is contraindicated for induction and first and second stages of labour, as powerful contraction caused by ergometrine may rupture the uterus or cause fetal asphyxia. It is not used in severe cardiovascular diseases, impaired pulmonary, hepatic and renal functions, sepsis and eclampsia.

Bromocriptine, a semisynthetic ergot alkaloid, acts as a stimulant of dopamine receptors in the brain. It inhibits both basal and stimulated prolactin and growth hormone secretion from the pituitary. It has less specific dopamine like actions in other areas of the central nervous system (basal ganglia and vomiting centre) and on blood vessels.

Bromocriptine is well absorbed and almost completely metabolized in the liver and is excreted in the bile.

Hyperprolactinaemia (increased production of prolactin by the pituitary) can cause impotence in men and anovulatory infertility in women. Bromocriptine restores prolactin concentrations to normal and ovulatory menstruation returns to normal. It is used in infertility or impotence due to hyperprolactinaemia, cyclical benign breast disease (danazol more effective), acromegaly (octreotide more effective), and inhibition of lactation (more effective than estrogen) and Parkinsonism in patients intolerant to levodopa.

Nausea and vomiting are common side effects. Others include dizziness, postural hypotension and constipation. Neuropsychiatry side effects are uncommon except in patients with Parkinson's disease.

Cabergoline and **quinagolide** are similar and can be used in patients intolerant to bromocriptine.

TOCOLYTIC AGENTS

These are the drugs that inhibit uterine contractions. β_2 agonists **salbutamol, terbutaline** and **ritodrine** diminish uterine activity and are used sometimes in the management of premature labour between 24 and 33 weeks of pregnancy.

10
Parathyroid Hormone and Calcium Metabolism

Calcium and phosphorus are the most important minerals of the bone with 98% of the 1–2 kg of calcium and 85% of the 1 kg of phosphorus stored in it.

Calcium and phosphorus are not only essential for bone's rigidity and strength, but are also two of the most important minerals for general cellular function. The body has evolved a complex set of mechanisms by which calcium and phosphorus homeostasis are carefully maintained with constant remodeling of bone and ready exchange of bone mineral with the extracellular fluid.

The abnormalities in bone mineral homeostasis can lead not only to a wide variety of cellular dysfunctions (e.g. tetany, coma, muscle weakness) but also disturbances in structural support of the body (e.g. osteoporosis with fractures) and loss of hematopoietic capacity (e.g. infantile osteopetrosis).

Calcium and phosphorus metabolism are chiefly regulated by three hormones:

- Parathyroid hormone (PTH)
- Fibroblast growth factor 23 (FGF23)
- Vitamin D (a prohormone rather than a true hormone)

These hormones contribute to bone mineral homeostasis mainly targeting intestine, kidney, and bone (Table 10.1). Other hormones: Calcitonin, prolactin, growth hormone, insulin, thyroid hormone, glucocorticoids, and sex steroids – influence calcium and phosphorus homeostasis under certain physiologic circumstances and can be considered secondary regulators. Deficiency or excess of these secondary regulators within a physiologic range does not

Table 10.1: Actions of parathyroid hormone (PTH), vitamin D, and FGF23 on gut, bone, and kidney

	PTH	Vitamin D	FGF23
Intestine	Increased calcium and phosphate absorption (by increased 1,25[OH]$_2$D production)	Increased calcium and phosphate absorption by 1,25 (OH)$_2$D	Decreased calcium and phosphate absorption by decreased 1,25(OH)$_2$D production
Kidney	Decreased calcium excretion, increased phosphate excretion	Calcium and phosphate excretion may be decreased by 25(OH)D and 1,25(OH)$_2$D*	Increased phosphate excretion
Bone	Calcium and phosphate resorption increased by high doses. Low doses may increase bone formation.	Increased calcium and phosphate resorption by 1,25(OH)$_2$D; bone formation may be increased by 1,25(OH)$_2$D and 24,25(OH)$_2$D	Decreased mineralization due to hypophosphatemia
Net effect on serum levels	Serum calcium increased, serum phosphate decreased	Serum calcium and phosphate both increased	Decreases serum phosphate

* Direct effect. Vitamin D often increases urine calcium owing to increased calcium absorption from the intestine and resulting decreased PTH.

produce the disturbance of calcium and phosphorus homeostasis that is observed in situations of deficiency or excess of PTH, FGF23, and vitamin D. However, certain of these secondary regulators – especially calcitonin, glucocorticoids, and estrogens are useful therapeutically.

Parathyroid hormone (PTH)

The four parathyroid glands lie behind the lobes of the thyroid. They produce PTH, which is the primary regulator of calcium metabolism. Serum PTH levels are tightly regulated by a negative feedback loop. Calcium, acting through the calcium-sensing receptor located on the surface of parathyroid chief cell reduces PTH release and synthesis. This feedback system is the critical homeostatic mechanism for maintenance of extracellular fluid (ECF) calcium (Fig. 10.1). Any tendency toward hypoglycemia is counteracted by an increased secretion of PTH, which restores serum calcium levels by (1) increasing the rate of dissolution of bone mineral, thereby increasing the flow of calcium from bone into blood, (2) reducing the renal clearance of calcium, and (3) increasing the efficiency of calcium absorption in the intestine by stimulating the production of $1, 25(OH)_2D$.

PTH regulates calcium and phosphates flux across cellular membranes in bone and kidney resulting in increased serum calcium and decreased serum phosphate.

In bone, PTH increases the activity and number of osteoclasts, the cells responsible for bone resorption.

The action of PTH on bone is an indirect one. PTH acts on osteoblast (the bone forming cell) to induce a membrane bound protein called RANK ligand (RANKL) which acts on osteoclast precursors to increase both the numbers and the activity of osteoclast to initiate bone remodeling for the renewal and repair of the skeleton during adult life.

PTH enhances both bone resorption and bone formation, the net effect of excess PTH is to increase bone resorption. The chronic effects of PTH are to increase the number of bone cells, both osteoblasts and osteoclasts, and to increase the remodeling of bone. Continuous exposure to elevated PTH leads to increased osteoclast

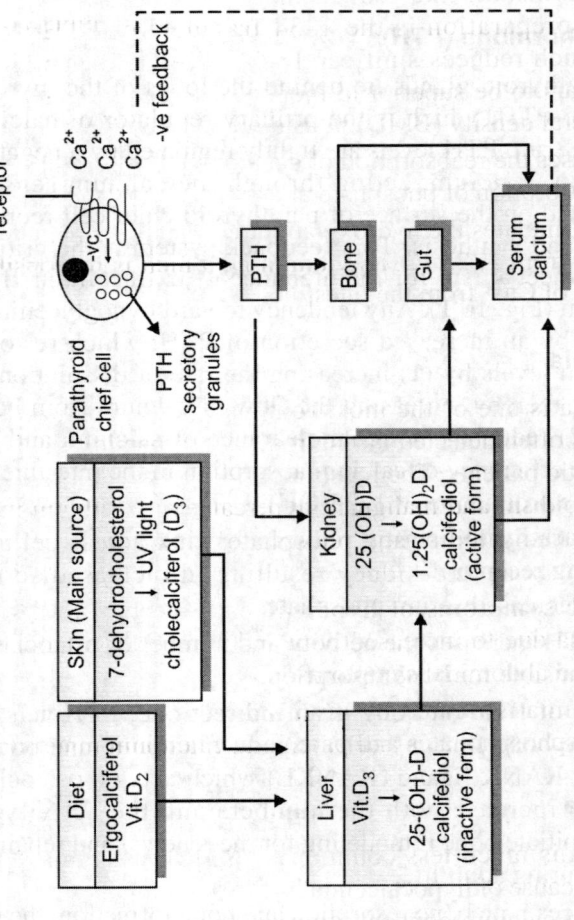

Fig. 10.1: Outline of calcium (Ca^{2+}) homeostasis showing interaction between parathyroid hormone (PTH), and vitamin D and calcium (Ca^{2+}). Calcium in serum exists as 50% ionized (Ca^{2+}), 10% non-ionized or complexed with organic ions such as citrate and phosphate, and 40% protein bond, mainly to albumin. It is the ionized calcium concentration which regulates PTH production.

mediated bone resorption. However, the intermittent administration of PTH, elevating hormone levels for 1-2 hours each day (pulsatile release of PTH) acts as an anabolic agent that works by stimulating new bone formation, without first stimulating bone resorption. This action may be indirect, involving other growth factor such as insulin-like growth factor 1 (IGF-1). The most widely used preparation is the 1–34 fragment of PTH (teriparatide), which reduces sinificantly fracture incidence. Teriparatide appears to be superior to biophosphonates in increasing the bone mineral density (BMD) in osteoporosis.

PTH increases the reabsorption of calcium and magnesium and reduces the absorption of phosphate and other ions by the kidney.

PTH also stimulates the hydroxylation of 25 hydoxy vitamin D into its active from $1, 25\ (OH)_2$ vitamin D, which is responsible for absorption of Ca^{2+} from the intestine.

Hypercalcemia

Hypercalcemia is one of the most common biochemical abnormalities and is often detected during routine biochemical analysis in asymptomatic patients. The most important causes are primary hyperparathyroidism and malignant hypercalcemia. Lithium may cause hyperparathyroidism by reducing the sensitivity of the calcium-sensing receptor.

The classic symptoms of hypercalcemia pertain to bones (osteitis fibrosa due to increased bone resorption), formation of renal stones and abdominal symptoms.

Hypercalcemia is treated by giving normal saline infusion, intravenous bisphosphonates and parenteral calcitonin injection.

Hypocalcemia

Hypocalcemia is much less common than hypercalcemia. The most common cause of hypocalcemia is a low serum albumin with normal ionized calcium concentration. It may also develop as a result of magnesium depletion, malabsorption, diuretic therapy or excess alcohol intake. Magnesium deficiency impairs the ability of parathyroid glands to secret PTH and may also impair the actions of PTH on bone and kidney.

VITAMIN D

Vitamin D is converted in the liver to 25 hydroxyvitamin D which is further hydroxylated in the kidneys to 1, 25 $(OH)_2D$, the active form of the vitamin, which activates specific intracellular receptors influencing calcium metabolism, bone mineralization and tissue differentiation. The synthetic form, ergocalciferol or vitamin D_2, is considered to be less effective than the endogenous 1, 25 $(OH)_2D$.

Calcium requirements depends on phosphorus intakes with an optimum molar ratio (Ca:P) of 1:1. Excessive phosphorus intake (1–1.5g/kg) with a Ca:P 1:3 causes hypocalcaemia and secondary hyperparathyroidism.

Vitamin D, like PTH induces RANK ligand in osteoblast and proteins such as osteocalcin which regulates the bone mineralization process.

Vitamin D receptors exist in a wide variety of tissue – not just bone, gut and kidney but have been found in most tissues in the body (e.g., brain, heart, and breast, prostate) that have nothing to do with calcium homeostasis. The function of these vitamin D receptors is unknown.

Vitamin D exerts a number of action including regulation of PTH secretion from parathyroid gland, insulin secretion from the pancreas, cytokine production by macrophages and T cells, and proliferation and differentiation of a large number of cells, including cancer cells.

Epidemiology studies have revealed an increased prevalence of cancer, diabetes mellitus, cardiovascular disease, and multiple sclerosis to lower serum levels of 25-hydroxyvitamin D (250 HD).

Thus, the functions of vitamin D receptors are unknown and the clinical utility of vitamin D is likely to expand.

The natural form of vitamin D, cholecalciferol or vitamin D_3 is formed in skin by the action of UV light on 7-dehydrocholesterol, a metabolite of cholesterol. Few foods contain vitamin D naturally but skin exposure to sunlight is the main source. Both forms of natural vitamin D are converted in the liver to 25-dihydroxy-vitamin D (25 OHD); 25 OHD is subsequently converted in various tissues (mainly kidney) to 1,25-dihydrooxyvitamins D

(1,25 [OH]$_2$D), the active hormone whose production is regulated by serum calcium, phosphorus and PTH. 1,25 (OH)$_2$D binds to cytoplasmic vitamin D receptors, increasing the absorption of dietary calcium from the intestine, and increasing the reabsorption of calcium in the renal tubule reducing calcium loss in the urine. 1,25 (OH)$_2$D also stimulates the osteoblasts to release RANKL that stimulates osteoclasts, which release calcium from the bone.

FIBROBLAST GROWTH FACTOR 23

Fibroblast growth factor 23 (FGF 23) is obtained from osteocytes, the cell that differentiates from osteoblast during bone formation and becomes embedded in bone matrix. Osteocytes play a crucial role in regulating phosphate metabolism by producing the hormone FGF 23 and are thought to be responsible for sensing and responding to mechanical loading of the skeleton. 1,25 (OH)$_2$D also stimulates the production of FGF23 which competes the negative feedback loop in that FGF23 inhibits 1,25 (OH)$_2$D production while producing hypophosphatemia, which in turn inhibits FGF23 production and stimulates that of 1,25 (OH)$_2$D. The net result of FGF23 is to decrease serum phosphate and maintain optimal molar ratio (Ca:P) of 1:1 by regulating phosphate metabolism.

Secondary hormonal regulators of bone mineral homeostasis

A large number of hormones affect bone mineral homeostasis and are used clinically in defective skeletal mineralization.

Calcitonin

Calcitonin is the hormone secreted by the parafollicular cells of the thyroid gland. Salmon calcitonin has a longer half-life than human calcitonin and is preferred therapeutically.

The main effect of calcitonin is to lower serum calcium and phosphate by actions on bone and kidney. Calcitonin inhibits osteoclastic bone resorption. Long-term administration inhibits both bone formation and resorption of bone.

Calcitonin reduces renal absorption of calcium and phosphate along with other ions including sodium, potassium and magnesium.

Therapeutically, calcitonin Salmon is used either as a nasal spray or parenterally in the treatment of Paget's disease, hypercalcaemia and osteoporosis due to its ability to block bone resorption and lower serum calcium levels.

Glucocorticoid

Glucocorticoid hormones alter bone mineral homeostasis by antagonizing vitamin D stimulated intestinal calcium absorption, by stimulating renal calcium excretion, and by blocking bone formation.

The negative impact of glucocorticoids on bone mineral homeostasis is employed in the management of hypercalcemia associated with lymphomas and granulomatous diseases such as sarcoidosis (in which production of $1,25\ (OH)_2D$ is increased) or in cases of vitamin D intoxication. Prolonged administration of glucocorticoids is a common cause of osteoporosis in adults and stunted skeletal development in children.

Estrogens

Estrogens play an important role in the bone mineral homeostasis by reducing the action of PTH and bone resorption and by increasing the $1,25\ (OH)_2D$ blood levels.

$1,25\ (OH)_2D$ increases the serum levels of calcium and phosphate by promoting their absorption and reducing excretion by the kidneys. Estrogens receptors have been found in bone and estrogen has direct effects on bone remodeling. Estrogens deficiency is responsible for postmenopausal osteoporosis.

Inadequate sex hormone production is a major cause of osteoporosis in men and women.

Estrogen therapy for postmenopausal osteoporosis, however, may be associated with adverse effects like malignancies, cardiovascular disease. Long-term use of estrogens is no longer advocated.

Selective estrogen receptor modulators (SERMs) have been developed to retain the beneficial effects on bone while minimizing the adverse effects on breast, uterus and the cardiovascular system.

METABOLIC BONE DISEASE

The term 'metabolic bone disease' denotes those conditions producing diffusely decreased bone density and diminished strength. It is categorized by histologic appearance: osteoporosis (abnormal loss of bone, remaining bone histologically normal), osteomalacia (abnormal bone formation due to inadequate mineralization) or osteitis fibrosa (excessive bone resorption with fibrotic replacement of resorption cavities and marrow).

Osteoporosis

Osteoporosis is characterized by a loss of bone osteoid that reduces bone integrity resulting in increased risk of fractures. It may occur as an adverse effect of long-term administration of glucocorticoids or other drugs; as a manifestation of endocrine disease such as thyrotoxicosis or hyperparathyroidism; as a feature of malabsorption syndrome; as a consequence of alcohol abuse and cigarette smoking: or without obvious cause (idiopathic). The postmenopausal form of osteoponsis may be accompanied by lower $1,25\ (OH)_2\ D$ levels and reduced intestinal calcium transport. This form of osteoporosis is due to estragen deficiency. Drug treatment prevents the vertebral and non-vertebral fractures in patients who have extensive involvement of the skull, long bones, or vertebrae.

Bisphosphonates

Bisphosphonates inhibit bone resorption by binding to hydroxyapatite crystals on the bone surface. When osteoclasts attempt to resorb bone that contains bisphosphonates, the drug is released within the cell, where it inhibits key signaling pathways that are essential for osteoclast function.

Bisphosphonates suppress the bone remodeling (due to inhibition of the normal activity of osteoclast and osteoblast), but the balance of effect of bone turnover is favourable, resulting in a gain in bone density due partly to increased mineralization of bone. Bisphosphonate leads to an increase in spine and hip bone mineral density (BMD) and prevent fractures.

Bisphosphonates are generally given orally once monthly or weekly. The half-life of bisphosphonates in bone is 10 years and therefore can be discontinued after a 5-year course of therapy.

Alendronate (70 mg) and **risedronate** (35 mg) orally once weekly reduces the risk of both vertebral and non vertebral fractures.

Ibandronate sodium, in one monthly dose of 150 mg, reduces the risk of vertebral fractures but not non vertebral fractures.

These oral bisphosphonates can cause nausea, chest pain, hoarseness, erosive esophagus and increased risk of developing esophageal cancer.

Zoledronic acid (2-4 mg once yearly) and **pamidronate** (30–60 mg every 3–6 month) are intravenous preparations, which are indicated when oral bisphosphonates cannot be tolerated or contraindicated. They are highly potent, especially zoledronic acid and are liable to cause serious side effects.

Bisphosphonates therapy can cause several side effects that are collectively known as the acute-phase response most commonly occurring after the first dose. Symptoms include GIT disorders, fever, musculoskeletal pain, dyspepsia, headache and edema.

Osteonecrosis of the jaw (ONJ) is rare but can occur spontaneously or after tooth extraction.

Atypical "chalk-like" fractures of the femur have occurred especially in patients concurrently taking high dose corticosteroids and those receiving bisphosphonate therapy for more than 5 years.

Calcium and vitamin D

Calcium and vitamin D have limited efficacy and can be used as adjunct to other treatment.

Strontium ranelate

Strontium ranelate (2 g daily orally) is useful in the treatment of osteoporosis. It has a weak inhibitory effect on bone resorption, stimulates biochemical markers of bone formation and is incorporated within hydrooxyapatite crystals in place of calcium. There is significant increase in bone mineral density (BMD) due to substitution of heavier strontium atoms for calcium atoms in bone mineral. The most common adverse effect is diarrhea. There is a slight increased risk of venous thromboembolism. Rarely, a severe rash occurs, and this is an indication to stop treatment.

Parathyroid hormone

PTH is an anabolic agent that works by stimulating new bone formation. Teriparatide (1:34 fragment of PTH) appears superior to bisphosphonates in increasing bone mineral density in corticosteroid induced and male oesteoporosis and is reserved for patients with severe osteoporosis or who fail to respond adequately to other treatment. It should not be given with bisphosphonates as this blunts its anabolic effects.

Teriparatide is given by single subcutaneous injection of 20 µg for 24 months followed by an anti-resorptive drug such as bisphosphonates.

Teriparatide should not be used in patients with Paget's disease of bone, past history of osteosarcoma or chondrosarcoma or patients with open epiphysis or hyperkalemia. Side effects may include dizziness and leg cramps.

Calcitonin

This osteoclast inhibitor is occasionally used for treatment of postmenopausal osteoporosis.

Calcitonin also has analgesic effect in bone pain from fractures. It can be given pareterally (100–200 U daily) or as intranasal spray (200 U daily).

Adverse reaction include flu-like symptoms, allergy, arthralgias, back pain. Nasal administration may cause rhinitis and epistaxis.

Selective estrogen receptor modulators

Raloxifene (60 mg/d/orally) is useful in postmenopausal osteoporosis. It causes a reduction in LDL cholesterol but not the rise of HDL. It is less effective than estrogen but has the advantage of not causing endometrial hyperplasia, uterine bleeding, breast soreness with reduced risk of breast cancer.

Raloxifene increases the risk for thromboemolism and may cause leg cramps.

Denosumab

This is a monoclonal antibody that inhibits the proliferation and maturation of preosteoclasts into mature osteoclast bone-resorbing cells. It does this by binding to osteoclast receptor activator RANKL.

Denosumab increases bone mineral density more than oral alendronate. It is relatively well tolerated. It can decrease serum calcium and should not be used in patients with hypocalcemia. Adverse side effects include flu-like symptoms, skin diseases, serious infections, new malignancies, and pancreatitis. Its long-term safety remains unknown, so it is reserved for patients with severe osteoporosis not responding to bisphosphonates.

Calcium and vitamin D

Calcium and vitamin D have limited efficacy in the prevention of osteoporotic fractures when given in isolation but are widely used as an adjunct to other treatment, most often as combination preparations containing 500 mg calcium and 800 U vitamin D (e.g., Ad Cal D_3 Calchew D_3). They are of greatest value in preventing fragility fractures in elderly or institutionalized patients who are at high risk of calcium and vitamin D deficiency.

11
Antibacterial Drugs

Sulfonamides were the first chemotherapeutic group of antibacterial drugs to be synthesized in 1935. The discovery by Fleming, Flory and Chain in 1941 led to the isolation of penicillin from the fungus Penicillium notatum and this was the first of the antibiotics. Since then a large number of antibiotics have been produced from various sources. Further, the structures of antibiotics have been modified in the laboratory to improve their antibacterial potency and these drugs are known as semisynthetic antibiotics.

MECHANISM OF ACTION

Antibacterial (chemotherapeutic or antibiotic) drugs broadly can be grouped into:
- Bacteriostatic agents that inhibit the growth/multiplication of the bacteria, but do not kill them (e.g. sulfonamide, tetracycline and chloramphenicol)
- Bactericidal agents that kill the bacteria (e.g. penicillin, aminoglycoside, vancomycin and polymyxin)

Antibacterial drugs mainly act by disrupting bacterial metabolism or directly on the bacterial cell wall protein molecules to prevent its synthesis.

Classification of bacteria

Bacteria are classified as gram-positive and gram-negative on the basis whether they stain or not with Gram's stain. Gram-positive and gram-negative bacteria differ in several respects particularly in respect of the structure of the cell wall.

Gram-positive have a simple cell wall, withstand better desiccation than gram-negative bacteria and many form spores which resist drying. Gram-negative bacteria have a complex cell wall; multiply rapidly in the presence of moisture even when provided with minimal nourishment, which may be relevant in their relative insusceptibility to the antibacterial therapy. Some of the bacteria responsible for commonly seen infectious diseases are:

Gram-positive	Gram-negative
Staphylococcus aureus	Neisseria gonorrhoeae
Streptococcus pyogenes	Neisseria meningitidis
Streptococcus viridans	Escherichia coli
Streptococcus pneumoniae	Proteus
Enterococcus	Pseudomonas aeruginosa
	Klebsiella pneumoniae
	Salmonella,
	Haemophilus influenzae
	Vibrio cholerae

Anaerobes. These are bacteria that can live and multiply in the absence of free oxygen. Anaerobic bacteria (such as gram-positive cocci *Streptococcus* anaerobic species, gram-positive rods Clostridia and gram-negative bacilli of the Bacteroides "family") may cause severe infections like bacteremia, endocarditis, brain, lung and intra-abdominal abscess.

Choice of antibacterial drug

The choice of antibacterial treatment depends on two factors – the patient and the known or likely causative organism.

The patient

The factors that influence the choice of antibacterial drug or its dose should include history of allergy, renal and hepatic functions, site of infection (e.g. in meningitis not all drugs enter cerebrospinal fluid) and pregnancy status.

The causative organism

The ideal approach is to have a bacteriological confirmation of the organism and its antibacterial sensitivity before starting therapy, but in practice this is not always possible and may even be not necessary. The initial treatment is usually based on the knowledge of the prevalent organisms from the nature of the disease and their current sensitivity.

Antibacterial combination therapy

The indications for use of two or more antibacterial drugs are:
- To provide coverage, when infection is due to more than one organism
- For the initial therapy, when the patient is seriously ill and the results of culture are pending
- To provide synergism, when organisms are not effectively eradicated with a single drug alone (e.g. in enterococcal endocarditis, both penicillin and gentamycin are given)
- To prevent the emergence of resistant organism, as in the treatment of tuberculosis
- To minimize adverse effects, when the organism is fully sensitive to both the drugs.

The disadvantages of combination therapy lie in antagonism between antibacterial drug action and increase in the number of severity of adverse reactions.

Duration of treatment

Treatment should be continued until apparent cure has been achieved and thereafter for about 3 days to avoid relapse. It should not be unduly prolonged, as it may encourage emergence of resistant strains and lead to side effects. In many cases, a 7-day course is sufficient. In certain chronic infections such as tuberculosis or osteomyelitis, the treatment requires long periods.

Drug resistance

The major cause of failure in the treatment of infectious disease is emergence of drug resistant bacteria, which includes *Staph.aureus, Strep.pneumoniae, N.meningitidis*, Enterococci, *E.coli, P.aeruginosa,* and *M. tuberculosis*.

Resistance may be produced in several ways such as emergence of mutant (changes in genetic makeup) resistant organisms, hydrolysis of drug by enzymes produced by bacteria (β lactum antibiotics), development of alternate metabolic pathway (sulfonamides) and incorporation of foreign DNA for protein synthesis (streptomycin).

The development of resistant organisms can be minimized, if antibacterial drugs are used only when really necessary, if prophylactic use of antibacterial drugs is avoided, if given a complete course of therapeutic doses and, if combination therapy is used for diseases like tuberculosis.

Antibacterial drugs and pregnancy

Most of the antibacterial drugs are contraindicate in pregnancy because of their teratogenic effects during first trimester or their toxic effects in the second and third trimester mainly because of blood disorders.

The antibacterial drugs not known to be harmful which can be used when necessary during pregnancy include penicillins, cephalosporins, erythromycin, clarithromycin, clindamycin, vancomycin, teicoplanm, linezolid and meropenem.

11.1 CHEMOTHERAPEUTIC ANTIBACTERIAL DRUGS

SULFONAMIDES

Sulfonamides are rarely used, because of increasing bacterial resistance. They have been replaced by antibiotics, which are generally more potent and less toxic.

Mechanism of action

Sulfonamides are bacteriostatic. They, being structural analogues of para-amino benzoic acid (PABA), are taken up by bacteria instead of PABA (competitive inhibition) and prevent bacterial folic acid synthesis, which is necessary for their multiplication.

Susceptible bacteria are those, which need PABA, because they are incapable of using folic acid directly. Human cells use exogenous folic acid and thus, a lack of PABA does not affect them.

Pharmacokinetics

Sulfonamides, with exceptions, are readily absorbed following oral administration. They are widely distributed into body fluids and cross blood brain barrier to enter cerebrospinal fluid. They are metabolized by acetylation in the liver, which negates the antibacterial activity, but not the adverse effects. The acetylated fraction is very poorly soluble and tends to precipitate in the urine, unless an adequate flow in maintained.

Antibacterial spectrum

Sulfonamides are effective against a fairly wide range of bacteria, which includes gram positive bacteria and some gram-negative bacteria such as *E.coli* (the organism responsible for acute urinary tract infection), *Haemophilus influenzae* and *Shigella*. Other susceptible organisms include *B. anthrax, Nocardia, Toxoplasma*. Activity is poor against anaerobes.

Therapeutic uses

Sulfonamides are rarely used in urinary tract infections and chronic bronchitis, provided the causative organisms are susceptible and for the prophylaxis of rheumatic fever.

Sulfasoxazole (1 g every 6 hours) or long acting sulfametopyrazine (2 g once weekly) are the preferred sulfonamides.

Silver sulfadiazine is applied locally as a cream to prevent infections in burns and sodium sulfacetamide ophthalmic solution or ointment is effective in the treatment of bacterial conjunctivitis and as adjunctive therapy for trachoma. Sulfasalazine is used for ulcerative colitis, Crohn's disease and rheumatoid arthritis.

Sulfonamides are infrequently used as single agents. Many strains of formerly susceptible species of microorganisms are now resistant.

Combination of sulfonamides with trimethoprim or pyrimehtamine is synergistic and bacteriocidal. Combinations in use include trimethoprim/sulfamethoxazole (co-trimoxazole) and pyrimethamine with either sulfadoxine (used to treat malaria) or sulfadiazine (used in toxoplasmosis). Co-trimoxazole is the first line drug for pneumocystis jiroveci (formerly P carinii) infection in HIV diseases. The clinical use of these agents is limited by adverse effects. Folate supplements should be given if these agents are used in pregnancy.

Adverse effects

Severe side effects of sulfonamides are rashes, Stevens-Johnson syndrome, renal failure, bone marrow depression and agranulocytosis.

Sulfonamides may provoke hemolytic reactions in patients with glucose-6-phosphate dihydrogenase deficiency. Sulfonamides taken near the end of pregnancy increases the risk of kernicterous in newborns.

Sulfonamides are contraindicated in hepatic or renal failure and in porphyria.

TRIMETHOPRIM

Trimehoprim is chemically related to the antimalarial drug pyrimethamine. It is bacteriostatic in action and acts by interfering with folic acid metabolism at the phase when folic acid is converted to folinic acid to build up the cell nucleus. Trimethoprim selectively inhibits the enzyme dihydrofolate reductase which converts the folic acid to folinic acid resulting in the death of the bacterial cell.

The pharmacological aspects of trimethoprim are very similar to sulfonamides. Trimethoprim can be used alone for urinary and respiratory infections, prostatitis, shigelliosis and invasive salmonella infection.

CO-TRIMOXAZOLE

It is a combination of a sulfonamide (sulfamethoxazole) and trimethoprim in the proportion of 5 parts to 1 part and is bactericidal because of their synergistic activity. It has excellent tissue penetration, including bone, prostate and brain. Co-trimoxazole is the drug of choice in *Pneumocystis crainii* and *Nocardia* infection. It can also be used in acute exacerbation of chronic bronchitis, urinary tract infections and acute otitis media in children, provided the causative organism is susceptible. It is given in doses of 500 mg twice daily. Side effects are essentially that of sulfonamides.

NITROFURANTOIN

Nitrofurantoin has a fairly wide antibacterial spectrum against gram-negative bacteria responsible for urinary tract infections. It is well absorbed and is considerably concentrated in the urine. It is bactericidal and is used in uncomplicated lower urinary tract infections (especially in vancomycin-resistant *Enterococcus faecium*) except those caused by *Proteus* and *P. aeruginosa*. Prolonged therapy with nitrofurantoin should be avoided, as it is associated with chronic pulmonary syndromes that can be fatal. Nausea is the most common adverse effect and others include rashes, fever and blood disorders. It should not be used in impaired renal function, as accumulation will occur.

METHENAMINE

Mehtenamine is a urine/bladder antiseptic that is converted to formaldehyde in the urine when the pH is less than 6.0. It is rarely used because of the large number of antibiotics that are available. However, it has a limited role in uncomplicated UTI caused by multiple drug-resistant bacteria or yeast.

Side effects include bladder irritation, dysuria, and hematuria with prolonged use. It is contraindicated in glaucoma, renal insufficiency, and acidosis and should not be used concomitantly with sulfonamides.

METRONIDAZOLE

Metronidazole (500 mg orally or by IV infusion every 8 hours) is one of the most important antimicrobial drug and is extensively used in diverse clinical conditions. It kills anaerobic bacteria and some protozoa.

Pharmcokinetics

Metronidazole is well absorbed orally (bioavailability 90%) and is widely distributed in the body tissues, attaining therapeutic concentrations in vaginal secretions, semen, saliva, breast milk and CNS. It penetrates into bone and abscess cavities. More than 50% of the drug is metabolized in the liver.

Antimicrobial spectrum

Metronidazole is highly effective against anaerobic bacteria and protozoa. It has greater activity against gram-negative than gram-positive anaerobes but is active against *Clostridium perfringens* (causative organism for gas gangrene, colitis and food poisoning) and *C. difficile* (causes pseudomembranous colitis).

Protozoa that respond to metronidazole include *Giardia lamblia, Entamoeba histolytica, and Trichomonas vaginalis*. It has no direct effect on helminth *Dracunculus medinensis*, but helps in the elimination of guinea worm.

Therapeutic uses

Metronidazole is one of the most widely used drugs in diverse clinical disorders, which includes;

Protozoal infections

Amoebiasis. Acute invasive intestinal amoebic dysentery and extra-intestinal amoebiasis including amoebic liver and brain abscess. (800 mg 6 hourly/ 5–10 days).

Urogenital trichomoniasis. (2 g as a single dose or 200 mg 8 hourly/ 7 days.)

Giardiasis (2 g daily/ 3 days).

Anaerobic infections

Metronidazole is highly effective against anaerobic infections in;

Leg ulcers and pressure sores

Bacterial vaginosis

Acute ulcerative gingivitis

Acute dental infections
Antibiotic associated colitis (pseuomembranous colitis)
Intra-abdominal infections
Surgical and gynaecological sepsis in which its activity against colonic anaerobes, especially *B. fragilis* is important.
Surgical prophylaxis
Intravenous (500 mg every 8 hours) metronidazole together with human tetanus immunoglobulin in established cases of tetanus

Other infections

H. pylori eradication along with omeprazole (proton pump inhibitor) and clarithromycin

Topical metronidazole gel 0.75% used in the management of rosacea and for reduction of the odour produced by anaerobic bacteria in fungating tumors.

Adverse effects

Metronidazole may cause GIT disturbances. Rarely, it may cause neurological and blood disorders and anaphylaxis. With alcohol, it produces disulfiram like reactions.

QUINOLONES

Nalidixic acid was the first quinolone to be introduced in 1960 for the treatment of GIT and urinary infections, but bacterial resistance and side effects limited its use.

The development of fluorinated derivatives called fluoroquinolones resulted in antibacterial activity with extended spectrum, higher potency, better tissue penetration and lesser bacterial resistance.

FLUOROQUINOLONES

Mechanism of action

Floroquinolones are rapidly bactericidal. They interfere with an enzyme (DNA gyrase) which is necessary for the cell division (DNA replication) of bacteria.

Antibacterial spectrum

Fluoroquinolones have a wide range of antibacterial activity. They are active against both gram-positive and gram-negative bacteria. They are particularly active against gram-negative bacteria, including *Salmonella, Shigella, Campylobacter, Neisseria* and *Pseudomonas*. They are moderately active against gram-positive bacteria such as *Strep. pneumoniae* and *Enterococcus fecalis*, *Chlamydia, Mycoplasma* and some Mycobacteria. Most anaerobic organisms are not susceptible.

Pharmacokinetics

Fluoroquinolones are well absorbed orally. The maximum serum levels are similar irrespective of the route (oral or IV) of administration. They are widely distributed throughout the body. Concentrations in lung, sputum, muscle, bone, prostate and phagocytes exceed that in plasma. They are excreted in urine. Antacids, sucralfate, bismuth, iron, calcium and zinc preparations markedly impair oral absorption.

Therapeutic uses

Norfloxacin is the least active of the fluoroquinolones against both gram negative and gram-positive organism. **Lomefloxacin** (400 mg daily) orally is useful in urinary tract infections caused by gram-negative organisms, but is not the fluoroquinolone of choice. They are not useful for systemic infections. They should not be used in children and pregnancy, in cases of porphyria and renal impairment.

Ciprofloxacin (500 mg orally once a day or 200–400 mg IV 12 hourly) and **ofloxacin** (200–400 mg orally or IV 12 hourly) are active against gram-positive aerobes including many β lactamase producing organisms. These drugs are commonly used for urinary tract infections, typhoid, prostatitis, gonorrhea (single-dose therapy) and intra-abdominal infections (with metronidazole). They are the preferred drug in adults as a prophylactic for close contact with meningococcal meningitis.

Ciprofloxacin is the most active quinolone against *P. aeruginosa* and is the quinolone of choice for serious infections with this organism. It has relatively poor activity against gram-positive cocci and should not be used as empiric monotherapy for community-acquired pneumonia, skin and soft-tissue infections or intra-abdominal infections.

Levofloxacin (250–750), **gatifloxacin** (400 mg), **sparfloxacin** (200–400 mg) and **moxifloxacin** (400 mg) are newer fluoroquinolones, which can be used orally or IV, given every 12 hourly. They are effective in aerobic infections, but less against gram-negative bacteria (especially *P. aeruginosa*) as compared to ciprofloxacin. Moxifloxacin and gatifloxacin have reasonable anaerobic activity, making them useful in mixed aerobic/anaerobic infections.

The important therapeutic uses on newer fluoroquinolones are:
- sinusitis, bronchitis and community acquired pneumonia
- urinary tact infections (except moxifloxacin, since it is minimally eliminated in the urine)
- soft-tissue infections as an alternative to β-lactum antibiotics
- post-operative surgical, obstetrical/gynecological infections
- multidrug resistant TB and atypical mycobacterial infections.

Adverse effects

Fluoroquinolones are extremely well tolerated. The principal adverse reactions with fluoroquinolones are gastrointestinal upsets (nausea) and skin rashes. They should be avoided, if possible, in patients with epilepsy as they have the potential to cause seizures, and in children they may cause damage to developing weight-bearing joints. They can also cause pain and inflammation of tendons, especially in older people.

Gatifloxacin has been associated with hyperglycemia in diabetic patients and with hypoglycemia in patients receiving oral hypoglycemic drugs. Because of these serious effects (including some fatalities), gatifloxacin is no longer available in USA.

Fluoroquinolones should be discontinued if psychiatric, neurological or hypersensitivity symptoms occur.

NSAIDs and theophylline increase the risk of convulsions and anticoagulant action of warfarin is enhanced, if used with fluoroquinolones.

11.2 ANTIBIOTICS

Antibiotics are soluble compounds that are derived from certain micro-organism and that inhibit the growth of other micro-organisms. Large number of chemically unrelated antibiotics are available and they can be grouped under following heads:
- β lactum group
- Aminoglycosides
- Tetracyclines
- Chloramphenicol
- Macrolides
- Miscellaneous antibiotics

β LACTUM ANTIBIOTICS

The β lactum antibiotics contain a β lactum ring, which is the key structural feature essential for their antibacterial activity. The β lactum includes penicillins, cephalosporins and other β lactum antibiotics.

PENICILLINS

The penicillins are bactericidal. They inhibit the synthesis of the bacterial cell wall by causing lysis of the bacterial cell membrane.

Pharmacokinetics

Natural penicillin (**benzylpenicillin**) is broken down by the gastric acid and is not effective orally. It is rapidly excreted by renal tubular secretion and the bactericidal levels are maintained for 4 to 6 hours after parenteral administration.

Penicillins diffuse well into body tissues and fluids, but penetration in cerebrospinal fluid is poor except, when meninges are inflamed.

They are excreted in urine in therapeutic concentrations. Probenecid blocks the renal tubular excretion of the penicillin, producing higher and more prolonged concentrations.

Antibacterial Drugs

Antibacterial spectrum

Benzylpenicillin (penicillin G) is effective against many streptococcal, pneumococcal and meningococcal infections and also for syphilis, anthrax, gas gangrene, tetanus, leptospirosis, actinomycosis and infections caused by Listeria monocytogenes. Most staphylococci and some strains of meningococci and gonococci have become resistant to penicillin G.

Therapeutic uses

Penicillins have a somewhat diminished role in therapy, because of acquired resistance in many bacterial species through alterations in penicillin-binding proteins or hydrolysis by enzyme β lactamase. However, penicillins remain the drug of first choice in streptococcal infections (such as endocarditis, dental infections, throat infections, and erysipelas), meningococcal meningitis, syphilis, anthrax, actinomycosis and Listeria infections. It is also useful in pneumonia, gas gangrene and tetanus and for prophylaxis in rheumatic fever and in limb amputation.

Penicillin G is generally given in doses of 1.2 g daily in 4 divided doses (2.4 g or more in severe cases) by intramuscular route or by intravenous infusion. It is contraindicated in penicillin hypersensitivity.

Adverse effects

The most important side effect of the penicillins is *hypersensitivity, which causes rashes and anaphylaxis and can be fatal.*

Penicillin allergic patients occasionally have allergic reactions to cephalosporins.

Penicillin, rarely, may cause encephalopathy due to cerebral irritation when very high doses are given or in patients with renal failure. This is the reason *penicillin should not be given by intrathecal injection.* Oral penicillin frequently causes diarrhea. Penicillins reduce the efficacy of oral contraceptives.

The only contraindication to the use of penicillin is penicillin hypersensitivity.

Procaine benzylpenicillin

Procaine penicillin G is a sparingly soluble salt of benzylpenicillin. It is used by intramuscular route and provides therapeutic blood levels up to 24 hours. It is the drug of choice for treatment of neurosyphilis in doses of 2 ml (procaine benzylpenicillin 600 mg and benzylpenicillin sodium 10 mg) daily for 10–14 days in combination with probenecid.

Procaine penicillin G is no longer used for pneumococcal pneumonia or gonorrhea as many strains are penicillin resistant.

Benzathine Penicillin

Benzathine penicillin is a long acting IM repository form of penicillin G that is used for the treatment of syphilis. In early latent syphilis one dose and in late latent syphilis three doses of 2.4 million units are given by deep intramuscular route. It is occasionally given for group A streptococcal pharygitis and prophylaxis after acute rheumatic fever or poststreptococcal glomerulonephritis.

Benzylpenicillin has a narrow antibacterial spectrum, is orally ineffective and certain organisms develop resistance to its antibacterial action due to production of an enzyme penicillinase, which inactivates penicillin by hydrolysis of the β lactum ring. To overcome the disadvantages of natural penicillin G, a number of semisynthetic penicillins have been produced. The available penicillins are:

- Oral penicillin
- Penicillinase resistant penicillin
- Broad spectrum penicillins
- Extended-spectrum penicillins (ureidopenicillins)

ORAL PENICILLIN

Phenoxymethyl penicillin (penicillin V) is less potent than penicillin G, but is gastric acid stable. It is used orally (250–500 mg 4 times a day) principally for group A streptococcal pharyngitis in children and for prophylaxis against rheumatic fever. It should not be used for severe infections.

PENICILLINASE RESISTANT PENECILLINS

These are semi synthetic penicillins that are not inactivated by penicillinase and are used extensively for the treatment of infections caused by staphylococcus aureus, such as otitis externa, impetigo, cellulites and staphylococcal endocarditis.

Flucloxacillin is not inactivated by penicillinase and is used extensively for treating infections caused by staphylococci, such as otitis externa, impetigo, cellulites, and staphylococcal endocarditis in doses of 250–500 mg every 6 hours orally or by injection.

Strains of staphylococci are emerging, which are even resistant to flucloxacillin. They are named methicillin (now discontinued) resistant staphylococcus aureus (MRSA) and respond to only vancomycin or teicoplanin.

Flucloxacillin, in addition to general side effects of natural penicillin, may cause cholestatic jaundice several weeks after stoppage of the treatment.

Nafcillin and **oxacillin** (2 g IV 4–6 hourly) are the semi synthetic penicillinase-resistant penicillins that are the drugs of choice for treating oxacillin sensitive staphylococcus (OSSA) infections. These drugs have little activity against enterococci or gram-negative bacteria.

Dicloxacillin and **cloxacillin** are oral (250–500 mg 4 hourly) antibiotics with a spectrum of activity similar to that of nafcillin and oxacillin and are typically used in the treatment of localized skin infections.

β LACTAMASE INHIBITORS

Clavulanic acid, sulbacctum and tazobactum are substances that irreversibly bind β lactamase (penicillinase) and, thus prevent the breakdown of β lactum ring.

β lactamase inhibitors have no significant antibacterial activity of their own, but are used in combination with broad spectrum and antipseudomonal penicillins against resistant organisms.

BROAD SPECTRUM PENICILLINS

These are aminopenicillins and include ampicillin and amoxicillin. These penicillins tend to be active against many gram-negative bacilli and have the same activity as natural penicillin against gram-positive bacteria. They are effective against *Salmonella, E. coli, Shigella* and *H. influenzae* but they are inactivated by penicillinase producing organisms.

Ampicillin is given orally or by injection. Orally, less than half is absorbed and absorption is further decreased by the presence of food in the gut. It is well excreted in the bile and urine.

Ampicillin (2–3 g IV 4–6 hourly) is the drug of choice for treatment of infections caused by enterococcus species (gram-positive anaerobic cocci: *E. faecalis* and *E. faecium*), which are normal inhabitant of the human intestinal tract and occasionally cause urinary tract infections, infective endocarditis and bacteremia, and *L. monocytogenes* (Gram-negative bacteria causing infections like meningitis, endocarditis, and disseminated granulomatous lesions). Oral ampicillin (250–500 mg 6 hourly) is very useful in chronic bronchitis, uncomplicated sinusitis, pharyngitis, otitis media, urinary infections and typhoid.

Many gram-negative species produce β lactamases and are resistant, precluding use of ampicillin for empirical therapy of urinary tract infections, meningitis, and typhoid fever, Ampicillin is not active against, *Klebsiella, Enterobacter, P. aeruginosa*, serratia, indole-positive proteus species, and other gram-negative aerobes that are commonly encountered in hospital-acquired infections.

Ampicillin/sulbactum (1.5–3.0 g IV 6 hourly) is effective against OSSA, anaerobes, and enterobacter and is used for the treatment of the upper and lower respiratory tract, genitourinary tract, and abdominal, pelvic, and polymicrobial soft-tissue infections and is the *drug of choice* for serious cellulites due to human or animal bites.

Amoxicillin is a derivative of ampicillin and has a similar antibacterial spectrum. It is better absorbed and its absorption is not affected by the presence of food in the stomach. It also produces higher plasma and tissue concentrations and is preferred to ampicillin.

Amoxicillin in doses of 250–500 mg orally every 8 hours is commonly used in chronic bronchitis, urinary infections, otitis media, sinusitis, dental infections and typhoid fever.

Amoxycillin is also indicated along with gentamycin in endocarditis caused by enterococci and meningitis caused by Listeria and as an adjuvant for H. pylori eradication.

Amoxicilin/clavulanic acid (Augmentin) is an oral antibiotic similar to ampicillin/sulbactum and is used in doses of 875 mg every 12 hourly as a *step-down therapy* from IV ampicillin/sulbactum. It is useful for treating complicated sinusiis, otitis mdia, and skin infections and is the *oral antibiotic of choice* for prophylaxis in human and animal bites after appropriate local treatment.

Broad spectrum penicillins give rise to gastrointestinal disorders, rarely antibiotic associated colitis and rashes.

EXTENDED-SPECTRUM PENICILLINS (UREIDO-PENICILLINS)

These are extended spectrum penicillins (ureidopenicillin) that have the antibacterial spectrum as ampicillin, but are also effective against pseudomonas aeruginosa and proteus morgani. They are inactivated by β lactamases and are not active against penicillin resistant staphylococci. They are not absorbed from the gut and must be given by injection.

Azlocillin, piperacillin and **ticarcillin** (4 g IV 6 hourly) have reasonable antipseudomal activity but generally require co-administration of an aminoglycoside for treatment of serious infections.

Ticarcillin/clavulanic acid (3.1 g IV 6 hourly) combination extends the spectrum to include most Enterobacteriaceae, OSSA, and anaerobes, making it a useful antibiotic for intra-abdominal and complicated soft-tissue infections.

Piperacillin is a ureido penicillin and is more active against P. aeruginosa than ticarcillin and is given in a dos of 4 g every 6–8 hours. **Zosyn** is a preparation that combines piperacillin with tazobactum (β lactamse inhibitor) and the dose is 2.25 g.

Exended-spectrum penicillins are reserved for serious infections with pseudomonas and in polymicrobial infection, where the causative organisms are not known such as peritonitis from ruptured viscous, osteomylitis in a diabetic patient or traumatic. They are usually combined with an aminoglycoside (gentamycin), since they have a synergistic action. As these drugs are excreted via the kidney, the dose should be reduced in renal impairment. Side effects and contraindications are the same as with other penicillins.

Adverse reactions of penicillins

Penicillins are generally free from toxic effects. However, they may cause rarely pain and abscess at the site of injection. Urticarial rash is common, which is sometimes resistant to treatment. Broad-spectrum penicillins may cause erythematous rash, which may even occur after the drugs have been stopped. Rarely, penicillin causes an *acute anaphylactic reaction with collapse*, which may be *fatal*. The incidence of allergic reactions in small children is negligible.

CEPHALOSPORINS

The cephalosporins are safe and reliable broad spectrum antibiotics and consist of large group of antibiotics with marked differences in activity, pharmacokinetics and toxicity. Like penicillin, they also contain β lactum ring and are amenable to inactivation by the enzyme β lactamase. All currently available cephalosporins are devoid of activity against enterococci and *L. monocytogenes*. They are synificantly associated with, *C. difficile* infection. Cephalosporins are arranged in generations and more active compounds are only available in intravenous form. Most of them can be given by injection only. They are divided into five groups:

The *first-generation cephalosporins* have a spectrum that include penicillinase-producing, methicillin-susceptible Staphylococci and most Streptococci, but are not the drugs of choice for infections with gram-positive bacteria. They have excellent activity against *E. coli, K. pneumoniae,* and *P. mirabilis* and are among the drugs of choice for community-acquired urinary tract infections.

Cefazolin (1–2 g IV/IM 8 hourly) is a parenteral preparation, while **cefadroxil, cefalexin,** and **cefradine** are oral preparations, which are given in doses of 500 mg every 6 hourly.

The *parenteral second-generation cefalosporins* extend the gram-negative spectrum of first generation compounds. No second-generation cephalosporin is active against *Pseudomonas* and *Acinetobacter*. The various second-generation agents have different activities and can be divided into above-the-diaphragm and below the-diaphragm agents.

Above the diaphragm

Cefuroxime (1.5 g IV/IM 8 hourly) and **cefamandole** (1–2 g IV/IM 4–6 hourly) have good activity against gram-positive (Staphylococci and Streptococci) and gram-negative aerobes that include *Klebsiella, Proteus, H. influnzae,* and *Serratia* and *N. gonorrhoeae*. They are not effective against *B. fragilis*. They are useful in:

- Skin/soft- tissue infections
- Community acquired pneumonia (cefuroxime)
- Complicated urinary tract infections

Below the diaphragm

Cefoxitin (1–2 g IV 4–8 hourly), **cefotetan** (1–2 g IV/IM 12 hourly) and **cefmetazole** (2 g IV every 6–12 hourly) do not have dependable activity against gram-positive organisms, but have an extended spectrum against gram-negative aerobes and anaerobes including *B. fragilis*. They are useful for surgical prophylaxis and treatment of:

- intra-abdominal prophylaxis and infections
- gynecological prophylaxis and infections
- diverticulitis
- pelvic inflammatory diseases

Oral second-generation cephalosporins include **cefuroxime axetil, cefprozil** and **cefaclor** and are given in doses of 250–500 mg twice a day. They have fair activity against gram-positive cocci and *H. influenzae* and are widely used in outpatient therapy for otitis media, bronchitis, sinusitis, and lower respiratory tract infections, urinary tract infections, local soft-tissue infections and step-down therapy for pneumonia or cellulites responsive to parenteral cephalosporins.

Loracarbef is chemically classified as a carbapenem rather than a cephalosporin but is generally used for the same indications as the oral second-generation cephalosporins.

The *parenteral third-generation* cephalosporins have broad coverage against enteric, aerobic gram-negative rods and retain significant activity against streptococci other than enterococci. They have moderate anaerobic activity but do not reliably cover *B. fragilis*.

Ceftazidime is the only third generation cephalosporin that is useful for treating serious *P. aeruginosa* infections. Several of these agents have substantial CNS penetration and are useful in treating meningitis.

Third-generation cephalosporins are not reliable for treatment of serious infections caused by organisms producing ampicillin-inducible beta-lactamases regardless of the results of susceptibility testing. These microbes should be treated with cefepime, carbapenems, or quinolones.

Ceftriaxone (1–2 g IV/IM 12–24 hourly), **cefotaxime** (1–2 g IV/IM 4–12 hourly), **ceftazidime** (1–2 g IV/IM 6 hourly), **ceftizoxime** (1–4 g IV/IM 8–12 hourly) and **cefoperazone** (2–4 g IV 12 hourly) are very similar to one another in spectrum and efficacy. They are used when the causative organism is not known (empiric therapy) or other antibacterial drugs are contraindicated. Their main indications are:

- pyelonephritis, urosepsis and pneumonia (cetriaxone or cefotaxime)
- intra-abdominal infections in combination with metronidazole
- gonorrhea and meningitis (ceftriaxone and cefotaxime)
- osteomyelitis, septic arthritis, endocarditis and soft-tissue infections, if the organism has been identified.

Oral third-generation cephalosporins include **cefpodoxime proxetil** (100–400 mg), **cefdinir** (300 mg), **ceftibuten** (400 mg), and **cefditoren pivoxil** (200–400 mg). They are given twice a day for the treatment of bronchitis and complicated sinusitis, otitis media, and urinary tract infections. They can also be used as step-down therapy for pneumonia that is responsive to third-generation parenteral cephalosporins. Cefpodoxime can be used as single-dose therapy for uncomplicated gonorrhea.

The *parenteral fourth-generation cephalosporin.*

Cefepime (500 mg–2 g IV/IM 8–12 hourly) is a fourth generation cephalosporin with excellent all-round activity including *P. aeruginosa* and other bacteria producing β lactamases. It is routinely used for empiric therapy in febrile neutropenic patients. It is used for serious antibiotic-resistant gram-negative bacillary and some polymicrobial infections (involving gram-negatives and gram-positives) in most sites.

The parenteral fifth-generation cephalosporins

Ceftobiprole and ceftaroline are the first of a new generation extended spectrum cephalosporins with similar anti-bacterial spectrum, pharmacokinetics and therapeutic uses. Ceftaroline is approved by FDA for clinical use. **Ceftaroline** is a broad-spectrum antibiotic active against a wide range of pathogens including gram-positive cocci: methicillin resistant *S. aureus* (MRSA) and *S. epidermidis*, penicillin resistant activity to third generation cephalosporins such as ceftazidime and cetriaxone against most gram-negative pathogens.

Caftaroline fosamil is given in doses of 600 mg by intravenous route lasting over 1 hour every 12 hourly for 5 to 14 days. It has low protein binding (< 20%) and serum half life of 2.6 hours. No drug accumulation occurs with multiple doses and elimination occurs primarily through renal excretion, no dose adjustment is needed for mild renal impairment.

Ceftaroline is approved for the treatment of complicated skin and soft structure infections and community-associated pneumonia. Ceftaroline is the sixth antibiotic to be approved by FDA for the treatment of cSSSI caused by MRSA. It is the first cephalosporin with this indication.

Ceftaroline has the potential to be used as monotherapy for polymicrobial infections, because of its broad-spectrum activity. However, the use of ciftaroline in absence of a proven or strongly suspected bacterial infection should be avoided to prevent the risk of development of drug-resistant bacteria.

Ceftaroline is well tolerated. The most common adverse effects include diarrhea, nausea and rash. *Clostridium difficile*-associated diarrhea (CDAD), common with nearly all broad-spectrum antibacterial drugs, my occur ranging in severity from mild diarrhea to fatal colitis. It is contraindicated in patients hypersensitive to cephalosporins. Anaphylaxis and anaphylactic reactions have been reported with ceftaroline.

Pharmacokinetic drug interaction does not occur with caftaroline because it does not inhibit major cytochrome P 450 enzymes.

Mechanism of action

Cephalosporins, like penicillins, inhibit bacterial cell wall synthesis and are bactericidal.

Bacterial resistance

Cephalosporins are highly resistant to penicillinase. Some bacteria elaborate a β lactamase called cephalosporinase that acts on cephalosporin nucleus to destroy its antibacterial activity. However, many newer cephalosporins are resistant to cephalosporinase.

Adverse effects

The principal side effect is hypersensitivity reactions and about 10% of patients, who are allergic to penicillin, will also be allergic to cephalosporins.

Gastrointestinal disorders are seen and rarely may lead to antibiotic associated colitis. Other side effects include blood disorders, hemorrhage due to interference with blood clotting factors and renal and hepatic impairment.

Cephalosporins are contraindicated in hypersensitivity and porphyria.

OTHER β LACTUM ANTIBIOTICS

Aztreonam is only effective against gram-negative aerobic bacteria including *P. aeruginosa, N. meningitides, H. influenzae* and *N. gonorrhoeae*. It has no activity against gram-positive organisms or anaerobes and should not be used for blind therapy. Usual dose is 1–2 g IV every 6–8 hours. It is useful in patients allergic to penicillin or cephalosporin, as no apparent cross hyersensitivity is present.

Carbapenems

These have the broadest antibiotic activity of the β-lactum antibiotics and include activity against anerobes. They are available in intravenous formulation only.

Imipenem (500 mg-1 g IV/IM 6–8 hourly) and **meropenem** (1 g IV 8 hourly) are short acting and **ertapenem** (1 g IV 24 hourly) is long-acting carbapenem. They are bactericidal and act by interfering with cell wall synthesis.

Carbapenems have a broad antibacterial spectrum of activity, which includes most gram-positive and gram-negative bacteria, anaerobes as well as organisms producing ampicillin/cephalosporin β lactamases. Notable bacteria that are resistant include amipicllin resistant enterococci and methicillin-resistant *S. aureus* (MRSA) and *C. difficile*.

Carbapenems are generally used for empiric treatment of antibiotic-resistant nosocomial (hospital acquired) infections at most body sites. Some of the common uses of carbapenems include severe polymicrobial infections, gangrene, intra-abdominal catastrophes, and sepsis in compromised patients. Meropenem is the dug of choice for the treatment of CNS infections.

Carbapenems should be avoided in patients with CNS pathology or renal insufficiency, as they may cause convulsions. Ideally, they are used unless no reasonable therapy is available. Cross-hypersensitivity is present with penicillin and like cephalosporin; carbapenems have been associated with anaphylaxis, nephritis, and blood disorders.

AMINOGLYCOSIDES

This group of antibiotics includes gentamycin, kanamycin, tobramycin, amikacin, netilmicin, spectinomycin, neomycin and

streptomycin. They have a number a number of common properties:
- They are bactericidal and are generally used as a component of combination therapy.
- They are not orally absorbed and have to be given intramscularly for systemic effects
- They are excreted by kidneys and accumulation occurs with impaired renal function
- They have potential ototoxicity and nephrotoxicity, especially in elderly and patients with renal failure
- They impair neuromuscular transmission

Antibacterial spectrum

Aminoglycosides are effective against a wide range of gram-positive and gram-negative organisms. Susceptible organisms include *S. aureus, S. viridans, Enterococci, H. influenzae, Brucella abortis, E. coli, Proteus, Pseudomonas, Klebsiella*. Streptomycin is also effective against *Mycobacterium tubrculosis* (all forms of tuberculosis).

Aminoglycosides are not particularly effective against *Streptococcus pneumoniae* or *Streptococcus pyogenes*.

Aminoglycosides are not effective against anaerobes and their activity is impaired in low pH/low oxygen environment of abscesses.

Mechanism of action

Aminoglycosides inhibit protein biosynthesis and are bactericidal. In normal cell RNA is bound to ribosomes, which are essential for protein synthesis. Aminoglycosides bind onto ribosomes, excluding the RNA and thus protein synthesis is inhibited. They also disrupt the bacterial cytoplasm membrane.

Bacterial resistance

Bacteria produce several enzymes that inactivate the aminoglycoside molecule. Amikacin and netilmicin are not affected by most aminoglycoside inactivating enzymes that cause bacterial resistance in some species.

Pharmacokinetics

Aminoglycosides are not absorbed from the gut. They are distributed in all extracellular fluids, but tissue concentrations are low except in the kidney and ear. Penetration in the cerebrospinal fluid is poor unless the meninges are inflamed. Excretion is principally by glomerular filtration and accumulation occurs in renal impairment. All the aminoglycosides are more active in alkaline environment

Gentamycin is the most important of the aminoglycosides and is widely used, especially in the treatment of severe staphylococcal infections and those caused by various gram-negative organisms. It is given by intramuscular or intravenous and intrathecal injection or as eye/ear drops. Excretion is fairly rapid so that it is usually given three times daily. The dose of gentamycin for most infections is up to 5 mg/kg daily given in divided doses every 8 hours and normally the treatment should not exceed 7 days. By intrathecal route, it is given in a dose of 1mg (increased, if necessary to 5 mg) along with intramuscular therapy.

Kanamycin is rarely used in gram-negative infections. It is not effective against pseudomonas.

Tobramycin, amikacin and **netilmicin** have similar activity as that of gentamycin. However, they are sometimes effective against gram-negative organisms, which are resistant to gentamycin. They are only indicated in the treatment of serious infections caused by gentamycin resistant gram-negative bacilli. Netilmicin is less liable to cause ototoxicity.

Tobramycin is also available as an inhalatonal agent for adjunctive therapy for patients with cystic fibrosis or bronchiectasis complicated by P. aeruginosa infection.

Amikacin has an unique role in mycobacterial and Nocardia infections.

Spectinomycin has only one use, the treatment of gonorrheal infection due to organisms, which have become resistant to penicillin.

Neomycin is too toxic for parenteral administration. It is very poorly absorbed from the gut and is only used to sterilize the gut prior to surgery or in hepatic failure.

Streptomycin. The development of resistance to streptomycin is relatively common. It is rarely used for infections other than drug resistant tuberculosis and as an alternative to gentamycin resistant enterococcal endocarditis

Therapeutic uses

Gentamycin is the drug of choice and used in:
- Peritonitis and biliary tract cephalosporin resistant infections (with ampicillin)
- Endocarditis caused by *Strept. viridans* or *Strep. faecalis* and hospital acquired pneumonia (with penicillin)
- Meningitis caused by listeria (with amoxicillin)
- Acute pyelonephritis or prostatitis (with ampicillin)
- Septicemia community or hospital acquired (with amoxicilin)
- Prulent conjunctivitis – gentamycin eye drops

Adverse effects

Aminoglycosis may cause vestibular and auditory damage (ototoxicity), nephrotoxicity and antibiotic associated colitis. Streptomycin is unique in that it causes more ototoxicity with a lower risk of nephrotoxicity.

Aminoglycosides are contraindicated in pregnancy and myasthenia gravis.

Frusemide increases the risk of ototoxicity.

TETRACYCLINES AND GLYCYLCYCLINES

Tetracyclines have similar pharmacological properties. They are **chlotetracycline, oxytetracycline, tetracycline, doxycycline, minocycline** and **demeclocycline**.

Mechanism of action

Tetracyclines are primarily bacteriosatic. They inhibit protein synthesis by binding to ribosomes.

Antibacterial spectrum

Tetracyclines are broad spectrum antibiotics. They inhibit not only the bacteria, but also some of the large viruses. The important organisms, which respond to tetracyclines include H. influenzae, *Strep. pneumoniae, Mycoplasmas, Chlamydia, Rickettsiae, Nocardia, Brucella abortus, Helicobacter pylori, Treponema pallidum,* and against some protoza (e.g. amebas). However, their general use is limited because of widespread resistance among most common bacterial pathogens.

Pharmacokinetics

Tetracyclines are well absorbed from the GIT, particularly from the stomach and upper small intestine. Blood levels are maintained with 6 hourly doses. Absorption is decreased by milk, antacids and calcium, iron and magnesium salts. They are widely distributed to tissues and body fluids. The penetration, across the meningeal barrier into CSF is variable (about 20%), unless the meninges are inflamed. They undergo enterohepatic circulation and are primarily excreted via the kidneys, although there is some fecal excretion. Tetracyclines are deposited in growing bones and teeth, causing staining and dental hyperplasia.

Doxycycline and minocycline are slowly excreted, so that only one dose is required daily. Unlike, other tetracyclines, doxycycline and minocycline absorption is not affected by food and calcium. Doxycycline does not exacerbate renal failure and can be used when renal function is impaired.

Therapeutic uses

Tetracycline and oxytetracycline are given in doses of 250–500 mg every 6 hours, while doxycycline and minocycline are given in doses of 100–200 mg once a day. Chlortetracycline is only available as eye drops or as an ointment.

Tetracyclines are the drug of choice for the treatment of infections caused by *Chlamydia* (trachoma, psittacosis, salpingitis, urethritis and lymphoganuloma inguinale), rickettsia (including Q fever), *Brucella* (doxycycline with either streptomycin or rifampin), the spirochaetes and *Borrelia burgdorferi* (lyme disease).

Tetracyclines are also used in respiratory and genital mycoplasma infections, in acne, in destructive (refractory) periodontal disease, in exacerbations of chronic bronchitis and leptospirosis in penicillin sensitive patients (as an alternative to erythromycin). Tetracyclines are used in combindation regimens to treat peptic ulcer caused by *Helicobacter pylori*. They are also used in infection caused by *Entamoeba histolytica*. Doxycycline is used for the prophylaxis against malaria and for treatment of community-acquired pneumonia. Minocycline is second-line therapy for pulmonary nocardiosis and cervicofacial actinomycosis.

Adverse effects

The most common side effect of tetracyclines is superinfection due to their broad antibacterial spectrum, which causes considerable changes in the bacterial flora in the intestine and elsewhere. This may result in antibiotic associated colitis, due to multiplication of resistant organisms, usually a *Staphylococcus*. *Candida* is the other troublesome organism, which may emerge causing "thrush" in the mouth or vaginal candidiasis.

Tetracyclines damage and colour developing teeth and depress bone growth and should be avoided from the fourth month of pregnancy until the child is 12 years old.

Other toxic effects include exacerbation of renal failure, rarely skin rashes and drug sensitization.

Doxycycline can be used in renal impairment.

Glycylcyclines (tigecycline)

Chemical modification of tetracycline has produced tigecyline, a broad-spectrum antibiotic with activity especially against resistant gram-positive and gram-negative pathogens. Many tetracycline-resistant strains are susceptible to tigecycline. Its spectrum is very broad. Coagulase-negative staphylococci and S. aureus, including methicillin resistant and vancomycin resistant strains, streptiococci, penicillin/vancomycin resistant enterococci, gram-positive rods, extended spectrum β-lactamoses (EBSL) excluding pseudomonas spp., multi-drug-resistant strains of acinetobactor; anaerobics, both gram-positive and gram-negative; atypical agents, rickettsiae, chlamydia and legionella, and rapidly growing mycobacteria all are susceptible.

Given intravenously as 100 mg loading dose; then 50 mg every 12 hours, tigecycline has excellent intracellular penetration. Elimination is biliary and can be given safely in renal insufficiency. Main side effect is nausea is addition to usual side effects of tetracyclenes.

Tigecycline is mainly indicated in skin and soft tissue infection and intra-abdominal infections due to multidrug resistant organisms.

CHLORAMPHENICOL

Chloramphenicol (chloromycetin) is a potent and cheap antibiotic, which is rarely used because of its potential toxicity, bacterial resistance and the availability of many other effective alternatives. Its use is increasingly reserved for severe and life-threatening infections where other antibodies are either unavailable or impractical. It is bacteriostatic to most organisms but apparently bacteriocidal to *H. influenzae, Strep. pneumoniae* and *N. meningitides*. It has a very broad-spectrum of activity against aerobic and anaerobic organisms, spirochaetes, rickettsia, and *Mycoplasma* spp. It also has useful activity against anaerobes such as *B. fragilis*.

It is well absorbed orally and unlike tetracycline crosses the meningeal barrier and diffuses widely into the CSF. It crosses placenta and reaches breast milk.

The main indications of chlorphanicol include serious rickettsial infections, as an alternative to a β-lactum antibiotic for meningococcal meningitis or bacterial meningitis caused by penicillin resistant preumococci..

Chloramphenicol is used topically in the treatment of eye infections because of its board spectrum and its penetration of ocular tissues and the aqueous humor. It is ineffective for chlamydial infections.

Dose-dependent adverse effects include 'grey baby' syndrome in infants (cyanosis and circulatory collapse due to inability to conjugate drug and excrete active form in urine) and reversible bone narrow depression in adults.

Severe idiopathic aplastic anemia, unrelated to dose, duration of therapy or route of administration, occur very rarely (1:25000–40000 patients).

MACROLIDES

This group of antibiotics consists of azithromycin, clarithromycin, and dirithromycin. erythromycin

Mechanism of action

The macrolides inhibit bacterial protein synthesis by binding to ribosomes of sensitive micro-organisms. They are bacteriostatic, but can be bactericidal in some situation.

Pharmacokinetics

Erythromycin is absorbed rather erratically and diffuses into most body tissues except cerebrospinal fluid. It is concentrated in the liver and is excreted primarily in bile and feces.

Antibacterial spectrum

Erythromycin has a antibacterial spectrum, that is similar but not identical to penicillin. It is effective against some strains of *S.aureus* that are penicillin G resistant, *Strep. pyogenes, Strep. pneumoniae, Strep. viridans, M. catarrhalis, Legionella, Mycoplasma pneumoniae, Chlamydia* and atypical mycobacteria. It is, however, not always effective against *H. influenzae*, a common cause of respiratory infection. Bacteria readily become resistant to erythromycin, but do not show cross-resistance to other antibiotics.

Therapeutic uses

Erythromycin (250–500 mg orally or 0.5–1.0 g IV every 6 hours) possesses activity against gram-positive coci (except enterococci) and can be used to treat bronchitis, pharyngitis, sinusitis, otitis media, and skin-soft tissue infections in penicillin allergic patients. It is effective for treatment of atypical respiratory tract infections.

It is, however, not always effective against *Haemophilus influenzae*, a common cause of the respiratory infection.

Erythromycin is also used for treatment of *Chlamydia trachomatis* infections (500 mg orally every 6 hours for 7 days) and as an alternate therapy for syphilis in penicillin allergic patients.

Clarithromycin (250–500 mg oral twice daily) has the same antibacterial activity as erythromycin, but a higher concentration is found in the tissues and has enhanced activity against *H. influnzae* species than erythromycin. It has the same uses against infections caused by gram-positive cocci as erythromycin.

Clarithromycin has a unique role in the treatment and prophylaxis of *Mycobacterium avium* complex infections in HIV patients and is an important component of regimens used to eradicate *H. pylori* infections in peptic ulcer.

It is also active against *M. leprae* and toxoplasma gondii. Except for lower incidence of GIT intolerance and less frequent dosing, clarithromycin and erythromycin are therapeutically very similar except for the organisms noted above.

Azithromycin (500 mg) appears to be similar to clarithromycin. It differs from clarithromycin in pharmacokinetic properties. A 500 mg dose of azithromycin produces tissue concentrations exceeding serum concentrations by 10 to 100-fold. The drug is slowly released from tissues (tissue half-life 2–4 days) to produce an elimination half-life approaching 3 days. These unique properties permit once-daily dosing and shortening of the duration of treatment in many cases. For example, a single 1-g dose of azithromycin is as effective as a 7-day course of doxycycline in chlamydial cervicitis and urethritis.

Community acquired pneumonia can be treated with azithromycin given as a 500-mg loading dose, followed by a 250 mg single daily dose for the next 4 days. Another advantage of azithromycin is that it does not inactivate cytochrome P450 enzymes and therefore is free of the drug interactions that occur with erythromycin and clarithromycin.

Dirithromycin (500 mg) has a similar spectrum of activity and clinical application as erythromycin with the convenience of once-a-day dosing. Like azithromycin, it also does not have the numerous drug interactions.

Adverse effects

Macrolides are well tolerated, but can cause vomiting and diarrhea and rarely jaundice (particularly erythromycin estolate), if injected. Intravenous administration is liable to cause thrombophlebitis.

Drug interactions

Erythromycin and clarithromycin inhibit the hepatic metabolism of a large number of drugs, resulting in an increase in their plasma concentrations and consequent toxicity. Some of the drugs whose plasma concentration is increased by these macrolides include analgesics (alfentanil), anticoagulants (warfarin), antiepileptics (carbamzepine), antihistamines (terfenadine), anxiolyics and hypnotics (midazolum and zopiclone), calcium antagonists, cardiac glycosides, cisapride, ergotamine, and theophylline.

Azithromycin is free of the drug interactions that occur with erythromycin and clarithromycin.

MISCELLANEOUS ANTIBIOTICS

Clindamycin

Clindamycin (150–450 mg orally 4 times or 600–900 mg IV 8 hourly) is effective against many gram-positive organisms similar to that of erythromycin. Unlike macrolides, clindamycin is active against most anaerobes, including *B. fragilis*, enterococci but gram-negative aerobic organisms are resistant. It inhibits bacterial protein synthesis and essentially has a bactriostatic action.

Clindamycin has excellent oral bioavailability and appears to penetrate into bone and abscesses. The important indications of clindamycin are:

- Aspiration pneumonia and lung abscesses
- MRSA and streptococal infections
- Osteomyelitis
- Anaerobic infections (peritosillar/retropharyngeal abscesses, necrotizing fasciitis). For intra-abdominal infections, metroni-

dazole is preferred because of its more reliable activity against *B. fragilis.*

- Toxoplasmosis (with pyrimethamine)
- *Pneumocystis crainii* (with primaquine)

Side effects are not common; diarrhea may be a problem and rarely takes the form of a serious colitis (pseudomembranous colitis). Clindamycin enhances the actions of non-depolarising muscle relaxants and antagonizes the effect of neostigmine and pyridostigmine.

Ketolides

The ketolides were developed in response to the emergence of penicillin and macrolide resistance in respiratory pathogens. Cross resistance with macrolides is uncommon. **Telithromycin** has useful activity against common bacterial causes of respiratory infection, as well as mycoplasma, chlamydia and legionella spp.

Telithromycin is given as once-daily dose of 800 mg and has good tissue and intracellular penetration. It is partly metabolized in the liver and eliminated by biliary and urinary routes of excretion.

The main indications of telithromycin are respiratory tract infections, sinusitis, and streptococcal pharyngitis. Rare cases of hepatitis and liver failure have been reported.

Sodium fusidate

Sodium fusidate, the salt of antibiotic fusidic acid, active against gram-positive bacteria is available in intravenous, oral or topical formulation. It is lipid soluble and distribute well to tissues. However, its antibacterial activity is unpredictable. It is given orally in doses of 0.5–1 g every 8 hours in osteomyelitis and staphylococcal endocarditis. A second antistaphylococcal antibiotic (flucloxacillin) is usually combined to prevent emergence of resistance. Sodium fusidate is relatively free of side effects, though high doses may cause jaundice, which recovers when the treatment is stopped.

Dalbavancin and telavancin

These antibiotics have been developed for treatment of gram-positive bacteria, including strains with reduced susceptibility/resistant to vancomycin.

Dalbavancin has an extremely long half-life of 6–11 days, permitting once-weekly intravenous administration and is still under clinical trials.

Telavancin has a half-life of approximately 8 hours and requires once-daily intravenous dosing for the treatment of complicated skin and skin structure infections due to methicillin-resistant strains of S aureus.

Vancomycin

Vancomycin is bactericidal for most aerobic and anaerobic gram-positive bacteria, particularly staphylococci and streptococci and bacteriostatic for enterococci. It is not effective orally for systemic infections and is given by slow intravenous infusion in doses of 1g every 12 hours.

The most serious problem with vanomycin is the emergence of vacomycin-resistant *Enterococcus faecium* and vancomycin-resistant *Staphylococcus aureus*. To avoid it, vancomycin should not be used routinely for surgical prophylaxis, empiric therapy for non-specific neutropenic fever, minor localized infections (e.g. .cellulitis, carbuncle) and in topical application or irrigation. The main indications for its use include:

- serious infections caused by methicillin-resistant *Staphylococcus aureus*
- serious infections caused by ampicillin-resistnt enterococcal endocarditis in combination with gentamycin.
- serious infections caused by gram-positive bacteria in patients allergic to all other antibacterial drugs
- oral first-line treatment of severe pseudomembranous colitis that has not responded to metronidazole
- empirically in suspected gram-positive meningitis along with third generation cephalosporins
- MRSA endocarditis

Adverse effects. Vanomyin is ototoxic and nephrotoxic, and is often given slowly (lasting for at least 1 hour) into a central vein as it can cause venous thrombosis. Rapid IV infusion of gentamycin can cause "red-man syndrome", which is a histamine-mediated reaction that is typically manifested by flushing and redness of the upper body.

Drug interactions. Anaesthetics with concomitant vancomycin infusion can cause hypersensitivity-like reactions. Aminoglycosides, capreomycin and loop diuretics increase the risk of ototoxicity and nephrotoxicity.

Teicoplanin

Teicoplanin is very similar to vancomycin, but has a longer duration of action, can also be given by intramuscular injection and has considerably less adverse effects. It is used for potentially serious infections such as *Staphylococcus aureus*, for dialysis-associated peritonitis and in orthopaedic surgery where there is a risk of infection with gram-positive organisms.

Adverse effects. Teicoplanin may cause angio-edema, anaphylaxis, blood disorders, hearing loss and injection abscesses. It is contraindicated in pregnancy, breast-feeding, renal impairment and in patients with adverse effects with vancomycin.

Polymyxin

Polymyxin is effective against a wide range of gram-negative organisms including *P. aeruginosa*. It is not absorbed by mouth and is rarely used for systemic effects, because of its toxicity. It is particularly useful in topical applications for the eye and ear infections.

Colistin

Colistin is active against gram-negative bacteria such as P. aeruginosa. It is not absorbed orally, and is only used with antifugal nystatin for bowel sterilization in neutropenic patients.

Quinupristin and **dalfopristin.** This is a mixture of two antibiotics. The anti-bacterial spectrum consists of antibiotic resistant gram-positive organisms, especially vancomycin-resistant *E. faecum* and S. aureus. MRSA, and antibiotic resistant strains of *Strept. pneumoniae*. It is ineffective against *E. faecalis*.

Quinupristin/dalfopristin is used via an IV infusion into central vein in serious infections caused by gram-positive organisms resistant to vancomucin as an alternative treatment. Most common side effects are arthralgia aand myalgia, which may require discontinuation of therapy. Drug interactions are similar to those with erythromycin.

Linezolid

Linezolid is effective against antibiotic-resistant gram-positive organisms, especially vancomycin-resistant *E. faecium* and *S.aureus*. MRSA, and *Strpt. pneumoniae*. Its use should be restricted to serious infections in patients, who are intolerant to vancomycin.

Linezolid is well absorbed orally (bioavailability 90%) and can be given by oral or IV route.

Linezolid is well tolerated and its principal side effects are diarrhea, nausea, disturbances of taste and headache. Rarely, it may cause hypertension, tinnitus and various blod disorders.

Linezoid is contraindicated in breast-feeding and other MAOI drugs.

Daptomycin

Daptomycin is available only for IV administration. It has a rapid bactericidal activity against a wide varietyof gram-positive organisms including enterococi, staphylocoi,and streptococci. It is effective against the bacteria which have become resistant to methicillin and vancomycin. Presently, the use of the drug is mainly confined to treatment of complicated soft-tissue infections and infective endocarditis, where options are not available.

The common side effects include muscle weakness and pain which may necessitate discontinuation of the drug.

Fostomycin

Fostomycin is bactericidal against most urinary tract pathogens that include *P. aeruginosa, Enterobacter* species, and vancomycin-resistant enterococci. It is used as a single-dose therapy for treatment of uncomplicated lower urinary-tract infections, particularly in women. Diarrhea is the most common side effect.

Mupirocin

Mupirocin is available only as topical antibiotic for use against staphylococci and streptococci. Its major applications are for impetigo and for eradication of the staphylococcal carrier state. It is the drug of choice for the elimination of carriage of both methicillin-susceptible and methicillin-resistant Staphylococci.

Bacitracin

Bacitracin is active against gram-positive organisms. It is bacteriocidal and shows no cross-resistance with other antimicrobial drugs.

Bacitracin is available only for topical use, since it is highly nephrotoxic.

Bacitracin (often combined with polymyxin or neomycin) ointment is used for suppression of mixed bacterial flora in surface lesions of the skin, in wounds, or on mucous membranes. It can also be used for irrigation of joints, wounds, or the pleural cavity.

11.3 ANTITUBERCULOUS DRUGS

Tuberculosis remains a major cause of mortality and morbidity world over. This is particularly so in our country, where resistance of the population is lowered by poverty, malnutrition and more recently by AIDS.

Tuberculosis is caused by bacteria *Mycobacterium tuberculosis* complex and usually affects the lungs, although other organs are involved in up to one-third of cases. If properly treated, TB caused by drug-susceptible strains is curable virtually in all cases.

Multidrug resistant TB (**MDR-TB**), a form of the disease caused by bacilli resistant at least to isoniazid and rifampin is on increase in India due to infection with HIV; social problems, such as increased urban poverty, drug abuse, and lack of proper organized TB services like lack of culture and drug-susceptibility testing capacity. Overall, 60% of all MDR-TB cases are in India, China and Russia.

Extensively drug-resistant TB **(XDR-TB)** in which MDR-TB is compounded by additional resistance to the most powerful second-line anti-TB drugs (fluoroquinolones and at least one of the injectable drugs amikacin, kanamycin, and capreomycin) are emerging and about 10% of the MDR-TB cases worldwide are XDR-TB.

FIRST-LINE ANTITUBERCULOSIS DRUGS

Isoniazid, rifampin, pyrazinamide, and ethambutol are considered as first-line drugs for the treatment of initial tuberculosis. These drugs are well absorbed after oral administration, with peak serum levels at 2–4 hours and nearly complete elimination within 24 hours. These drugs are recommended on the basis of their bactericidal activity (i.e., their ability to rapidly reduce the number of viable organisms and render patients noninfectious), their sterilizing activity (i.e., their ability to kill all bacilli and thus sterilize the affected tissues, measured in terms of the ability to prevent relapses) and their low rate of induction of drug resistance.

Rifabutin, rifapentine and streptomycin are also considered as **first-line supplemental drugs**, because of their use in certain special circumstances.

FIRST-LINE DRUGS

Isoniazid (INH)

Isoniazid is a critical drug for treatment of TB because of its excellent bactericidal activity against both intracellular and extracellular actively dividing tubercular bacilli. The drug has bacteriostatic action against slowly dividing organisms. It is well tolerated, highly effective and is inexpensive. It is taken daily or thrice weekly. It is always included in the standard treatment of TB in DOT regimen unless tubercle bacilli is resistant or there is a specific contraindication (e.g. drug induced liver disease).

The exact mode of action is not known. It probably interferes with cellular metabolism, specially the synthesis of mycolic acid, an important constituent of the myobacterial cell wall.

INH is rapidly absorbed from the intestine and is largely excreted by the kidneys. It diffuses widely throughout the body, it enters into the cells, crosses the meningeal barrier with therapeutic effective concentrations in the CSF. Isoniazid is metabolized in the liver and the plasma concentration depends on whether the patient is a fast or slow acetylator of the drug (a genetically determined characteristic). However, the acetylator status does not matter, because the drug is given daily.

INH is given daily in dose of 300 mg/day or thrice weekly in doses of 600 mg (maximum 900 mg). It does not require dosage adjustment in patients with renal diseases.

The incidence of development of resistance is very low (−7%).

Drugs-induced liver injury and peripheral neuropathy are significant adverse effects. Other adverse reactions include rash, fever, anemia, acne, arthritic symptoms, a systemic lupus erythematosus-like syndrome, optic atrophy, seizures and psychiatric symptoms.

Pyridoxine (25–50 mg/d) is given prophylactically to prevent peripheral neuropathy.

Rifampin

Rifampin is a key antibiotic of any antitubercular regimen and like isoniazid should always be included, unless there is a specific contraindication (e.g. jaundice).

Rifampin inhibits RNA synthesis in bacteria and chlamydiae by binding to DNA dependent RNA polymerase.

Rifampin is effective against several gram-positive and gram-negative organisms and in particular against the tubercle bacillus. As an antitubercular drug, it is as effective bacteriocidal as INH. The use of the drug as a single therapeutic agent always promotes the emergence of resistant organism. Apart from tuberculosis, it is also used in brucellosis, Legionnaires disease, serious staphylococcal infections and leprosy in combination with other appropriate drugs. There is no cross-resistance to other classes of antimicrobial drugs, but there is cross-resistance to other rifamycin derivatives, e.g. rifabutin and rifapentine.

Rifampin is well absorbed orally and is widely distributed in the body tissues including CSF and is mainly excreted in the bile. It is given orally in a dose of 600 mg either daily or thrice weekly. No adjustments of dose or frequency are necessary in patients with renal insufficiency.

Side effects are uncommon, but it should be used with caution in hepatic impairment (requires reduction of doses). Liver function tests and blood counts should be monitored in hepatic disorders. Persistent nausea, vomiting or jaundice requires discontinuation of the drug. It may cause red colouration of urine and sputum.

Rifampin induces hepatic enzymes, which accelerate the metabolism of several drugs including estrogens, glucocorticoids, phenytoin, sulphonylureas, warfarin, cyclosporine, protease inhibitors, some nonucleoside reverse transcriptase inhibitors, and a host of others.

Pyrazinamide

Pyrazinamide is a powerful bactericidal drug only active against intracellular dividing forms of tubercle bacillus. It is principally used in individuals with severe, possibly life-threatening forms of TB, e.g., meningitis and disseminated disease, and in the treatment of infections resistant to other drugs. Initially it is given daily for several weeks, followed by two or three times weekly for several months. It is absorbed orally and has good penetration into tubercular lesions. It is particularly useful in tubercular meningitis, because of good meningeal penetration. It is given in daily doses of 25 mg/kg with a maximum of 2 g orally or 35 mg/kg with a maximum of 3 g thrice weekly.

Pyrazinamide is an important first-line drug used in conjunction with INH and rifampin in short-course (i.e, 6 month) regimens as "sterilizing" agent active against residual intracellular organisms that may cause relapse. Tubercle bacilli develop resistance to pyrazinamide fairly rapidly.

Pyrazinamide may cause liver damage with jaundice, light sensitization and attacks of gout. It is contraindicated in liver disease.

Ethambutol

Ethambutol is also commonly used in a treatment regime, when resistance to isoniazid is suspected. It can be omitted, if the risk of resistance to INH is low.

Mode of action of ethambutol is not known. It is bacteriostatic and resistance occurs rapidly, when used alone. It is given in daily oral doses of 15 mg/kg or 30 mg/kg thrice weekly.

Ethambutol is well absorbed orally and is widely distributed in the body, except the CSF. It is partly metabolized and partly excreted by kidney.

The most important side affect of ethambutol is damage to optic nerve leading to deteoriation of visual acuity and colour vision. Other side effects include peripheral neuritis and rarely rashes.

FIRST-LINE SUPPLEMENTAL DRUGS

Rifabutin

Rifabutin is derived from rifamycin and is related to rifampin.

Rifabutin is both substrate and inducer of cytochrome P450 enzymes. Because it is less potent inducer, rifabutin is indicated in place of rifampin for the treatment of tuberculosis in HIV infected patients who are taking protease inhibitors or non nucleoside reverse transcriptase inhibitors, particularly efavirenz, that also are cytochrome P450 substrates.

The typical dose of rifabutin is 300 mg/d, unless the patient is receiving a protease inhibitor, in which case the dose should be reduced to 150 mg/d. If efavirenz (also a P450 inducer) is used; the recommended dose of rifabutin is 450 mg/d.

Clarithromycin and fluconazole appear to increase rifabutin levels by inhibiting hepatic metabolism.

Rifabutin is generally well tolerated with adverse effects occurring at higher doses. The most common adverse effects include gastrointestinal asthenia, chest pain, myalgia and insomnia. Less common adverse reactions are flulike syndrome, anterior uveitis, hepatitis, clostridium difficile-associated diarrhea.

Rifapentine

Rifapentine has the same mechanism of action as rifamipin. Because of higher rates of relapse, rifapentine is not recommended for patients with HIV diseases.

Rifapentine 600 mg once weekly is indicated for treatment of tuberculosis caused by rifampin-susceptible strains during the continuation phase only (i.e. after the first sputum cultures to negative).

The adverse effects are similar to that of other rifamycins. Rifapentine is teratogenic and is contraindicated in pregnancy.

Streptomycin

Streptomycin is an aminoglycoside that can be used as substitute for ethambutol and for drug-resistant MTB. It is bactericidal against actively multiplying tubercle bacilli. It is principally used in individuals with severe, possibly life-threatening forms of TB, e.g., meningitis and disseminated disease, and in the treatment of infections resistant to other drugs. Initially it is given daily for several weeks in dosage of 15 mg/kg followed by 1–1.5 g two or three times weekly for several months.

The main disadvantage of streptomycin lies in its administration by intramuscular injection and its toxicity (especially ototoxicity and sensitization phenomena, which may even occur to the person handling the drug). Streptomycin should not be used in pregnancy because of auditory or vascular damage to the fetus. Strains of *M. tuberculosis* resistant to streptomycin generally are not cross resistant to capreomycin or amikacin.

Streptomycin, because its low cost, is used in developing country.

TREATMENT REGIMEN FOR INITIAL TREATMENT OF TUBERCULOSIS

Standard short-course regimens are divided into an initial or bactericidal, phase and a continuation, or sterilizing phase (Table 11.1).

Table 11.1: Recommended treatment regimens for initial treatment of tuberculosis[2]

Indication	Initial Phase		Continuation Phase	
	Duration, Months	Drugs	Duration, Months	Drugs
Culture-positive[1]	2	Isoniazid[4], Rifampin, Pyrazinamide, Ethambutol[3]	4	Isoniazid, Rifampin
Culture-negative	2	Isoniazid, Rifampin[5], Pyrazinamide, Ethambutol	4	Isoniazid, Rifampin
Pregnancy	2	Isoniazid, Rifampin, Pyrazinamide, Ethambutol	7	Isoniazid, Rifampin
Relapses	3	Isoniazid, Rifampin, Pyrazinamide, Ethambutol, Streptomycin	5	Isoniazid, Rifampin

[1] extension of continuation phase by three months (total 7 months) in patients with cavity pulmonary TB who remain sputum-culture positive after the initial phase of treatment.
[2] all drugs given orally except for streptomycin.
[3] streptomycin can be used in place of ethanbutol but is no longer considered to be first-line drug.
[4] prophylactically 25–50 mg/d pyridoxine to prevent peripheral neuropathy.
[5] rifabutin in HIV co-infected patients because of less interaction with protease inhibitors.

DIRECTLY OBSERVED TREATMENT (DOT)

Failure to comply with the treatment regimen is a major factor in prolonged infections illness, risk of relapse and the emergence of drug resistant TB. DOT involves the supervised administration of therapy and has become an important control strategy in resource-poor nations.

DOT should be adopted in rural population and especially for patients, who are thought unlikely to be adherent to therapy, who are homeless, alcohol or drug addicts, drifters, those with serious mental illness and those with a history of non-compliance.

SECOND-LINE DRUGS

These are indicated for treatment of drugs resistant TB, for patients who are intolerant or allergic to first-line drugs.

Fluoroquinolones

The later-generation fluoroquinolones moxifloxacin and levofloxacin are the most active while ciprofloxacin is not recommended because of its poor efficacy against TB. The dosage of moxifloxacin is 400 mg once a day.

Fluoroquinolones are well absorbed orally, widely distributed into body tissues and fluids. Adverse effects are relatively infrequent and include GI intolerance, rashes, dizziness and headache.

Drug resistance can develop rapidly if fluoroquinolone is used alone.

Capreomycin

Capreomycin is an important second-line drug, particularly when additional resistance to aminoglycoside is present. It is administered by the IM route in a dose of 15 mg/kg per day given 5 to 7 times per week. A minimal duration of 3 months is recommended for MDR-TB treatment.

Penetration of capreomycin into the CSF is poor. Cross-resistance to kanamycin and amikacin is common.

Adverse effects are relatively common. Significant hypokalemia and hypomagnesemia as well as oto- and renal toxicity have been reported.

Amikacin and Kanamycin

These are aminoglycosides highly active against M. tuberculosis. They are used only infrequently because of their significant side effects. Cross resistance among kanamycin, amikacin and capreomycin is common. Isolates resistant to streptomycin are frequently susceptible to amikacin and kanamycin. Adverse effects of amikacin include ototoxicity with auditory dysfunction occuring more commonly than vestibulotoxicity) nephrotoxicity and neurotoxicity. Kanamycin causes less frequent and less severe side effects.

Ethionamide

Ethionamide is a tuberculocidal drug chemically related to isoniazid. It acts on both extra and intracellular organisms. It is absorbed orally, widely distributed including CSF and is completely metabolized. Side effects include gastrointestinal disorders, hepatitis and neurologic symptoms. Neurologic symptoms may be alleviated by pyridoxine.

Para-amino salicylic acid (PAS)

PAS is only active against tubercle bacilli. It is one of the least active tuberculostatic drug and only delays development of resistance to other antitubercular drugs. It is used infrequently now because other oral drugs are better tolerated.

PAS is completely absorbed by oral route and distributed all over except CSF. It competes with the acetylation of isoniazid. It is partly acetylated and rest excreted by kidney. Side effects include diarrhea, hepatitis and hypersensitivity reactions.

Cycloserine

Cycloserine, an antibiotic, acts as bacteriostatic against tubercle bacilli, some gram-positive bacteria, *E. coli* and chlamydial infections. It is absorbed orally, widely distributed including CSF, partly metabolized and rest excreted unchanged by kidney. It is a toxic drug and gives rise to high incidence of neurological disorders including depression, personality changes, psychosis and convulsions.

Pyridoxine should be given with cycloserine because this ameliorates neurologic toxicity. Cycloserine is contraindicated in severe renal impairment, epilepsy, psychotic states and alcohol dependence.

Multi-drug resistant tuberculosis

The regimens for treatment of MDR-TB are given in Table 11.2.

Table 11.2: Regimens for treatment of MDR-TB

Indication	Duration	Drugs
Resistance (or intolerance) to isoniaizid	Throughout for 6 months	Rifampin, pyrazinamide, ethambutol
Resistance (or intolerance) to rifampin	Throughout for 12–18 months	Isoniazid, pyrazinamide, ethambutol, moxifloxacin
Resistance to isoziazid and rifampin	Throughout for at least 20 months	pyrazinamide, ethambutol, moxifloxacin, streptomycin
Resistance to all first-line drugs	Throughout for at least 20 months	Moxifloxacin, ethionamide, cycloserine, streptomycin
Resistance to pyrazinamide	Isoniazid, rifampin, ethambutol for 2 months plus isoniazid, rifampin for 7 months	

WHO management guidelines for strongly suspected XDR-TB

- Use any first-line oral agents that may be effective.
- Use an injectable agent to which the strain is susceptible, and consider an extended duration of use (12 months or possibly the whole treatment period). If the strain is resistant to all injectable agents, use of an agent that the patient has not previously received is recommended.

- Use a later-generation fluoroquinolone, such as moxifloxacin.
- Use all second-line oral agents (para-aminosalicylic acid, cycloserine, ethionamide, or pyrazinamide) that have not been used extensively in a previous regimen or any that are likely to be effective.
- Use two or more of the following drugs of unclear role: clofazimine, amoxicillin/clavulanic acid, clarithromycin, imipenem, linezolid, thiacetazone.
- Consider treatment with high-dose isoniazid if low-level resistance to this drug is documented.
- Consider adjuvant surgery if there is localized disease.
- Enforce strong infection-control measures.
- Implement strict directly observed therapy and full adherence support as well as comprehensive bacteriologic and clinical monitoring.

NEWER ANTITUBERCULOSIS DRUGS IN CLINICAL TRIALS

Linezolid

Linezolid is an oxazolidinone used primarily for the treatment of gram-positive infections.

Several studies have suggested that linezolid may help clear organisms relatively rapidly when included in a regimen for the treatment of complex MDR – and XDR – TB.

Linezolid has nearly 100% bioavailability, with good penetrations in tissues and fluids, including CSF. Clinical resistance to the drug has been observed.

Adverse effects include optic and peripheral neuropathy, pancytopenia, and lactic acidosis.

11.4 ANTILEPROTIC DRUGS

Leprosy, first described in ancient Indian texts from the sixth century BC, is a nonfatal, chronic infectious disease caused by *Mycobacterium leprae*. The clinical manifestations of leprosy are largely confined to the skin, peripheral nervous system, upper respiratory tract, eyes, and testicles.

Leprosy is labeled as a social stigma because of disfigurement, loss of digits, bone resorption etc and the belief that the disease is communicable from person to person. Early diagnosis and appropriate and effective antimicrobial therapy can lead the patients a productive life in the community, and deformities and other visible manifestation can largely be prevented.

The route of transmission of leprosy remains uncertain and transmission routes in fact are multiple. Nasal droplet infection, contact with infected soil, and even insect vectors have been considered the prime candidates.

ANTIMICROBIAL THERAPY

Established agents used to treat leprosy include dapsone (50–100 mg/d), clofazimine (50–100 mg/d, 100 mg three times weekly, or 300 mg monthly), and rifampin (600 mg daily or monthly). Of these drugs, only rifampin is bactericidal.

The sulfones (folate antagonists), the foremost of which is dapsone, were the first antimicrobial agents found to be effective for the treatment of leprosy and are still the mainstay of therapy.

Other antimicrobial agents active against *M. leprae* in clinical trials include ethionamide/prothionamide; the aminoglycosiders (except gentamycin and tobramycin); minocycline: clarithromycin; and several fluoroquinolones, particularly ofloxacin. Most recently rifapentine and moxifloxacin have been found to be especially potent against *M. leprae* in mice. In a clinical trial in lepromatous leprosy, moxifloxacin was profoundly bactericidal, matched in potency only by rifampin.

Dapsone

Dapsone is the principal drug to treat leprosy and is chemically related to sulfonamides It is bacteriostatic for *M. leprae* and its mechanism of action is similar to that of sulfonamides.

Dapsone is slowly, but completely absorbed from the gut. It undergoes intestinal reabsorption from the bile, resulting in a sustained level of the drug in the circulation. It is concentrated in skin (especially lepromatous skin), muscle, liver and kidney. It is metabolized and excreted by kidney.

Dapsone is generally safe and inexpensive. Individuals with glucose-6-phosphate dehydrogenase deficiency who are treated with dapsone may develop severe hemolysis; those without this deficiency also have reduced red cell survival and a hemoglobin decrease averaging 1 g/dl. Dapsone's usefulness is limited occasionally by allergic dermatitis and rarely by the sulfone syndrome (including high fever, anemia, exfoliative dermatitis, and a mononucleosis-type blood picture).

Clofazimine

Clofazimine is a dye with leprostatic and anti-inflammatory properties. It binds to mycobacterium DNA, thereby inhibiting template function.

Clofazimine is orally active, 50% of an oral dose reaches the systemic circulation. It is lipophilic and accumulates in adipose tissue and reticuloendothelial cells. The elimination half life after repeated oral dosing is 70 days.

Clofazimine causes dose related nausea, vomiting and abdominal pain. A brownish-black discolouration of lesions and skin including areas exposed to light and red discolouration of hair and body secretions may occur. Atropine like symptoms can occur.

TYPES OF LEPROSY

The disease is divided clinically and by laboratory tests into two distinct types: lepromatous and tuberculoid.

The **lepromatou**s type (also referred to multibacillary leprosy) occurs in persons with defective cellular immunity. The course is progressive and malignant; with nodular skin lesions, slow, symmetric nerve involvement, abundant acid-fast bacilli in the skin lesion,, and a negative lepromin skin test.

In the **tuberculoid** type (pancibacillary leprosy), cellular immunity is intact and the course is more benign and less progressive, with macular skin lesions, severe asymmetric nerve involvement of sudden onset with few bacilli present in the lesions, and a positive lepromin skin test. Intermediate ("borderline" cases are frequent.

TREATMENT REGIMES FOR LEPROSY

Combination therapy is recommended for the treatment of all types of leprosy. Single-drug treatment is accompanied by emergence of resistance, and primary resistance to dapsone also occurs.

WHO in 1982 made recommendation for the chemotherapy of leprosy for control programmes which involves a triple drug regimen, although longer courses may be needed for patients with high burden of disease. Table 11.3 gives the antimicrobial regimen for the treatment of leprosy.

Table 11.3: Leprosy antimicrobial regimen

Forms of leprosy	More intensive regimen	WHO recommended regimen (1982)
Tuberculoid (paucibacillary)	Dapsone 100 mg daily for 5 years.	Rifampin 600 mg once a month plus dapsone 100 mg daily for 6 month.
Lepromatous (multibacillary)	Rifampin 600 mg daily for 3 years plus dapsone 100 daily indefinitely	Rifampin 600 mg once a month, dapsone 100 mg daily and clofazimine 300 mg once a month and 50 mg daily for 1–2 years.

Two reactional states–erythema nodosum leprosum and reversal reactions – may occur as a consequence of therapy.

The reversal reaction, typical of borderline lepromatous leprosy, probably results from enhanced host immunity. Skin lesions and nerves become swollen and tender, but systemic manifestations are not seen.

Erythema nodosum leprosum, typical of lepromatous leprosy, is a consequence of immune injury from antigen-antibody complex deposition in skin and other tissues; in addition to skin and nerve manifestations, fever and systemic involvement may be seen. **Prednisone**, 60 mg/d orally, or **thalidomide**, 300 mg/d orally (in the nonpregnant patient only), is effective for erythema nodosum leprosum. Improvement is expected within a few days after initiating prednisone, and thereafter the dose may be tapered over

Antibacterial Drugs 427

several weeks to avoid recurrence. Thalidomide is also tapered over several weeks to a 100 mg bedtime dose.

Erythema nodosum leprosum is usually confined to the first year of therapy, and prednisone or thalidomide can be discontinued.

Thalidomide is ineffective for reversal reactions, and prednisone, 60 mg/d, is indicated. Reversal reactions tend to recur, and the dose of prednisone should be slowly tapered over weeks to months.

Therapy for leprosy should not be discontinued during treatment of reactional states.

12

Antifungal Drugs

Fungal infections have assumed an increasing important role as advances in surgery, cancer treatment, treatment of patients with solid organ and bone marrow transplantation, the HIV epidemic, and increasing use of broad-spectrum antibiotics have resulted in increased number of patients at risk of fungal infections.

Fungal organisms are eukaryotic cells that contain most of the same organelles (with many of the same physiological functions) as human cells. The identification of drugs that selectively kill or inhibit fungi but are not toxic to human cells has been highly problematic. Far fewer antifungal than antibacterial drugs are available for use into clinical medicine.

The antifungal drugs presently available fall into several categories: systemic drugs (oral or parenteral) for systemic infections, oral drugs for mucocutaneous infections, and topical drugs for mucocutaneous infections.

SYSTEMIC ANTIFUNGAL DRUGS

Amphotericin

Amphotericin B (AmB) is fungicidal and is the most important drug for severely ill patients with systemic fungal infections, such as systemic candidiasis, cryptococcal meningitis and histoplasmosis.

AmB is not absorbed orally and is given only by IV infusion. It is highly protein bound and penetrates poorly into body fluids. The drug is excreted very slowly in the urine and has a plasma half-life of 24 hours.

AmB remains the broadest-spectrum antifungal agent but carries several disadvantages, including significant nephrotoxicity, lack of an oral preparation, and unpleasant side effects (fever, chills, and nausea) during treatment. To circumvent nephrotoxicity and infusion side effects, lipid formulations of AmB were developed which have virtually replaced the original colloidal deoxycholate formulation in clinical use. The lipid formulations include liposomal AmB and AmB lipid complex.

AmB is often used as the initial induction regimen in order to rapidly reduce fungal burden in immunosuppressed patients and is then replaced by one of the newer azole drugs for chronic therapy or prevention of relapse. Therapy may be lifelong in patients at high risk for disease relapse. It is also used in lozenges that are given four times daily in, the treatment of oral candidiasis.

The major adverse effect of amphotericin B including the lipid form is nephrotoxicity. Common infusion-related effects (fever/chills, nausea, headache and myalgias) can be prevented by premedication with antihistamine and glucocorticoid.

Flucytosine

Flucytosine is less often used with the discovery of newer antifungal drugs. Development of resistance to this drug has limited its use as a single agent. Flucytosine is nearly always used in combination with AmB. Its good penetration into the CSF has led it to be used with AmB for the treatment of cryptococcal and candidal meningitis.

Adverse effects include dose related bone-marrow suppression and bloody diarrhea. It should be used cautiously in patients with impaired renal and hepatic functions.

AZOLES

This class of antifungal drugs offers important advantages over AmB: the azoles cause little or no nephrotoxicity and are available in oral preparations. Early azoles included ketoconazole and miconazole, which have been replaced by newer agents for the treatment of deep organ fungal infections. The azole's mechanism of action is inhibition of ergosterol synthesis in the fungal cell wall. Unlike AmB, these drugs are considered fungistatic, not fungicidal.

Itraconazole

Itraconazole is a broad-spectrum antifungal drug and is the drug of choice in systemic candidiasis, histaplasmosis, blastomycosis and dermatophyte infections. Orally, it is well absorbed and requires adequate gastric acidity for absorption and, therefore, should be taken with food to ensure maximum absorption. In serious cases, it is given by IV route. It is equally and sometimes more effective than toxic antifungal amphotericin and flucytosine drugs. It should not be used in patients with liver disease, severe heart failure and renal impairment.

Fluconazole

Fluconazole is an extremely important drug for the treatment of a wide variety of serious fungal infections. Its major advantages are the availability of oral and IV formulations, a long half-life, satisfactory penetration of most body fluids (including ocular fluid and CSF), and minimal toxicity. Its disadvantages include hepatotoxicity and at large doses alopecia, muscle weakness, and dry mouth with a metallic taste.

Fluconazole has become the agent of choice for the treatment of coccidioidal meningitis. In addition, it is useful for both consolidation and maintenance therapy of cryptococcal meningitis. Fluconazole is effective as AmB in the treatment of candidemia.

Fluconazole is considered effective as fungal prophylaxis in bone marrow transplant recipients and high-risk liver transplant patients.

Voriconazole

Voriconazole is a new triazole antifungal with broad-spectrum activity against a wide range of pathogenic fungi. Unlike, other azoles, it is active against all clinically important species of aspergillus. It is even superior to the conventional amphotericin B therapy of invasive aspergillosis.

Voriconazole has the advantage of easy transition from IV to oral therapy, because of its excellent oral bioavailability.

Voriconazole has the disadvantage of numerous interactions with many of the drugs used in patients predisposed to fungal infections.

Hepatotoxicity, skin rashes, and visual disturbances are relatively common. Skin cancer surveillances are recommended in patients taking voriconazole.

Posaconazole is the latest triazole with the broadest spectrum member of the azole family, with activity against most species of candida and aspergillus. It is the only azole with significant activity against the agents of zygomycosis and mucormycosis. Presently, its main indications include invasive aspergillosis, prophylaxis of fungal infections during induction chemotherapy for leukemia, and for allogeneic bone marrow transplant patients with graft-versus-host disease.

Posaconazole is given orally with meals high in fat to improve its absorption. Visual changes as seen with voriconazole have not been reported.

Table 12.1 summarizes the major properties of currently available antifungal drugs for the treatment of systemic fungal infections.

Echinocandins

Echinocandins are the antifungal agents active against candida and aspergillus, and include caspofungin, micafungin and anidulafemgin. The echinocandins are amongst safest antifungal drugs.

Caspofungin

Caspofungin acetate is a fungicidal drug against most *Aspergillus* and *Candida* species, including azole-resistant *Candida* strains. It is not effective against *Cryptococcus, Histoplasma* or Mucor (Mucor is a genus of fungus found on decaying organic matter). It is not absorbed from GI tract and has to be given by IV route. It is metabolized by the liver, but does not involve cytochrome P-450 system significantly.

Caspofungin is effective in patients who do not respond to amphotericin B or itraconazole. It is better tolerated than amphotericin B for the treatment of infections caused by Candida species.

Caspofungin is well tolerated. Fever, rash, nausea and phlebitis at the injection site are infrequent side effects. In liver diseases, the doses should be reduced.

Table 12.1: Drugs for systemic fungal infections

Drug	Dose	Uses	Toxicity
Amphotericin B	0.3–1.5/kg daily intravenously	All major pathogens except scedosporium	Rigors, fever, azotemia, hypokalemia, hypomagnesemia, renal tubular acidosis, anemia.
Liposomal amphotericin B	3–6 mg/kg daily intravenously	All major pathogens except scedosporium	Fever, rigor, nausea, hypotension azotemia, anemia, tachypenea, chest tightness.
Itraconazole	100–400 mg daily	Histoplaomosis, coccidioidomycosis, blastomycosis, para-coccidioidomycosis, mucosal candidiasis, sporotrichosis, aspergillosis, chromomycosis.	Nausea, hypokalemia, edema, hypertension.
Fluconazole	100–180 mg daily intravaneously or orally	Mucosal candidiasis, cryptococcosis, histoplasmosis, coccidioidomycosis	Nausea, rash, alopecia, headache, hepatic enzyme elevations.
Voriconazole	200–400 mg daily orally or 12 mg/kg daily intravenously	All major pathogens except zygomycetes and sporotrichosis	Transient visual disturbances, rash, hepatic enzyme elevations.
Posaconazole	400–800 mg daily orally	Broad range of activity including zygomycetes	Nausea, vomiting, abdominal pain, diarrhea and headache.

(Contd.)

Table 12.1: Drugs for systemic fungal infections (Contd.)

Drug	Dose	Uses	Toxicity
Caspofungin acetate	70 mg followed by 50 mg daily intravenously	Aspergillosis, mucosal and invasive candidiasis, empiric antifungal therapy in febrile neutropenia	Transient neutropenia, hepatic enzyme elevations when used with cyclosporine.
Anidulafungin	100 mg followed by 50 mg daily intravenously	Mucosal and invasive candidiasis	Diarrhea, hepatic enzyme elevations, allergic reactions.
Flucytosine	100–150 mg/kg daily orally	In combination with AmB in cryptococcosis and candidiasis, chromomycosis	Leukopenia, diarrhea, hepatitis, renal damage.

Micafungin

Micafungin is licensed for esophageal candidiasis and candidemia and prophylaxis of candida infection in bone marrow transplant patients.

Anidulafungin

Anidulafungin is approved for use in esophageal candidiasis and invasive candidiasis, including candidemia.

SYSTEMIC DRUGS FOR MUCOCUTANEOUS INFECTIONS

Terbinafine

Terbinafine is given orally and is the drug of choice for fungal nail and ringworm infections. It is not used for systemic infections. Side effects include GIT upset and rashes. Serious skin reactions and rarely liver toxicity have also been reported.

Griseofulvin

Griseofulvin is given orally for the ringworm infections of nail, skin and scalp where local treatment is inadequate. It is a slow-acting drug and requires several weeks of therapy. It is not used for systemic infections. Adverse effects include an allergic syndrome much like serum sickness, hepatitis and drug interaction with warfarin and phenobarbital.

Griseofulvin has been largely replaced by newer antifungal medications such as itraconazole and terbinafine.

TOPICAL ANTIFUNGAL DRUGS

Nystatin

Nystatin is too toxic for parenteral administration and is only used topically. It is available in creams, ointments, suppositories, and other forms for application to skin and mucus membranes, or GIT. Its oral use is limited by the unpleasant taste. It is active against most candida species and is most commonly used for suppression of local candidal infections. Some common indications include oropharyngeal thrush, vaginal candidiasis and intertriginous candidal infections.

Topical azoles

The two azoles most commonly used topically are **clotrimazole** and **miconazole**. Oral clotrimazole troches are available for treatment of oral thrush and are a pleasant tasting alternative to nystatin. In cream form, both agents are useful for dermatophytic tinea infections. Absorption is negligible and adverse effects are rare.

Topical and shampoo form of ketoconazole are useful in the treatment of seborrheic dermatitis and pityriasis versicolor.

Topical allylamines

Terbinafine and **naftifine** are allylamines available as topical creams. Both are effective for treatment of dermatophytic infections.

13

Antiviral Drugs

The specific therapy of virus infections is generally unsatisfactory, because viruses live within human cells, where they are not readily accessible to the drugs. Furthermore, a great deal of virus replication takes place before the patient develops symptoms. The majority of viral infections is of minor importance (e.g. the influenza), but may become virulent and life threatening in subjects who are immunosupressed (e.g. by AIDS or treatment with cytotoxic drugs).

The drugs available for different type of viruses are;

Virus	Drug
Herpes simplex and varicella-zoster virus	Acyclovir, famciclovir and valacyclovir, penciclovir, docosanol, trifluridine
Cytomegalovirus	Ganciclovir, valganciclovir, foscarnet and cidofovir
Respiratory syncytial virus	Tribavirin
Influenza virus	Amantidine and zanamivir
Human immunodeficiency virus (HIV)	Antiretroviral drugs

The antiviral drugs act mainly by inhibiting viral DNA synthesis or inhibition of vital proteins, which are essential for virus replication.

Acyclovir

Acyclovir is active against herpes viruses, but does not eradicate them. It is effective only if started at the onset of infection. Orally, acyclovir is about 20% absorbed and is widely distributed including the CSF.

Acyclovir, by intravenous infusion is the drug of choice for treatment of herpes simplex in the immunosuppressed, severe initial genital herpes, varicella zoster (chickenpox) and herpes meningoencephalitis.

Oral acyclovir is effective in accelerating the healing of genital herpes, in preventing damage to the eye on involvement of ophthalmic branch of the trigeminal nerve by herpes zoster (shingles) and chickenpox in immunocompetent adults.

Topical acyclovir is used to treat ulceration of the cornea due to herpes simplex virus and labial herpes.

Acyclovir, intravenously, can cause severe local inflammation, hallucinations, tremors. psychosis, convulsions and coma. Orally, acyclovir is well tolerated, however GIT disturbances, rashes, neurological reaction including dizziness and headache can occur. Topical applications can cause local discomfort and pruritis. It is contraindicated in pregnancy.

Famciclovir and valacyclovir

These are pharmacologically similar and are given orally to treat herpes simplex, herpes zoster and suppression of initial and recurrent genital herpes. They have the advantage of less frequent oral administration.

Penciclovir

Penciclovir, the active metabolite of famciclovir is available as a cream (1%) for local application in the treatment of herpes labial. Adverse effects are uncommon, though skin reactions may occur rarely.

Docosanol

Docosanol prevents the entry of HSV into cells and its replication by inhibiting the fusion between the virus and the cell membrane. Topical docosamol 10% cream shortens the healing time in recurrent labial herpes.

Trifluridine

Trifluridine is available for topical use as 1% solution in the treatment of keratoconjunctivitis and recurrent epithetial keratitis due to HSV. Cutaneous application of trifluridine solution, alone or in combination with interferon alfa, is effective in acyclovir resistant HSV infection.

DRUGS FOR CYTOMEGALOVIRUS (CMV)

Ganciclovir

Ganciclovir is related to acyclovir, but is more active against cytomegalovirus (CMV). It is used in life threatening or CMV retinitis in immunosuppressed patients only (e.g. those with AIDS). It is available for intravenous infusion. It can be inserted surgically into the eye as slow release ocular implants. Orally, it is used for maintenance treatment of CMV retinitis, following intravenous therapy. The most serious side effect is suppression of white cell count and of the platelets. It is contraindicated during pregnancy.

Valganciclovir

Valganciclovir is prodrug of ganciclovir and is indicated for the oral treatment of CMV retinitis as well as for its prophylaxis. Adverse effects and rest of the pharmacological consideration are the same as with ganciclovir.

Foscarnet

Foscarnet is reserved for CMV retinitis in AIDS patients and mucocutaneous herpes simplex virus infections, non-responsive to amantadine or acyclovir in immunosuppressed patients. It is given by intravenous infusion and is highly nephrotoxic.

Cidofovir

Cidofovir is used in the treatment of CMV retinitis in AIDS patients, when ganciclovir and foscarnet are contraindicated. It is given in combination with probenecid. It is nephrotoxic.

Tribavirin

Tribavirin is used in the treatment of severe respiratory syncytial virus (RSV) bronchiolitis in infants and children. It is given by nebulizer or aerosol inhalation. Side effects include worsening of respiration, bacterial pneumonia and rarely anemia and hemolysis.

Amantadine

Amantadine has some action against the influenza virus and can be used for prophylaxis during an outbreak of influenza A only. It can be used in Parkinson's disease when levodopa is contraindicated, as it increases the concentration of dopamine in basal ganglia. Side effects include nausea, central effects and swelling of the ankles.

Zanamivir

Zanamivir is used in the treatment of influenza A or B within 48 hours after onset of symptoms, when influenza is epidemic in the community. It is given by nebulizer or aerosol inhalation. It is doubtful, if it prevents complications in high-risk patients, who are better immunized. Side effects include GIT disturbances, bronchospasm and rashes.

HIV infection and AIDS

Human immunodeficiency virus (HIV) type 1 is a retrovirus that infects predominantly lymphocytes that bear the CD4 surface protein as well as co receptors belonging to the chemokine family (CCR5). The sequence of events in life cycle of HIV and drugs blocking the steps in replication are given in Fig. 13.1 and Table 13.1.

Modes of transmission

HIV is present in blood, semen and other body fluids such as breast milk and saliva.

The mode of transmissions are sexual, parenteral (blood or blood product ecepients, injection drug-users and those experiencing occupational injury) and during pregnancy and vaginal/elective caesarean delivery and breast feeding.

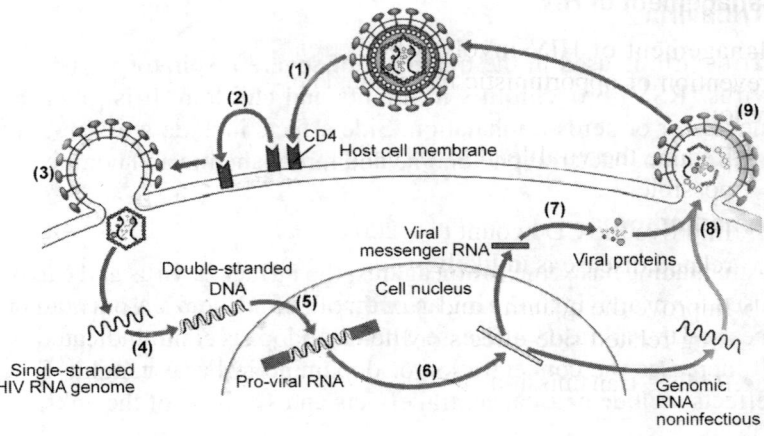

Fig. 13.1: Life cycle of HIV.

Table 13.1: Drug targets on steps of replication of HIV

Stage	Steps in replication	Blocked by	
1.	Attachment to CD4 receptor		
2.	Blinding to Chemokine receptors	CCR5 receptor antagonists	Entry inhibitors
3.	Fusion and uncoating	Fusion inhibitors	
4.	Reverse transcription	Nucleoside and non-nucleoside reverse transcription inhibitors	
5.	Integration	Integrase inhibitors	
6.	Transcription		
7.	Translation		
8.	Virion assembly, budding and maturation	Protease inhibitors	
9.	Viral release		

Acquired immunodeficiency syndrome (AIDS)

AIDS is defined by the development of specified opportunistic infections, tumours and HIV-associated wasting and dementia. The predominant opportunistic seen in HIV disease are intracellular parasites (e.g. *Mycobacterium tuberculosis*) or pathogens susceptible to cell-mediated rather than antibody-mediated immune responses.

Management of HIV

Management of HIV involves both treatment of the virus and prevention of opportunistic infection. The aims of HIV treatment are to:

- Reduce the viral load to an undetectable level for as long as possible.
- Improve the CD4 count to > 200 cells/mL, so the severe HIV-related disease is unlikely.
- Improve the quantity and quality of life without unacceptable drug-related side-effects or life-style alteration.
- Reduce transmission.

Antiretroviral therapy

The prognosis in persons with HIV/AIDS has dramatically improved due to the introduction of highly active antiretroviral therapy (HAART). The life expectancy of HIV-infected persons with HAART therapy may approach that of uninfected person when the treatment is initiated early in the course of the disease.

The greater potency and the improved side effect profile have led to recommendations to start treatment earlier in the course of HIV disease. Treatment should be initiated for all symptomatic patients, and for asympatomatic person who have:

- CD4 cell count below 500 cell/mcL.
- Rapidly dropping CD4 counts (> 100 cells/mcL/yr) or very high viral loads (> 100,000/mcL)
- Active infection with hepatitis B or C (rapid HIV replication is thought to hasten progression of hepatitis B and C).
- Risk factors for cardiac disease (ongoing HIV replication may increase the risk of cardiac disease).
- HIV-related renal impairment or pregnancy.
- Or risk factors for non-AIDS related cancers (rapid HIV replication may increase such cancers).

Five groups of antiretroviral drugs are available (Table 13.2).

Table 13.2: Antiretroviral drugs and their different groups

NRTIs	NNRTIs	Protease inhibitors (PIs)	Entry inhibitors	Integrase inhibitor
Zidovudine	Nevirapine	Saquinavir	Enfuvirtide	Raltegravir
Didanosine	Delavirdine	Ritonavir	Maraviroc	
Zalcitabine	Efavirenz	Indinavir	**Fixed-dose combinations**	
Stavudine	Etravirine	Nelfinavir	Zidovudine/Lamivudine.	
Lamivudine		Amprenavir	Emtricitabine/Tenofovir.	
Emtricitabine		Fosamprenavir	Lamivudine/Abacavir.	
Abacavir		Lopinavir	Zidovudine/Lamivudine/	
Tenofovir		Atazanavir	Abacavir.	
		Darunavir	Emtricitabine/Tenofovir/	
		Tipranavir	Efavirenz.	

Nucleoside and nucleotide reverse transcriptase inhibitors (NRTIs)

The NRTIs act through intracellular phosphorylation to the triphosphate form and incorporation into the DNA, where they inhibit further lengthening of the complementary strand to the viral RNA template. Each drug specifically competes with a natural nucleoside (e.g. Zidovudine with thymidine). CNS penetration is good with all NRTIs and ZDV has been demonstrated to be benefit in AIDS dementia. Tenofovir is a nucleotide drug which only requires two phosphorylation steps to triphosphate form. The inclusion of two NRTIs or one NRTI and tenofovir remains the cornerstone of HAART.

Resistance occurs to all NRTIs unless they are a part of a maximally suppressive HAART regimen, resistance to lamivudine (3TC) and emtricitabine (FTC) is rapid and of high level. Occasionally, certain single mutations in the viral reverse transcriptase may result in broad resistance to several or all of the NRTIs and tenofovir.

The common side effects of nucleoside reverse transcriptase inhibitors are given in Table 13.3.

Table 13.3: Common sides effects of NRTIs

Drug	Characteristic adverse effects	Comments
Zidovudine	Anemia, neutropenia nausea, headache, insomnia, asthenia, myopathy	Avoid stavudine and myclosuppressive drugs.
Didanosine (ddl)	Peripheral neuropathy pancreatitis, hepatitis hyperuricemia	Avoid stavudine, zalcitabine isomazid, ribavirin and alcohol. Do not administer with tenofovir.
Zalcitabine	Peripheral neuropathy oral ulceration, pancreatitis, arthralgias	Avoid cimetidine, neuropathic drugs. Do not administer with lamivudine
Stavudine	Peripheral neuropathy pancreatitis, lipodystrophy, hepatitis	Avoid concurrent zidovudine and neuropathic drugs.
Lamivudine	Rash, peripheral neuropathy	Do not administer with zalcitabine.
Embricitabine	Headache, diarrhea, nausea, asthenia, skin hyper pigmentation	Do not administer concurrent lamivudine. Avoid metronidazole
Abacavir	Rash, possible increase in myocardial infraction	Avoid alcohol
Tenofovir	Gastrointestinal distress, renal insufficiency	Single fixed dose combination pill (efavirenz + emtricitabine + tenofovir (initial choice)

Nonnucleoside reverse transcriptase inhibitors (NNRTIs)

The NNRTIs bind directly to HIV-1 reverse transcriptase resulting in allosteric inhibiton of RNA- and DNA-dependent DNA polymerase. The binding site of NNRTIs is near to but distinct from that of NRTIs. Unlike the NRTI agents, NNRTIs neither compete with nucleoside triphosphates nor require phosphorylation to be active. In addition, they lack in vitro activity against HIV-2. All have good bioavailability.

The major advantage of NNRTIs is that two of them (nevirapine and efavirenz) have potencies comparable to PIs – with lower pill burden and fewer side effects. In particular they do not appear to cause lipodystrophy; patients with cholesterol and triglycerides elevations who are switched from a PI to an NNRTI may have improvement in their lipids. The major disadvantage of NNRTIs is the rapid development of resistance with virological failure. There is no therapeutic reason for using more than one NNRTI at the same time.

The common side effects of nonnucleoside reverse transcriptase inhibitors are given in Table 13.4.

Table 13.4: Common side effects of NNRTIs

Drugs	Characteristic adverse effects	Comments
Nevirapine	Rash, nausea, headache, hepatitis (occasionally fulminant)	Only indicated in Efavirenz in tolerant patient because of potential fatal hepatotoxicity.
Delavidine	Rash headache, nausea, diarrhea, ↑ liver enzyme	NNRTIs inhibits P450 cytochrome, first generation, least used.
Efavirenz	Neurologic disturbances, rash, ↑ liver enzyme, headache nausea teratogenic	Efavirenz + tenofovir + emtricitabine in a single pill best choice for initial treatment
Etravirine	Rash, nausea, diarrhea peripheral neuropathy	2nd generation drug*

* Should not be used in patients with severe liver disease. Do not administer with other NNRTIs or PIs.

Rilpivirine

A fifth NNRTI is currently in late stage of clinical development and will be co formulated with tenofovir/emtricitabine in a new single tablet regimen.

Protease inhibitors (PIs)

PIs have been shown to potently suppress HIV replication and are administered as part of a combination regimen.

Currently used PIs should always be boosted by low-dose ritonavir, which is a potent inhibitor of liver metabolism. This increases drug exposure by prolonging the PIs half-life, allows reduction in pill burden and dosing frequency and so optimizing adherence. It also limits the development of resistance. PIs prevent post-translational cleavage of polypeptides into functional viral proteins. When they are given with two NRTIs, the combination controls viral replication in plasma and tissues and allows reconstitution of the immune system.

Unfortunately all PIs, with the exception of unboosted atazanavir have been linked to a constellation of metabolic abnormalities, including elevated cholesterol and triglyceride levels, insulin resistance, diabetes mellitus, and changes in body fat composition (e.g. buffalo lump, abdominal obesity).

Protease inhibitors are metabolized by the P450 cytochrome system (mainly the CYP3A4 isoenzyme) giving rise to the potential for multiple drug interactions. Commonly use drugs that interact with PIs (in particular ritonavir) are rifampicin, midazolam and simvastatin. Monitoring plasma levels and dose adjustments may be necessary to optimize the antiviral effect and to reduce toxicity.

The common side effects of protease inhibitors (PIs) are given in Table 13.5.

Entry inhibitors

Currently two classes of entry inhibitors exist. Those which block the entry of HIV into cells by blocking the fusion of HIV particle to the cell membrane and those that binds to the CCR5 coreceptor. Both are used in patients with advanced disease with triple-class failure or resistant virus. They are used in combination with other three active agents.

Because 95% of patients with early disease harbor CCR5-tropic virus, maraviroc is indicated in the primary treatment of HIV infection.

These drugs are generally well tolerated.

Table 13.5: Common side effects of PIs*

Drug	Characteristic drug effect	Comments
Indinavir	Nephrolithiasis, nausea, indirect hyperbilirubinemia, headache, asthenia, blurred vision.	Avoid efavirenz
Saquinavir	Nausea, diarrhea, rhinitis, abdominal pain, dyspepsia, rash	Avoid in severe hepatic insufficiency.
Ritonavir	Nausea, diarrhea, paresthesias, hepatitis	Widely used in lower doses as a booster of other PIs.
Nelfinavir	Diarrhea, nausea, flatulence	Ritonavir boosting not recommended
Fosamprenavir	Diarrhea, nausea, vomiting, rash, headache, perioral paraesthesias, ↑ liver enzymes	Avoid in severe hepatic insufficiency, metromidazole vitamin E, alcohol.
Lopinavir/ritonavir	Diarrhea, abdominal pain, nausea headache, ↑ liver enzyme.	Avoid fosamprenavir, metranidazole, alcohol.
Atazanavir	Nausea, vomiting, diarrhea, abdominal pain, peripheral neuropathy, skin rash, indirect hyperbilirubinemia, prolonged PR interval.	Avoid in severe hepatic insufficiency.
Tipranavir	Diarrhea, nausea, vomiting abdominal pain, ↑ liver enzyme rash	Avoid concurrent fosamprenavir, saquinavir.
Darunavir	Diarrhea, nausea, headache, rash ↑ liver enzyme ↑ serum amylase.	Avoid in patients with sulfa allergy.

* Contraindicated concurrent drugs include anti-arrhythmics, antihistamines, statins, sedative-hypnotics, anticonvulsants, oral contraceptives, rifampin and rifapentine

Integrase inhibitors

Raltegravir is an HIV integrase inhibitor that blocks the HIV integrase enzyme needed for the virus to multiply. It inhibits the third and final step of proviral DNA integration: that of strand transfers.

Raltegravir in combination with tenofovir/emtricitabine has been found to be as effective as the current first-line choice of efavirenz/tenofovir/emtricitabine for early treatment and has fewer side effects. Common side effects are diarrhea, nausea, and headache.

Antiretroviral therapy

A combination of three or more drugs from at least two different groups is necessary to achieve long-term suppression of HIV RNA to below the threshold of detection (viral load to < 50 copies ml) and to improve CD4 cell count. The drugs of choice for initial and subsequent antiviral therapy are given in Table 13.6.

Problems of ART therapy

- Adherence to the drug treatment regimen.
- Drug resistance. Despite the prevalence of resistance in patients who have not responded to multiple prior treatment regimens and given the availability of new class drugs and new generation drugs, virtually all patients – no matter how much resistance is present – can be treated with a combination of ART that should be fully suppressive.

Complication of ART

The long term use of ART has been associated with toxicity which mainly include.

- Lipodystrophy syndrome consist of an alteration in body fat leading to the accumulation of visceral fat in the abdomen, neck (buffalo lump), and pelvic areas, and/or the depletion of subcutaneous fat, causing facial or peripheral washing.

  Lipodysytrophy has been associated in particular with PIs and NRTIs.

- Hyperlipidemia, especially hypertriglycemia, is associated with PIs (especially ritonavir).

Table 13.6: Approach to initial and subsequent antiretroviral therapy

Initial			Subsequent		
(Regimen should consist of one drug from each column)			(Regimen should include two fully active new agents from different classes)		
PIs and NNRTIs	NRTI-1	NRTI-2	PIs and NNRTIs	Entry inhibitors	Integrase Inhibitors
Preferred Efavirenz	Tenofovir Abacavir	Lamivudine Emtricitabine	Darunavir Tipranavir Etravirine	Maraviroc Enfuvirtide	Raltegravir
Alternative Lopinavir Fosamprenavir Darunavir Atazanavir Saquinavir Nevirapine	Didanosine Zidovudine				

Other preferred initial regimens

Emtricitabine/tenofovir Atazanavir Ritonavir	Emtricitabine/tenofovir Darunavir Ritonavir
Emtricitabine/tenofovir Raltegravir	

- Peripheral insulin resistance, impaired glucose tolerance, and hyperglycemia have been associated with the use of PI-based regimens, mainly indinavir and ritonavir.
- Lactic acidosis with liver steatosis is a rare but sometimes fatal complication associated with NRTIs.
- Osteopenia and osteoporosis are common in HIV infections. The role of ART is not clear.
- Osteonecrosis, particularly of the hip, has been increasingly associated with HIV infection.

Prevention of HIV

Sexual

- Safe sex practices (avoiding penetrative intercourse, delaying sexual debut, condom use, fewer sexual partners)
- Control of sexually transmitted infections
- Effective treatment of HIV-infected individuals.
- Post-sexual exposure prophylaxis

Parenteral

- Blood product transmission: routine screening of donated blood, blood substitute use.
- Injection drug use: needle/syringe exchange, sharing and needles.

Prenatal

- Routine 'opt-out' antenatal HIV antibody testing
- Treatment of HIV in pregnancy
- Ritonavir-boosted PI (e.g. lopinavir) with zidovudine and lamivudine from 20 weeks.
- Zidovudine monotherapy who are willing to have caesarian section.

- Zidovudine intravenous infusion at onset of labor or administered to the infant within 48 hours of birth.
- Avoid breast-feeding.

Occupational

- Education/training: universal, precaution, needle stick avoidance.
- Post-exposure prophylaxis.

13.1 ANTIHEPATITIS AGENTS

Treatment for hepatitis B virus (HBV) and hepatitis C virus (HCV), available at present, is only suppressive and not curative.

INTERFERONS

Interferons are cytokines produced by natural T cells, macrophages and large granular lymphocytes which exert complex-antiviral, immunomodulatory, and antiproliferative actions.

Interferon alfa acts on all the stages of viral life cycle leading to inhibition of viral penetration to release of viral particles from T lymphocytes. Injectable preparations of interferon alfa are available for treatment of both HBV and HCV infections. Psegylated interferon alfa is long acting and require less frequent dosing. Interferon does not induce antiviral resistance.

Common adverse effects of interferon alfa include a flu-like syndrome. Potential adverse effects during chronic therapy include neurotoxicity, myelosuppression, retinopathy, pneumonitis and cardiotoxicity.

Hepatic decompensation, autoimmune disease and history of cardiac arrhythmias contraindicate the use of interferon alfa.

HEPATITIS B VIRUS INFECTION

The goals of antiviral therapy in patients with chronic HBV infection are suppression of HBV DNA to undetectable levels, seroconversion from hepatitis antigen (HBeAg) from positive to negative, and reduction in elevated hepatic transaminase levels. These end points are correlated with improvement in microinflammatory disease, a decreased risk of hepatocellular carcinoma and cirrhosis, and a decreased need for liver transplantation.

The current available drugs suppress HBV replication rather than eradicate the virus. The covalently closed circular (CCC) DNA exists in stable form indefinitely within the cell; serving as a reservoir for HBV throughout the life of the cell and resulting in the capacity to reactivate. Relapses are more common in patients co-infected with HBV and hepatitis D virus.

Five oral nucleoside/nucleotide analogs (lamivudine, adefovir dipivoxil, tenofovir, entecavir, telbivudine) and two injectable interferon drugs (interferon alfa-2b, pegylated interferon alfa-2a) are available for treatment of HBV. In general mucleoside/nucleotide analog therapies have better tolerability and incur a higher response rate than the interferons, but the response is less sustained after the discontinuation of nucleoside/nucleotide therapies, and emergence of resistance may be problematic.

The nucleotides are effective in nucleoside resistance and vice versa. In addition oral agents may be used in patients with decompensated liver disease, and the therapy is chronic rather than finite as with interferon therapy.

HEPATITIS C INFECTION

In contrast to the treatment of patients with chronic HBV infection, the primary goal of the treatment in patients with HCV infection is viral eradication.

Treatment of patients with chronic HCV infection is recommended for those with an increased risk of progression to cirrhosis. Pegylated interferon alfa-2 and -2b have replaced their unmodified interferon alfa counterparts because of superior efficacy in combination with ribavirin. The combination therapy is more effective than monotherapy with either interferon or ribavirin. Monotherapy with pegylated interferon alfa is recommended only in patients who cannot tolerate ribavirin.

Table 13.7 Summarizes the drug treatment of hepatitis virus.

Table 13.7: Drugs used treat viral hepatitis

Drugs	Significant side effect	Comments
Hepatitis B		
First line drugs		
Entecavir	Well tolerated, headache, fatigue, dizziness & nausea.	HBV DNA clearance < 90%, resistance very low
Tenofovir	Well tolerated, GIT disorders, headache and asthenia. Renal failure and Fanconi syndrome rare	HBV DNA clearance < 90% resistance practically negligible
Preglylated interferon alfa-2a	Poor tolerability profile	Parenteral agents. No antiviral resistance induction
Second line drugs		
Telbivudine	Excellent safety profile. Headache, nausea, and dizziness rare	Poor resistance profile. Not effective in antiviral resistance
Adefovir	Well tolerated, dose-dependent nephrotoxicity. Headache, diarrhea, asthenia and abdominal pain	Less effective viral suppression
Lamivudine	Excellent safety profile,	Diminished use due to high rates of resistant mutations
Hepatitis C		
Preglylated interferon alfa-2a/2b	Flu-like symptoms neuropsychiatric disorders, endocrine dysfunction and bone marrow suppression.	Induction of auto antibodies, exacerbation or unmasking of autoimmune disease. Non toxic.
Ribavirrin	Tcrotogenicity, hemolytic anemia, and pulmonary symptoms.	Contraindicated in end-stage renal failure, ischemic vascular disease.

14 Vaccines, Antisera, Immunoglobulins and Immunotherapy

Vaccines provide **active immunity** against diseases by production of antibodies or sensitized lymphocytes to certain microorganisms.

Vaccines sensitize B lymphocytes in the blood, which are specific for particular infecting organism. The sensitized B lymphocytes persist in blood as memory cells for varying periods, from a few months up to many years. This establishment of 'memory cells' by the B lymphocytes forms the basis of vaccination (active immunization) against infecting organisms and harmful toxins they produce.

Following infection after vaccination, the memory cells (sensitized B lymphocytes) become activated, multiply rapidly and release proteins (immunoglobins or antibodies) that destroy the infecting organism or its toxin and prevent the disease.

Vaccines are of three types:

LIVE ATTENUATED VACCINES

These consist of live virus or bacteria, which has been rendered avirulant. Immunization is generally achieved with a single dose (but 3 doses are required with oral poliomyelitis and oral typhoid vaccines), which provides a durable immunity.

Live vaccines should not be given to individuals with impaired immune response, whether caused by disease or as a result of radiotherapy or treatment with high doses of corticosteroids or other immunosuppressive drugs. They should not be given to those suffering from malignant conditions such as leukemia and tumors of reticuloendothelial system.

HIV positive patients should not receive BCG, yellow fever and typhoid (oral) vaccines.

INACTIVATED VACCINES

These consist of virus or bacteria killed by heat or chemicals. They may require a primary series of injections of vaccine to produce adequate antibody response, followed by booster injections in most of the cases. Immunity produced varies from months to many years.

TOXOIDS

These are extracts of or detoxified endotoxins produced by bacteria. They are more immunogenic, if adsorbed into an adjuvant (such as aluminium hydroxide) and require primary series of injections followed by booster doses.

VIRAL VACCINES

MMR vaccine is a combined live measles, mumps and rubella vaccine that has replaced measles vaccine and should be given to every child, irrespective of previous measles, mumps or rubella infection. The first dose is given to children aged 12–15 months, followed by a second (booster) dose at 4–5 years of age.

MMR vaccine occasionally produces malaise, fever, a rash and parotid swelling, about 1 week after injection. MMR vaccine should not be given within 8 weeks of administration of another live vaccine by injection and in children, who are allergic to neomycin or kanamycin (MMR vaccine contains small amounts of neomycin).

If given to women, pregnancy should be avoided for 1 month (as for rubella vaccine).

Poliomyelitis vaccine is of two types; oral attenuated live virus (Sabin vaccine) and injectable inactivated live virus (Salk vaccine). Oral Sabin vaccine is preferred as it avoids injections, provides a more prolonged immunity and by providing antibodies in the intestines, prevents the spread of infection. The dose is three drops given at an interval of 1 month, starting at two months of age. Two-booster doses of poliomyelitis oral vaccine are recommended the first before school entry and second before leaving school.

Oral poliomyelitis vaccine should not be given, if the child has vomiting and diarrhea and in immunodeficiency disorders.

Inactivated vaccine may be used, when oral (live) vaccine is contraindicated and for immunosppressed individuals. Vaccine associated poliomyelitis is extremely rare.

Rubella vaccine is an attenuated live virus vaccine. It is indicated for seronegative women of childbearing age. It is important to exclude pregnancy and to avoid it for 1 month thereafter, before giving the vaccine. The objective is to prevent fetal rubella infection, which can occur up to second trimester of pregnancy. Joint pain, low-grade fever and rash may occur after vaccination.

Hepatitis B vaccine contains inactivated hepatitis B virus surface antigen (HbsAg) adsorbed on aluminum hydroxide adjuvant. It is made biosynthetically using recombinant DNA technology. This vaccine is of particular importance to the health professionals, who have direct contact with blood or blood stained body fluids or with patients' tissues, as it can be spread by infected body fluids (blood and saliva). Immunization takes up to 6 months to confer adequate protection. Duration of immunity is not known, but it persists for at least for 2 years. A single booster dose after 5 years is recommended.

Passive immunization is also possible in individuals, who get accidentally infected by using a special serum containing large amounts of antibody (hepatitis B immunoglobulin, HBIG) against the hepatitis B virus.

Rabies vaccine is of three types:

Antirabic vaccine carbolized (simple vaccine) is a 5% suspension of brain substance containing carbolic acid fixed rabies virus. It is injected subcutaneously in the abdominal wall daily for 14 days for post dog bite prophylaxis. Vaccine associated encephalitis and neuroparalytic complications have been reported.

Purified chick embryo cells (PCEC) vaccine is inactivated rabies virus grown on chick fibroblasts. For, post exposure prophylaxis, a course of 6 injections of 1ml is given intramuscularly in the deltoid region, on days 0, 3, 7, 14, 30 and 90. It is highly effective and is less likely to cause neuroparalytic complications.

Merieux inactivated rabies vaccine (HDC) is freeze-dried inactivated Wister rabies virus strain cultivated in human diploid cells. For post exposure prophylaxis, a course of 5 injections is given on days 0, 3, 7, 14 and 30 in the deltoid region, as injections in the gluteal region produce poor response. This diploid vaccine is well tolerated and its use is not associated with neurological complications.

Other viral vaccines for *H. influenzae* type B, hepatitis A, yellow fever and other less common viral diseases, are available for use in special high-risk situations.

BACTERIAL VACCINES

BCG (Bacillus Calemette Guerin) vaccine is a live attenuated strain derived from mycobacterium bovis, which produces tuberculosis antibodies. It is given intradermally in the deltoid region in the newly born infants of up to 3 months. In children between 10 and 14 years of age, it should be given, if tuberculin test is negative. Within 2–6 weeks, a small swelling appears at the injection site, which progresses to a papule or to a benign ulcer of about 10–mm in diameter which heals in 6–12 weeks. It is contraindicated in tuberculin positive individuals and in individuals with impaired immune response.

Whooping cough (pertussis) vaccine is a suspension of killed B. pertussis. It is usually given combined with diphtheria and tetanus vaccine (triple vaccine), starting at 2 months of age. Pertussis vaccine immunization should not be carried out in children, who have a history of severe general reactions to preceding dose. In these children, immunization should be completed with absorbed diphtheria and tetanus vaccine. General reactions to a preceding dose, which contraindicates its continuation of subsequent immunization, include temperature of 39.5°C or more, anaphylaxis and convulsions within 72 hours.

Other bacterial vaccines for immunization against cholera, meningococcal group C, typhoid and pneumococci are available for use in special high-risk situations.

TOXOIDS

Tetanus toxoid (tetanus vaccine) is formalin treated exotoxin of tetanus bacilli, which stimulates the production of protective antitoxin. In general, adsorption on aluminium hydroxide, aluminium phosphate or calcium phosphate improves antigencity. Adsorbed tetanus vaccine is given routinely to babies in combination with adsorbed diphtheria and pertussis vaccine. In children, the triple vaccine, not only gives protection against tetanus in childhood, but also gives the basic immunity for subsequent booster doses of adsorbed tetanus vaccine at school entry and at school leaving (combined with adsorbed diphtheria vaccine) and also when a potentially tetanus contaminated injury takes place.

Tetanus vaccine is important for pregnant women (two doses during second and third trimester) and persons in older age groups for elective surgery, who may never, had a routine or complete course of earlier immunization. Apart from minor local reactions, complications are extremely rare.

Diphtheria vaccine is prepared from the toxin of *Corynebacterium diphtheriae*. Adsorbed diphtheria vaccine is used in combination with adsorbed tetanus vaccine for routine immunization schedule for children.

ANTISERA AND IMMUNOGLOBULINS

Unlike vaccines, antibodies are prepared by injecting an antigen, either vaccine or toxoid into an animal (antisera) or from the human blood after the subject has been actively immunized or has suffered a particular infection (immunoglobulin). These provide passive immunity which lasts for about 2 weeks.

Antisera

Antisera are purified concentrated preparations of serum of horses actively immunized against specific antigen. Antiserum carries a real risk of hypersensitivity reactions, which are of two types.

Immediate or anaphylactic reactions occur within a few minutes of injection and patient collapses with difficulty in breathing, low blood pressure, which can be fatal. A syringe of 1: 1000 adrenalin, an antihistamine and hydrocortisone hemisuccinate should be kept ready in case of immediate reaction.

Serum sickness occurs 7–12 days later. The patient develops fever, rash and arthritis. Spontaneous recovery is usual, but calamine lotion applied to rash and oral antihistamine and prednisolone in more severe case will relieve symptoms and speed recovery

The antiserum in use are diphtheria antitoxin, gas gangrene antitoxin and anti-snake venous polyvalent.

Immunoglobulin

Human immunoglobulin are safe and rarely produce a serious reaction, although, there may be discomfort at the injection site. There are two types of human immunoglobulin preparations— normal immunoglobulin and specific immunoglobulin.

Normal immunoglobulin (HNIG)

HNIG is prepared from pools of at least 1000 donations of human plasma. It contains antibody to measles, mumps, varicella, hepatittis A and other viruses that are currently prevalent in the general population.

HNIG is administered by intramuscular injection for the protection of susceptible contacts against hepatitis A virus and measles, and prevention of clinical attack of rubella in pregnancy. For replacement therapy, intravenous immunoglobulin is preferred for patients with congenital agammaglobulinemia, for the management of idiopathic thrombocytopenic pupura and Kawasaki syndrome and for the prophylaxis of infections following bone marrow transplantation.

Side effects of HNIG include malaise, chills, fever and rarely anaphylaxis. It is contraindicated in patients with known class specific antibody to immunoglobulin A.

Specific immunoglobulin

These are prepared from immunized donors or convalescent patients.

Anti-D immunoglobulin is used to prevent from forming antibodies to fetal rhesus-positive cells which may pass into the maternal circulation during childbirth or abortion. It is given within 72 hours after delivery/abortion to prevent Rh hemolytic disease in future offspring. It may be given at 26–28 weeks of pregnancy followed by a further dose within 72 hours of delivery.

Hepatitis B immunoglobulin (HBIG) can be given in association with the vaccine for the prevention of infection to the health professional, and in infants born to mothers, who had become infected with the hepatitis B virus in pregnancy.

Rabies immunoglobulin should be injected at the site of the bite and also intramuscularly along with vaccine to non-immunized individuals

Tetanus immunoglobulin (HTIG) is indicated in tetanus prone wounds along with adsorbed tetanus vaccine and chemotherapy prophylaxis.

Varicella zoster immunoglobulin (VZIG) is indicated in neonates of women not latter than 10 days after exposure to chickenpox.

Cytomegalovirus (CMV) immunoglobulin

CMV immunoglobulin is indicated for prophylaxis in patients receiving immunosuppressive drugs.

IMMUNOTHERAPY

MODULATING DRUGS

The development of drugs that modulate immune system function rather than suppress it has become an important area of pharmacology. The rationale underlying this approach is to design ways to specifically interrupt pathologic immune responses, leaving non-pathologic immune responses intact. Novel ways to interrupt pathologic immune responses, that are under investigations, include the use of anti-inflammatory cytokines or specific cytokine inhibitors as anti-inflammatory agents, the use of monoclonal antibodies against T or B lymphocytes as therapeutic agents, the induction of anergy (unresponsiveness) of T cells by the administration of tolerogens or inhibitors of immune cell co-stimulation. The use of intravenous 1 g for certain infections and immune complex-mediated diseases, the use of specific cytokines to reconstitute components of the immune system, and bone marrow transplantation to replace the pathologic immune system with a more normal immune system.

The major potential uses of these drugs are in immune deficiency diseases, chronic infectious diseases, and cancer. The AID epidemic has greatly increased interest in developing more effective immunomodulatory drugs.

CYTOKINES

The cytokines are a large and heterogenous group of proteins that act as multipurpose chemical messangers. They are produced by cells involved in innate and adaptive immune responses and by stromal tissues. More that 100 cytobines have been developed, with overlapping complex roles in modifying the immune microenvironment. Abnormal expression of cytokines may result in immune, inflammatory and injection discase states. The most important cytokines are listed in Table 14.1.

Recombinant cytokines

Cytokines are gaining popularity as immunomodulators. With the advent of genetic engineering cytokines can be produced in bulk and in purified forms.

Aldesleukin

This is recombinant IL-2 obtained from cultures of *E.coli*. Aldesleukin stimulates TH cells and Tc cells and thus enhances cellular immunity. It is used in the treatment of metastatic renal cell carcinoma and melanoma. Side effects include capillary leak syndrome, hypotension and concomitant infection due to decrease in neutrophil function.

Table 14.1: Important cytokines in regulation of immune responses

Cytokines	Source	Actions
Interferon-alpha (IFN-α)	T cells and macrophages	Antiviral activity Actirates NK cells CD8+ T cells and macrophages.
Interferon-gamma (IFN-γ)	T cells and NK cells	Increases antimicrobial and antitumor activity of macrophages. Determines cytokine production by T cells and macrophages
Tumor necrosis factor alpha (TNF-α)	Macrophages and NK cells	Pro-inflammatory Increases apoptosis and expression of cytokines and adhesion molecules. Directly cytotoxic.
Interleukin-1 (IL-1)	Macrophages and neutrophils	Acute phase reactant Stimulates neutrophil recruitment, fever, T-cell and macrophage activation, immunoglobulin production.
Interleukin-2 (IL-2)	CD4+ T cells	Stimulates proliferation and differentiation of antigen-specific T lymphocytes
Interleukin-4 (IL-4)	CD+ 4 T cells and mast cells	Stimulates maturation of B and T cells and production of 1gE antibody
Interleukin-6 (IL-6)	Monocytes and macrophages	Acute phase reactant Stimulates maturation of B cells into plasma cells.
Interleukin-12 (IL-12)	Monocytes and Macrophages	Stimulates IFN-γ and TNF-α release by T cells, activates NK cells

(NK: natural killer)

Other recombinant interleukins

rIL-1 is produced by macrophages and is essential for activation and proliferation of various immune cells. It is used for general augmentation of immune responses.

Oprelvekin (rIL-11) stimulates megakaryocytes and their precursors in the bone marrow and is used to prevent thrombocytopenia in patients receiving chemotherapy for cancer.

Recombinant interferons

Interferon-α (IFN-α). Human recombinant IFN-α as a immunostimulent, as it activates T-lymphocytes, natural killer cells and macrophages. Both IFN-α and IFN-α2b are indicated for a variety of cancers, and in the treatment of hapatitis-B and C virus infections. Side effects include flu like syndrome, blood dyscrasias, nephrotoxicity and neurological symptoms such as nervousness and confusion.

Interferon-β_{1a} and β_{1b} are used for the treatment of relapsing type multiple sclerosis.

Interferon γ recombinant human IFN-γ restores macrophages cytotoxicity by generating free radicals and is used for the treatment of chronic granulomatous disease.

Cytokine inhibitors

Tumor necrosis factor-α (TNF-α) inhibitors

TNF-α secreted by activated cytotoxic TH$_1$ cells, macrophages and mast cells binds to TNF receptor (TNFR, or TNFR2) present on fibroblasts, neutrophils, and vascular endothelial cells. Besides these, there are "soluble form of TNF-α receptor" present in serum and synovial fluid.

Activation of TNF-α results in the release of cytokines IL-1, IL-6 and adhesion molecules that promote leukocyte activation and trafficking (migration).

Infliximab is a humanized mouse (25% mouse and 75% human) anti-TNF-α monoclonal antibody (MAb). This drug cross-links with membrane bound TNF-α receptor on cell surface to inhibit T-cell and macrophage function and to prevent the release of other proinflammatory cytokines (1L-1, 6 and 8 along with collagenase and metalloproteinases) and is currently used in crohn's disease and rheumatoid arthritis.

Adalimumab, a human recombinant monoclonal antibody to TNF-α, is less antigenic than infliximab as it does not contain any foreign component.

Interleukin-1 (1L-1) inhibitors

IL-1 enhances the production of 1L-6 of adhesion molecule and the release of metalloproteinase. 1L-1 also stimulates cell proliferation. The role of metalloproteinase is to degrade the cellular matrix in preparation for their proliferation. The naturally occurring endogenous antagonists of 1L-1 receptor is 1L-1ra. Anakinra is a recombinant form of 1L-1ra which inhibits 1L-1 interactions with the immune cells and is used for the treatment of rheumatoid arthritis.

Interleukin-2 (IL-2) inhibitors

Daclizumab and Basiliximab are chimeric monoclonal antibodies that block the α-chain of IL-2 receptor (CD 25) located on the surface of activated T-cells and are used for the prophylaxis of acute organ transplant rejections.

Monoclonal antibodies to T and B cells

Muromonab-CD3 (anti-CD3 or OKT3) is a murine monoclonal antibody against CD3, one of an important signaling molecule for activation of T-cell receptor. As a result, treatment with muromonab depletes the total circulating T-cells from the blood. This depletion of T-cell is due to cell death (anergy in absence of signal) and antibody mediated activation of complement.

OKT3 is used for the prevention of allograft rejection after kidney, liver and heart transplant. Alemtuzumab (Anti-CD52), CD52 is a glycoprotein expressed on normal and malignant T- and B-lymphocytes, monocytes, NK cells and macrophages.

Alemtuzumab is a humanized anti CD52 monoclonal antibody that binds to CD52 and causes prolonged lymphopenia. It is used to treat B-cell lymphocytic leukemia.

It is important to realize the potential risk for these immunosuppressive monoclonal antibodies, which increases the risk of opportunistic infections.

Tolerogens or **inhibitors of immune cell costinulation**

Specific immunotherapy is now focused to induce T-cell tolerance in order to have immunosuppression without concomitant risk of developing opportunistic infections and secondary tumors with the induction of soluble CTLA-4 protein in clinical trials.

Tolerogens (none available at present) refers to drugs that have the capability to induce T cell "anergy or tolerance". The development of tolerance involves development of mature T-cell, which will not attack native proteins and abolish the signal that activates T-cells.

The activation of T-cells requires two activating signals. The first signal is provided by binding of antigen complex specific T-receptor (TCR) with foreign antigen (MHC class antigen). But for T-cell to become responsive a "second signal" is also needed, in absence of which the T-cells become "anergic" (unresponsive). In other words, "signal one" in absence of "signal two" leads to tolerance or a "functional silencing" of T-cells (anergy).

Soluble CTLA 4 (CD-152) protein expressed on T-cells dampens (down regulate an immune response) or block T-cell activation.

CTLA4-1g (a homologue of CTLA4, i.e. a part of immunoglobulin molecule and a part of CTLA-4) is undergoing clinical trials with promising results in bone marrow transplantation and autoimmune disease psoriasis.

Stem cell transplantation

Stem cell transplantation using hematopoietic stem cells is an extremely valuable treatment for a variety of hematologic malignancies. The basis of treatment with stem cell transplantation is the ability of the hematopoietic stem cells to completely restore bone marrow function and formation of all blood components, as well as to re-from the immune system.

Hematopoietic stem cells transplantation (SCT) is now being studied to re-form immune system in autoimmune disease syndrome to replace a dysfunctional immune system. Preliminary clinical trials with SCT have shown encouraging results in certain autoimmune diseases like systemic lupus erythematosus, multiple sclerosis and scleroderma.

Recent evidence suggests that hematopoietic stem cells can differentiate into non-hematological cells, such as nerve, skeletal muscle, cardiac muscle, liver and blood vessel's endothelium. This is termed stem-cell plasticity and may have exciting clinical applications in the future.

Thus, the possibility of replacement of dysfunctional immune system by SCT, induction of tolerogens and other developments may replace the existing toxic immunotherapy with non-toxic specific and functional therapies for immune and inflammatory diseases

15

Drugs for Malaria

Malaria is one of the most common and widespread disease. It is caused by the malarial parasite, plasmodium, which is injected by the bite of female anopheline mosquito. In man, the malarial parasite undergoes an asexual cycle, which consists of a pre-erythrocytic stage, an erythrocytic and an exo-erythrocytic cycle.

Pre-erythrocytic cycle takes place in the liver and accounts for the incubation period of 10–14 days.

Erythrocytic cycle. The parasites, released from the rupture of the liver cells, enter red blood cells and undergo erythrocyte cycle, which is either 48 hours or 72 hours. The red cells then rupture releasing the parasites, which re-enter fresh red cells and the cycle goes on. The clinical symptoms of malarial fever coincide with the rupture of red cells. Some parasites develop into gametocytes.

Exo-erythrocytic cycle. Some of the parasites re-enter the liver cells and form the resting forms of the parasites – dormant hypnozoite stages of *P. vivax* and *P. ovale* which can be reactivated to continue erythrocytic cycle of multiplication and thus causes relapses.

There are four varieties of human malarial parasites.

P. falciparum is the most dangerous of the malarias and patients are either 'killed or cured'. It has an erythrocytic cycle of less than 48 hours. The fever has no particular pattern. It does not have an exo-erythrocytic phase, so that relapse does not occur.

P. vivax and *P. ovale* have an erythrocytic cycle of 48 hours and are characterized by classical bouts of fever on alternate days. Exo-erythrocytic phase persists and relapses are frequent.

P. malariae has an erythrocytic cycle of 72 hours with no exo-erythrocytic phase.

Chemoprophylaxis and treatment

Clinical attacks of malaria are preventable with chemoprophylaxis and the choice of drugs used depend mainly on the degree of chloroquine resistance (Table 15.1).

Table 15.1: Chemoprophylaxis of malaria

Drug	Adult dose	Regimen
Chloroquine resistance high		
Mefloquine[1]	250 mg weekly	Begin 1–2 weeks before and continue until 4 weeks after travel
Or		
Doxycycline[2,3]	100 mg daily	Begin 1–2 days before and continue until 4 weeks after travel
Or		
Malarone[3]	1 tablet daily	Begin 1–2 before and continue until 1 week after travel
Chloroquine resistance absent		
Chloroquine and proguanil	300 mg base weekly 100 mg daily	Begin 1 week before and continue until 4 week after travel

[1] Contraindicated in the first trimester of pregnancy, lactation, cardiac conduction disorders, epilepsy, psychiatric disorders.
[2] Causes photosensitization.
[3] Avoid in pregnancy

The main problem encountered in the treatment of malaria is the potential for drug resistance. *P. falciparum* is now commonly resistant to chloroquine and sulfadoxine- pyremethamine in most areas. Recommendation for the treatment of uncomplicated falciparum malaria have undergone major changes in recent years, with artemisinin based combinations, all including a short-acting artemisinin and longer-acting partner drug as first-line therapies.

Regimens for treatment of malaria are given in Table 15.2.

QUININE AND QUINIDINE

Quinine is an alkaloid obtained from the bark of the Cinchonna tree and remains one of the best drugs for all complicated malaria, especially chloroquine resistant *P. falciparum* infection. Quinidine,

Table 15.2: Regimens for the treatment of malaria

Malaria status	Regimen(s)
Uncomplicated non-falciparum malaria[1]	
Known chloroquine-sensitive strains	Chloroquine 600 mg of base stat followed by 300 mg base in 6 hours, then 150 mg base 12-hourly for 2 more days *Or* Amodiaquine 600 mg of base for 3 days.
Radical treatment for *P. vivax* or *P. ovale* infection	In addition to chloroquine or amodiaquine as detailed above, a course of primaquine (15 mg daily for 14 days) destroys the hypnozoite phase in the liver to prevent relapse.
Mild *P. falciparum* malaria	Artesunate 240 mg daily for 3 days plus sulfadoxine 1.5 g and pyrimethamine 75 mg as a single dose *Or* Artesunate 240 mg plus amodiaquine 600 mg of base daily for 3 days.
Multidrug resistant *P. falciparum* malaria	Co-artemether (artemether 20 mg and lumefantrine 120 mg) four tablets twice daily for 3 days with food *Or* Artesunate 240 mg plus mefloquine 480 mg daily for 3 days[2]
Second-line treatment	Artesunate 120 mg daily for 7 days or quinine 600 mg thrice daily plus either doxycycline[3] 200 mg or clindamycin 600 mg daily for 7 days or Atovaquone–proguanil (20/8 mg/kg) daily for 3 days with food.
Severe falciparam malaria[4]	Artesunate 2.4 mg/kg stat IV followed by 2.4 mg/kg at 12 and 24 hours[4] and then daily if necessary *Or* Artemether 3.2 mg/kg stat followed by 1.6 mg/kg daily *Or* Quinine dihydrochloride 20 mg/kg infused over 4 hours, followed by 10 mg/kg infused over 2–8 hours every 8 hours *Or* Quinidine gluconate 10 mg/kg infused over 1–2 hours, followed by 1.2 mg/kg per hour[5].

[1] Many of non-falciparum malaria have developed resistance to chloroquine.
[2] Fixed-dose coformulated combinations are available. The world Health Organization now recommends artemisinin combination regimens as first-line therapy for falciparum malaria and advocates use of fixed-dose combinations.
[3] Doxycycline should not be given to pregnant women or to children < 8 years of age.
[4] Oral treatment should be substituted as soon as the patient recovers sufficiently to take fluids by mouth.
[5] Avoid loading doses in persons who have received quinine, quinidine or mefloquine in the prior 24 hours. Cardiac monitoring should be in place during intravenous administration of quinine or quinidine.

isomer of quinine is at least as effective as parenteral quinine in the treatment of severe falciparum malaria.

Pharrmacokinetics

Quinine is well absorbed orally, about 70% is bound to plasma proteins and CSF penetration is poor. It is mainly metabolized in the liver and excretion is complete within 24 hours. Quinidine has a shorter half-life than quinine, mostly as a result of decreased protein binding.

Pharmacological actions

Quinine suppresses the multiplication of the plasmodium in the blood stream. It does not have any action on exo-erythrocytic stage of malarial life cycle and relapses (symptoms) may occur, when quinine is stopped. Quinine has no action on gametes and does not prevent transmission of the infection.

Quinine has a number of other actions, which are responsible for the adverse effects seen with the drug. It is a cardiac depressant (action similar to quinidine), causes contraction of the uterus, decreases the excitability and contractility of the skeletal muscles and releases insulin.

Therapeutic uses

Quinine is not suitable for the prophylaxis of malaria. It is used for the treatment of falciparum malaria or if the infective species is not known or if the infection is mixed. It is given in dosage of 600 mg of quinine sulfate every 8 hourly for 7 days, followed by fansidar (combination of pyrimethamine 25 mg and sulfadoxine 500 mg), 3 tablets as a single dose. Doxycycline 200 mg daily for 7 days is an alternative to fansidar.

In cerebral malaria, quinine dihydrochloride is given by intravenous infusion in a loading dose of 20 mg/kg in 500 ml dextrose saline, followed by a maintenance dose of 10 mg/kg at 8 hourly intervals in IV drip until the patient can take it orally.

Quinine in dosage of 200–300 mg at bed time is used for nocturnal leg cramps.

Adverse effects

Cinchonism, hypoglycemia, giddiness, psychosis, visual disturbances, nausea and vomiting are common. Cardiac arrhythmia, hemolysis and renal failure may occur. It should not be given in hemoglobinuria and optic neuritis.

Antiarrhythmics, antihistmines, antipsychotics and cisapride increase the risk of ventricular arrhythmias.

Blackwater fever is a rare severe illness that includes hemolysis and hemoglobinuria in the setting of quinine therapy for malaria. It appears to be due to a hypersensitivity reaction to the drug, although its pathogenesis is uncertain.

MEFLOQUINE

Mefloquine is a synthetic quinoline methanol compound. Its antimalarial action is similar to quinine. Although toxicity is a concern, mefloquine is one of the recommended chemoprophylactic drugs for use in most malaria-endemic regions with chloroquine-resistant strains.

Pharmacokinetics

Mefloquine is well absorbed orally and is highly bound to plasma proteins. It is concentrated in many organs including lungs, liver and intestines. It undergoes extensive enterohepatic circulation and is primarily secreted in the bile.

Therapeutic uses

Mefloquine has the advantage of being given in a single dose of 1 g. It is used for chemoprophylaxis of malaria, treatment of uncomplicated falciparum malaria and chloroquine resistant vivax malaria.

Adverse effects

Dizziness, nausea and vomiting are common. Arrhythmia and acute brain syndrome consisting of fatigue, asthenia, convulsions and psychosis may occur

Mefloquine should not be given in patients with history of neuropsychiatric disorders including depression or convulsions or hypersensitivity to quinine.

Concomitant use of beta blockers, calcium channel blockers and cardiac glycosides increases the risk of bradycardia.

Mefloquine is generally considered safe in young children and pregnant women (excluding first trimester).

HALOFANTRINE

Halofantrine is a synthetic phenanthrene methanol compound, which is not suitable for the prophylaxis of malaria. It is effective in falciparum malaria, but owing to its side effects, it is seldom used.

Adverse effects

The most serious toxic effect is ventricular arrhythmia. Others include GIT disturbances and hypersensitivity reactions. It should not be used in cardiac disease associated with prolonged QT interval and with drugs that induce arrhythmia.

LUMEFANTRINE

Lumefantrine, related to halofantrine, is available only as a fixed-dose combination with artemether (Co-artemether), which is now the first-line treatment for uncomplicated falciparum malaria.

Lumefantrine does not possess the risk of dangerous arrhythmias seen with halofantrine and quinidine. It is well tolerated.

Adverse effects include GIT disturbance, headache, dizziness, rash, and pruritus which may even be due to underlying malaria or concomitant medication rather than to co-artemether.

ARTEMISININS

Artemisinin is the active component of a Chinese herbal medicine that is a very rapidly acting blood schizonticide against all human malaria parasites. It has no effect on tissue schizonts (hepatic stages).

Artemisinin is unstable and its analogs have been synthesized to increase solubility and improve antimalarial efficacy. The most important of these analogs are artesunate (water soluble, useful for oral, intravenous, intramuscular, and rectal administration), artemether (lipid-soluble, useful for oral, intramuscular, and rectal administration), and the active metabolite dihydroartemisinin (water soluble, useful for oral administration).

Artemisinins have short plasma half life and recurrence rates are high after short-course therapy, and they are best used in combination with another agent. Also because of their short-half life, they are not useful in chemoprophylaxis.

The WHO is encouraging availability of oral artemisinins only in co-formulated combination regimens. The artemisinins-based combination regimens, that are currently most advocated are artesunate plus amodiaquine (ASAQ) and artemether plus lumefantrine (Co-artemether). A third available co-formulated regimen that has performed well in clinical trials, and was added to the list of WHO recommended regimen for uncomplicated falciparum malaria in 2010, is dihydroartemisinin plus piperaquine. This is the first-line regimen in some countries in Southeast Asia.

Artesunate plus mefloquine has demonstrated excellent efficacy against multidrug resistant parasites in Thailand.

Intravenous artesunate is considered to be superior to intravenous quinine in the treatment of complicated falciparum malaria in terms of parasite clearance time and more importantly in patient survival. Further, it has a superior side-effect profile compared with that of intravenous quinine or quinidine. Artesunate and artemether are also effective when administered rectally, offering a valuable treatment modality when parenteral therapy in not available.

Artemisinins are well tolerated. The most common adverse effects include GIT disorders and dizziness and these may often be due to malaria rather than the medications. Serious toxicity is rare and includes blood and allergic disorders. Artemisinins are teratogenic in animals, and they should be avoided in first trimester of pregnancy. However, for severe malaria for which all available treatment entails some risk, the WHO endorses the use of intravenous artesunate or quinine while additional data are gathered on artesunate safety.

CHLOROQUINE

Chloroquine is a 4-aminoquinoline, which is a very useful drug to treat malaria, but resistant strains of *P. falciparum* and vivax are common. It is effective against all forms of the plasmodia in the blood stream, but has no effect on the exoerythrocytic stages.

Chloroquine has a number of other actions, which include anti-inflammatory, local anesthetic, antihistaminic and antiarrhythmic properties.

Pharmacokinetics

Chloroquine is rapidly absorbed orally and is stored in various organs of the body. Its selective accumulation in retina is responsible for the ocular toxicity seen with prolonged therapy. It is partly metabolized and partly excreted in urine.

Therapeutic uses

Chloroquine is no longer recommended for the treatment of falciparum malaria owing to widespread resistance. It is the drug of choice for chemoprophylaxis and clinical cure of benign malaria caused by sensitive *P. vivax* and less commonly by *P. ovale* and *P. malariae*. In an acute attack of malaria, an initial dose of 600 mg of chloroquine (of base) is followed by 300 mg after 6 hours and then 300 mg daily for 2 days. For prophylaxis 300 mg chloroquine base is given weekly. Chloroquine sulphate 300 mg contains 225 mg of chloroquine base.

Chloroquine is moderately effective against gametocytes of *P. vivax, P. ovale* and *P. malariae* but not that of *P. falciparum*. Chloroquine is not active against liver stage parasites, and for that reason primaquine must be added for the radical cure of *P. vivax* and *P. ovale* malaria.

Resistance to chloroquine is now very common among stains of *P. faleparum* and uncommon but increasing for *P. vivax*.

Chloroquine is concentrated in liver and may be used for amebic abbesses that do not response to metronidazole.

Other uses of chloroquine include rheumatoid arthritis, lupus erythematosus and hepatic amoebiasis.

Adverse effects

These are generally uncommon with doses employed for malaria. Chloroquine is liable to cause GIT disturbances, headache, convulsions, visual disturbances, skin rashes and rarely bone marrow depression.

Other side effects like retinal damage, keratopathy, ototoxicity, blood disorders, mental changes, myopathy, exfoliative dermatitis and hepatic damage are not usually associated with doses used for malaria prophylaxis or treatment.

Chloroquine is contraindicated in patients with psoriasis or porphyria, in which it may precipitate acute attacks of these diseases. It should generally not be used in patients with retinal or visual field abnormalities or myopathy.

Chloroquine is safe in pregnancy and for young children.

AMODIAQUINE

Amodiaquine is closely related to chloroquine, but may be effective against chloroquine-resistant strains of *P. falciparum* in some areas.

Amodiaquine use has been limited because of its toxicity such as agranulocytosis, aplastic anemia, and hepatotoxicity. However, recent revaluation has revealed that these toxicities are rare and World Health Organization recommends amodiaquine with artesunate for treatment of uncomplicated *P. falciparam* malaria in African counties.

Chemopophylaxis with amodiaquine is not indicated because of the dangerous toxicity associated with long-term use.

PIPERAQUININE

Piperaquinine, a bisquinoline, has a longer half life than other antemalarial drugs, which is an advantage for post-treatment prophylaxis. Piperaquinine in combination with dihydroartemisinin is the first-line therapy for the treatment of uncomplicated falciparum malaria in Vietnam, because of the excellent efficacy and safety, without apparent drug resistance.

PROGUANIL

Proguanil acts slowly against erythrocytic forms of susceptible strains of all four human malaria species. It has some activity against hepatic forms. It is neither adequately gametocidal nor effective against the persistent liver stage of *P. vivax*.

Proguanil is generally used either in combination with chloroquine or atovaquone for prophylaxis of malaria.

Proguanil is well tolerated. Adverse effects are rare, but it may cause mouth ulcers and alopecia. It is considered safe in pregnancy. Folate supplements should be routinely administered during pregnancy.

ATOVAQUONE PLUS PROGUANIL (MALARONE)

Atovaquone, a hydroxynaphthoquinone, is not effective when used alone, due to rapid development of drug resistance. However, Malarone, a fixed combination of atovaquone (250 mg) and the antifolate proguanil (100 mg) is highly effective for both the treatment and chemoprophylaxis of falciparum malaria. Unlike most other antimalarials, malarone provides activity against both erythrocytic and hepatic stage parasite.

For treatment, malarone is given in an adult dose of four tablets daily for 3 days. For chemoprophylaxis, it must be taken daily. It has an advantage over mefloquine and doxycycline in requiring shorter periods of treatment before and after the period at risk for malaria transmission, due to activity against liver-stage parasites. It should be taken with food.

Malarone is well tolerated. Adverse effects include GIT disorders, headache and rash.

Atovaquone can also be used for *P. jirovecii* pneumonia as an alternative to trimethoprim-suefamethoxazole, though it is less effective.

PYRIMETHAMINE

The antimalarial action of pyrimethamine resembles proguanil. It is not effective as a single drug for the prevention and treatment of malaria, because of development of resistance. Pyrimethamine (25 mg) is used in combination with sulfadoxine (500 mg). The combination preparation **Fansider** is a component of two combination regimens for uncomplicated malaria recommended by WHO.

Pyremethmine along with sulfadiazine is the treatment of choice for toxoplasmic encephalitis in patients with AIDS.

ANTIBIOTICS

The antibiotics that inhibit the bacterial protein synthesis are also effective against malaria parasites. None of the antibiotic should be used as single agents.

Doxycycline

Doxycycline is the most commonly used antibiotic. It is the standard chemoprophylactic drug, especially in areas of Southeast Asia with high rates of resistance to other antimalarials, including mefloquine.

Doxycycline is also used to complete treatment courses after initial treatment of severe malaria with intravenous quinine or artesunate, allowing a shorter and better tolerated course of these drugs.

Adverse effects include GIT symptoms candidal vaginitis and photosensitivity. It is not recommended for use in children and pregnancy.

Clindamycin

Clindamycin is slowly active against erythrocytic schizonts and can be used after treatment courses of quinine or artesunate in those for whom doxycycline is not recommended, such as children and pregnant women.

Azithromycin

Azithromycin also has antimalarial activity and is now under study for treatment and chemoprophylaxis.

PRIMAQUINE

Primaquine is an 8-aminoquinoline and is the only antimalarial, which is effective against the exoeryhrocytic stage in the dormant hypnozoite stage of P. vivax and P. ovale and the gametocytes. The only indication of primaquine is to achieve a radical cure of benign tertian malaria due to P. vivax and P. ovale, where resting forms of parasites exist in the liver and give rise to relapses. It is given in adult dose of 15 mg daily of 14 days following chloroquine treatment. It destroys the hypnozoite phase in the liver.

Primaquine may cause nausea vomiting and abdominal pain. The serious, though less common, side effect is methemoglobinemia and hemolytic anemia, especially in G6PD deficiency. It should be avoided in pregnancy, as fetus is G6PD deficient.

MALARIA VACCINE

Development of a fully protective malaria vaccine is still some way off, which is not surprising considering that natural immunity, is incomplete and not long-lived. There is, however, some evidence that vaccination can reduce the incidence of severe malaria in populations. Trial vaccines are being evaluated in Africa.

16
Antiamebic and other Antiprotozoal Drugs

Amebiasis is one of the most common infection of the lower bowel, which is endemic in India. It is caused by *Entamoeba histolytica*.

The vegetative forms (trophozites) of *E. hisolytica* live on the surface of the colonic mucosa and invade the mucosa, causing amoebic ulcers leading to acute amoebic dysentery or chronic diarrhea. Sometimes, tophozites enter the blood stream and invade other tissues, particularly liver, where they cause an abscess.

The cysts of *E. histolytica* remain in the bowel, produce no symptoms and pass in the stools, which propagates the infection.

EMETINE AND DEHYDROEMETINE

Emetine, an alkaloid obtained from Cephalis ipecacuanha and dehydroemetine, a synthetic analog, are effective against tissue trophozoites of *E. histolytica*, but because of major toxicity, their use is limited to unusual circumstances in which severe amebiasis requires effective therapy and metronidazole cannot be used.

Dehydroemetine is preferred because of its somewhat better toxicity profile. Serious toxicities include cardiac arrhythmias, heart failure, and hypotension. The drug should not be used in patients with cardiac or renal disease, in young children, or in pregnancy unless absolutely necessary.

MERTONIDAZOLE

Metronidazole is the drug of first choice in treating amoebic infection of the bowel and abscess of the liver since it is very effective against vegetative forms of *Entamoeba histolytica*. A 5 to 10 days course is often sufficient (metronidazole is also used to treat the protozoan parasite *Trichomonas vaginalis* and *Giardia lamblia* and anaerobic infections). Vomiting can be troublesome at the dose levels used to treat amoebic dysentery.

Metronidazole can be combined with diloxanide furoate, which is active against organisms in the bowel lumen, but not in the tissues. The combination appears to be even more efficient in eradicating the infection.

Adverse effects

Nausea, headache, dry mouth or a metallic taste are common side-effects. It has a disulfirm like effects, so that nausea and vomiting can occur if alcohol is taken during therapy.

Metronidazole should be avoided in pregnant or nursing mothers if possible.

TINIDAZOLE AND OTHER NITROIMIDAZOLES

Tinidazole or ornidazole has similar pharmacological properties as that of metronidazole, but is better tolerated and has a longer duration of action and are given in doses of 2 g daily for 3 days.

CHLOROQUINE

Chloroquine, an antimalarial, has little effect on intestinal amebiasis, but is highly effective in amebic liver abscess. It is used only in those cases of hepatic amebiasis, which fail to respond to metronidazole.

NITAZOXANIDE

Nitazoxanide, a broad spectrum anti-parasitic drug, is active against *E. histolytica* trophozoites in both tissues and gut lumen and may become an important addition for the management of amebiasis. Unlike metronidazole, nitazoxanide and its metabolites appear to be free of mutagenic effects.

DILOXANIDE FUROATE

Diloxanide furoate is effective against the non-invasive vegetative forms (trophozites) of *E. histolytica* in the intestinal lumen. It has no effect on amoebic ulcers or in systemic amoebiasis. It directly kills trophozites, responsible for cyst formation. It has no antibacterial action. It is partly absorbed, metabolized in the liver and excreted in the urine within 48 hours.

Diloxanide furoate is given orally in doses of 500 mg every 8 hours for 10 days in combination with metronidazole or tinidazole for eradication of amoebic infection (elimination of cysts).

Diloxanide furoate is relatively free from toxic effects. Flatulence, vomiting, urticaria and pruritis may occur. It is not recommended in pregnancy.

IODOQUINOL

Iodoquinol (diiodohydroxyquin) is an effective luminal amebicide that is commonly used with metranidazole to treat amebic infections. Its pharmacokinetic properties are poorly understood, ninety percent of the drug is retained in the intestine and excreted in feces.

Iodoquinol is effective against organism in the bowel, but not against trophozoites in the intestinal wall or extraintestinal tissues.

Infrequent adverse effects include diarrhea, anorexia, nausea, vomiting, abdominal pain, headache, rash and pruritis. Neurotoxicity can occur if doses exceed the recommended dosage.

Iodoquinol is taken with meals to limit gastrointestinal toxicity. It should be discontinued if it produces persistent diarrhea or signs of iodine toxicity. It is contraindicated in patients with intolerance to iodine.

PAROMOMYCIN

Paromomycin is an aminoglycoside antibiotic that is not significantly absorbed. It is used only as a luminal amebicide and has no effect against extra intestinal amebic infections. It is probably less toxic and even superior to diloxamide in clearing asymptomatic infections (Table 16.1).

Paromomycin is given in a dose of 500 mg orally 8-hourly for 10 days after treatment to eliminate luminal cysts. Adverse effects include occasional abdominal distress and diarrhea. Parenteral paromomycin is used to treat visceral leishmaniasis.

Table 16.1: Treatment of amebiasis

Clinical setting	Drugs of choice	Alternate drugs
Asymptomatic intestinal infection	Luminal agent: Diloxanide furoate, 500 mg 3 times daily for 10 days, Or Iodoquinol, 650 mg 3 times daily for 21 days, Or Paromomycin, 10 mg/kg 3 times daily for 7 days	
Mild to moderate intestinal infection	Metronidazole, 750 mg 3 times daily (or 500 mg IV every 6 hours) for 10 days, Or Tinidazole, 2 g daily for 3 days, Plus Luminal agent (see above)	Luminal agent (see above) Plus either Tetracycline, 250 mg 3 times daily for 10 days, Or Erythromycin, 500 mg 4 times daily for 10 days
Severse intestinal infection	Metronidazole, 750 mg 3 times daily (or 500 mg IV every 6 hours) for 10 days, Or Tinidazole, 2 g daily for 3 days, Plus Luminal agent (see above)	Luminal agent (see above) Plus either Tetracycline, 250 mg 3 times daily for 10 days, Or Dehydroemetine or emetine, 1 mg/kg SC or IM for 3–5 days
Hepatic abscess, ameboma, and other extraintestinal cisease	Metronidazole, 750 mg 3 times daily (or 500 mg IV every 6 hours) for 10 days, Or Tinidazole, 2 g daily for, 5 days, Plus Luminal agent (see above)	Dehydroemetine or emetine, 1 mg/kg SC or IM for 8–10 days, followed by (liver abscess only) chloroquine, 500 mg twice daily for 2 days, then 500 mg daily for 21 days, Plus Luminal agent (see above)

16.1 LEISHMANIASIS

Visceral leishmaniasis (Kala azar) is endemic in the eastern states of India. There are several varieties of Kala azar caused by closely related organisms, due to the bite of female sand fly, Phlebotomus. These organisms invade spleen, liver, lymph glands and bone marrow, producing a generalized disease with constitutional symptoms or produce a local ulcerative lesion. It may complicate HIV infection. Cutaneous leishmaniasis frequently heals spontaneously.

SODIUM STIBOGLUCONATE

Sodium stibogluconate, an organic pentavalent antimony compound, is no longer preferred because of the development of resistant to the drug in India. It is believed to act by interfering with enzymes within the parasites. It is given in a dose of 20 mg/kg by intramuscular or slow intravenous injection for 20–30 days. Sometimes, it may be necessary to repeat courses at intervals of 2 weeks.

Side effects are common and include arthnalgias, myalgias, raised hepatic transaminases, pancreatitis (especially in patients coinfected with HIV) and ECG changes. Severe cardiotoxicity and ventricular dysmythmias are not uncommon.

AMPHOTERICIN B

The antifungal drug liposomal amphotercin B given once daily or on alternate days at a dose of 3 mg/kg/d intravenously on days 1–5, 14 and 21 is the first-line drug for the treatment of visceral leishmaniasis in India because of significant level of antimony unresponsiveness. It has a cure rate of nearly 100%. Infusion – related side-effects, e.g. high fever with rigor, thrombophlebitis, diarrhea and vomiting are extremely common. Serious adverse effects, such as renal or hepatic toxicity, hypokalemia and thrombocytopenia are not uncommon.

Conventional amphotericin B is much less expensive and is given as a intravenous infusion of 1 mg/kg/d for 20 days. It is more toxic than lipid formulation and in rare cases elicits hypersensitivity reactions, bone marrow depression and myocarditis, all of which can be fatal.

MILTEFOSINE

Miltefosine, an alkyl phospholipid, is the first oral drug for the treatment for visceral leishmaniasis. It provides excellent results in India, where resistance to antimonials is increasing. A daily dose of 2.5 mg/kg/d for 28 days cures over 94% of patients. Because of its long half-life, milteposine is prone to induce resistance in Leishmania. Side effects include vomiting and diarrhea, which are generally short-lived toxicities. It may rarely cause skin allergy or renal or liver toxicity. Since it is a teratogenic drug, it cannot be used in pregnancy.

Miltefosine is best administered as directly observed theraphy to ensure completion of treatment and to minimize the risk of resistance induction.

Various drug combinations, including miltefosine with, amphotericin or paromomycin are under study, to circumvent the problem of development of resistance to miltefosine.

PAROMOMYCIN

Paromomycin, an a minoglycoside antibiotic has been found to possess excellent efficacy for the treatment of visceral leishmaniasis in daily intramuscularly dose of 11 mg/kg for 21 days. The cure rate has been reported up to 95%. Paromomycin appears to be well tolerated, but some patients develop hepatotoxicity, reversible ototoxicity, in rare instances nephrotoxicity and tetany. It has the same efficacy as that of amphotericin B in the treatment of visceral disease in India and is much less expensive.

PENTAMIDINE

Pentamidine isethionate a drug used for phenmocytosis (commonest cause of pneumonia in AIDS) is no longer used in visceral leishmamiasis, because of declining efficacy and serious side effects, such as type1 diabetes mellitus, hypotension, tachycardia, GIT disorder, and pancreatic, liver and kidney abnormalities.

17

Antihelmintic Drugs

Helminths (worms) are multicellular organisms that infect humans and cause a broad range of diseases. They include three groups of parasitic worms.

1. **Nematodes or roundworms**

    - *Intestinal human* nematodes   **Drugs of choice**

        Ancylostoma duodenale (hookworm)   Albendazole or mebendazole or pyrantal pamoate

        Strongyloides stercoralis (threadworm)   Ivermectin

        Ascaris lumbricoides (roundworm)   Same as hookworm

        Enterobius vermicularis (pinworm)   Same as for hookworm

        Trichuris trichiura (whipworm)   Mebendazole or albendazole

    - *Tissue-dwelling* human nematodes

        Wuchereria bancrofti (filariasis) loa loa (loiasis)   Diethylcarbamazine

        Onchocerca volvulus (onchocerciasis)   Ivermectin

        Dracunculus medinensis (guineaworm)   Metronidazole

        Trichinella spiralis (trichinosis)   Albendazole

2. **Trematodes or flukes**

    Blood flukes (Schistosomiasis)   Praziquantel or niclosamide

    Other flukes (lung, hepatobilliary and intestinal)   Praziquantel

3. **Cestodes or tapeworms**

    Intestinal tapeworms   Praziquantel or niclosamide

    Tissue-dwelling cysts or worms   Albendazole

ALBENDAZOLE

Albendazole, a broad-spectrum oral antihelminthic, is the drug of choice for the treatment of intestinal human nematodes, trichnosis, hydatid disease and cysticercosis.

Albendazole, undergoes first-pass metabolism in the liver to the active metabolite, is highly protein bound and well distributed including the bile, cerebrospinal fluid and hydatid cysts.

Albendazole is given on an empty stomach for intestinal parasites, but with a fatty meal against tissue parasites.

Therapeutic uses

- *Intestinal nematodes:*
  Albendazole is the drug of choice for roundworm, hookworm, pinworm, whipworm and trichuris infections. A single dose of 400 mg achieves good cure rates except for whipworm infection, where three daily doses are recommended. Albendazole is superior to mebendazole or pyrantel pamoate for treatment of hookworm infection.

- *Hydatid disease:*
  Albendazole in doses of 400 mg 12-hourly for three months is the treatment of choice with PAIR (percutaneous puncture, aspiration, injection of scolicidal agent and re-aspiration). Praziquantal 20 mg/kg 12-hourly for 14 days also kills larvae (protoscolices) in the cystic brood capsule.

- *Neurocysticercosis:*
  Albendazole, 15 mg/kg daily for a minimum of 8 days is the drug of choice for parenchymal neurocysticercosis. Praziquantel in another option. Prednisolone is also given for 14 days starting 1 day before albendazole. In addition, antiepileptic drugs should be given until the reaction in the brain has subsided.

The side effects are not of great significance, when used for intestinal worms, but prolonged treatment may cause liver damage, blood disorders, convulsions and meningism in cerebral disease. It should not be used in patients with cirrhosis. The safety of albendazole in pregnancy and children younger than 2 years age has not been established.

MEBENDAZOLE

Mebendazole, a congener of albendazole, has a wide spectrum of antihelminthic activity and a low incidence of adverse effects.

Oral absorption is only 10%, which increases if ingested with a fatty meal. It is highly protein bound and rapidly converted to inactive metabolites and has a short duration of action (half life 2 to 6 hours).

Mebendazole is indicated for use in roundworm, whipworm, hookworm and pinworm infections, and certain other helminthic infections. Cure rates are good for pinworm and roundworm infections, but are lower in hookworm infection and disappointing in trichuriasis.

Mebendazole is well tolerated when used for short-term therapy in intestinal nematodes, but may cause hypersensitivity reactions, blood disorders, liver damage, and alopecia with high-dose therapy.

It is contraindicated in pregnancy and may cause convulsions in children younger than 2 years of age.

PIPERAZINE

Piperazine is highly effective against threadworm and roundworm infections, but is not the drug of choice. It blocks the response of roundworm cell to acetylcholine and the flaccid worm is then expelled by peristalsis.

Piperazine may cause GIT disturbances and allergic reactions. Rarely, it may cause Stevens-Johnson syndrome, drowsiness and clonic convulsions. It is contraindicated in severe renal impairment, neurological disorders, epilepsy, pregnancy and peptic ulcer.

PRAZIQUANTEL

Praziquantel is effective treatment of schistosome infections of all species and most other trematode and cestode infections, including cysticercosis. The drug's safety and effectiveness as a single oral dose have made it as a drug of choice in mass treatment of several infections.

Pharmacokinetics

Praziquantel is rapidly and largely absorbed after oral administration. Antiepileptic and corticosteroids markedly decrease its bioavailability. The drug is rapidly metabolized and excretion is mainly via the kidney and bile.

Therapeutic uses

Schistosomiasis

Praziquantel is the drug of choice for all forms of schistosomiasis. Three doses of 20 mg/kg at intervals of 4–6 hours achieve a cure rate of up to 95%. The drug is well tolerated even in advanced hepatosplenic stage of the disease. Corticosteroids are generally given to limit inflammation from the acute immune response and dying worms.

Clonorchiasis, Opisthorchiasis, and Paragonimiasis

Praziquantel is given at a dose of 25 mg/kg thrice daily for 2 days for each of these fluke infection.

Taeniasis and Diphyllobothriasis

A single dose of praziquantel, 5–10 mg/kg results in 100% cure.

Neurocysticercosis

Praziquantel is as effective as albendazole and in doses of 100 mg/kg in three divided doses, followed by 50 mg/kg daily for 2 to 4 weeks causes dramatic improvements of seizures and neurologic findings and even progression of the disease.

H. nana

Praziquantel is highly effective and the drug of choice for *H. nana* infections in a single dose of 25 mg/kg, repeated after one week.

Hydatid disease

In hydatid diseases, it is used with albendazole before and after surgery.

Adverse effects

Common side effects include headache, drowsiness, GIT disorders, skin rashes, arthralgia, myalgia and low grade fever. Corticosteroids are commonly used with praziquantel therapy to decrease the inflammatory reactions and neurologic abnormalities occurring due to dying parasites.

Praziquantel is contraindicated in ocular cysticercosis, because parasites destruction in the eye may cause irreparable damage.

PYRANTEL PAMOATE

Pyrantel pamoate is a broad-spectrum antihelminthic highly effective for pinworm, hookworm, roundworm, and trichostrongylus orientalis infections. It is not effective in whipworm and threadworm infections.

Pyrantel pamoate in doses of 11 mg (base)/kg (maximum, 1g), repeated after 2 weeks yields cure rates of 85–100%.

Adverse effects are infrequent mild, and transient.

THIABENDAZOLE

Thiabendazole is an alternative to ivermectin or albendazole for the treatment of threadworm, cutaneous larva migrans and to metronidazole or mebendazole for guinea worm.

Thiabendazole is toxic and generally not a preferred antihelminthic since it may cause irreversible liver failure and fatal Stevens-Johnson syndrome.

NICLOSAMIDE

Niclosamide is the second-line antihelminthic for the treatment of tapeworms and intestinal fluke infections. Adverse effects are infrequent, mild, and transient and mainly confined to GIT disorders.

DIETHYLCARBAMAZINE CITRATE

Diethylcarbamazine citrate is the drug of choice for the treatment of filariasis, loiasis, and tropical eosinophilia because of its efficacy and lack of serious toxicity.

Diethylcarbamazine citrate taken after meals is rapidly absorbed, plasma half-life is 2–3 hours in the presence of acidic urine, but about 10 hours if the urine is alkaline. It is widely distributed including all tissues except fat. It is excreted mainly in the urine.

Therapeutic uses

Wuchereria bancrofti, Brugia malayi, Brugia timori, and Loa loa

Microfilaria of all these species are rapidly killed. Adult parasites are slowly killed, requiring several courses of treatment.

The initial dose is 50 mg on day 1 to minimize the incidence of allergic reactions due to dying microfilaria, followed by 50 mg three doses on day 2, and thereafter 100 mg three times daily for 2–3 weeks. Antihistamines are given routinely for the first few days of therapy to combat allergic reactions, which if become severe, may require corticosteroids or even interruption of the therapy. Several courses of treatment may be required for permanent cure.

In severe infections therapy may initially be started with albendazole (slower acting and better tolerated), before diethylcarbamazine. A single dose of diethylcarbamazine (300 mg) in combination with either albendazole (400 mg) or invermectin (200 mg/kg) has proved to be highly successful in the mass treatment to reduce the prevalence of *W. bancrofti* infection.

Tropical pulmonary eosinophilia

Diethylcarbamazine is given orally in doses of 100 mg thrice daily for 14 days.

Adverse effects

Diethylcarbamazine generally does not cause any significant toxicity. Adverse effects are mainly due to the release of proteins from dying microfilaria or adult worms. They are generally mild with *W. bancrofti*, more intense with *B. malayi*, and severe in *L. loa* infections. The main symptoms are fever, headache, nausea, vomiting, arthralgia and prostration. Retinal hemorrhages and, rarely, encephalopathy have been described.

Chronic manifestations of lymphatic filariasis require meticulous skin care to prevent secondary bacterial and fungal infections. Antibiotic therapy may be necessary for bacterial cellulitis to prevent further lymphatic damage and worsening of existing elephantiasis.

DOXYCYCLINE

Doxycycline has significant macrofilaricidal activity against W bancrofti, suggesting better activity than any other available drug against adult worms. Activity is also seen against onchocerciasis. Doxycycline acts indirectly by killing Wolbachia, an intracellular bacterial symbiont of filarial parasites.

Doxycycline may become an important drug for filariasis, both for treatment of active disease and in mass chemotherapy campaigns.

IVERMECTIN

Ivermectin is the drug of choice in strongyloidiasis (threadworm) and onchocerciasis. It is also an alternative drug for a number of other helminthic infections and parasitic infection scabies.

Ivermectin is orally rapidly absorbed and has a wide tissue distribution. The half-life is about 16 hours. The drug and its metabolites are almost exclusively excreted in the feces.

Ivermectin does not effectively kill the adult worm but blocks the release of microfilariae. With repeated doses of ivermectin, the drug appears to have a low-level macrofilaricidal action and to permanently reduce microfilarial production.

In onchocerciasis, it is given orally, initially 150 mcg/kg followed by monthly/6 monthly/12 monthly intervals until the adult worms die, which may take 10 years or longer.

Corticosteroids are given to prevent inflammatory eye reaction only with the initial dose.

Ivermectin also has a key role in the reduction of disease transmission.

Strongyloidiasis is treated by two daily doses of 200 mcg/kg of ivermectin. A single oral dose is required for the treatment of scabies.

Adverse effects are principally from the killing of the microfilariae.

18

Anticancer Drugs

The chemotherapy of cancer is a highly specialized field of pharmacology which should be carried out only in special units by medical oncologists. Chemotherapy may be given with a curative intent or it may aim to prolong life or to palliate symptoms (Table 18.1).

Table 18.1: Goals of non-surgical treatment	
Curative	
Choriocarcinoma	High-grade lymphoma
Teratoma	Cervical cancer
Seminoma	Head and neck cancer
Radical, occasionally curative	
Small cell lung cancer	Stage III ovarian cancer
Adjuvant (following surgery)	
Breast cancer	Colorectal cancer
Stage I-II ovarian cancer	Osteosarcoma
Palliative	
Metastatic breast cancer	Metastatic sarcoma
Stage IV ovarian cancer	Metastatic prostate cancer
Advanced gastrointestinal cancer	Advanced lung cancer

Chemotherapy, in most cases, is combined with radiotherapy or surgery or both as either neoadjuvant treatment (initial chemotherapy aimed at shrinking the primary tumor, thereby rendering local therapy less destructive or more effective) or adjuvant treatment after complete surgical or radiologic eradication of a primary malignancy to eliminate any presumed but immeasurable metastatic disease. All chemotherapy drugs cause side-effects and it is very important to weigh possible benefits against acceptable toxicity.

Cancer cell biology

Cancers are characterized by unregulated cell growth, tissue invasion, and metastasis.

Cancers are named based on their origin: Those derived from epithelial tissue are called carcinomas, those derived from mesenchymal tissue are sarcomas, and those derived from hematopoietic tissues are leukemias or lymphomas.

Cancer nearly always arises as a consequence of genetic alterations. The genes that can promote cell growth when altered are often called oncogenes.

Human cancers are characterized by multiple genetic abnormalities, each of which contributes to the loss of control of cell proliferation and differentiation and the acquisition of capabilities, such as tissue invasion and angiogenesis.

Cancer cell lose the signals that control the proliferation and differentiation of normal cells to acquire functional capability. Cancer behaves as organs that have lost their specialized function and stopped responding to signals that normally limit their growth. Signal transduction pathways in cancer cells.

The tyrosine kinase play critical role in signal transduction pathways. They may be receptor tyrosine kinases or they may be linked to other cell surface receptors through associated docking proteins.

Normally, tyrosine kinase activity is short-lived and reversed by protein tyrosine phoshatases (PTPs). However, in many human cancers, tyrosine kinases or components of their downstream pathways are activated by mutation, gene amplification, or chromosomal translocations. Because these pathways regulate proliferation, survival, migration and angiogenesis, they have been identified as important targets for cancer therapeutics.

Another strategy the antitumor effects of targeted agents are to use them in rational combination with each other.

The cell cycle

Proliferation of both normal cells and cancer cells is dependent on progression of the cell cycle, which consists of four phases. Briefly there are two functional (S phase and M phase) and two preparatory phases (G1 phase and G2 phase). In the S phase, DNA replication occurs, doubling the number of chromosomes and producing sister chromatids.

In the M phase, the nucleus divides and the chromosomes separate into two daughter cells during the process of mitosis. The G1 phase precedes the S phase, while G2 phase precedes the M phase, their function is primarily synthesis of the materials needed for the subsequent phase (Fig. 18.1).

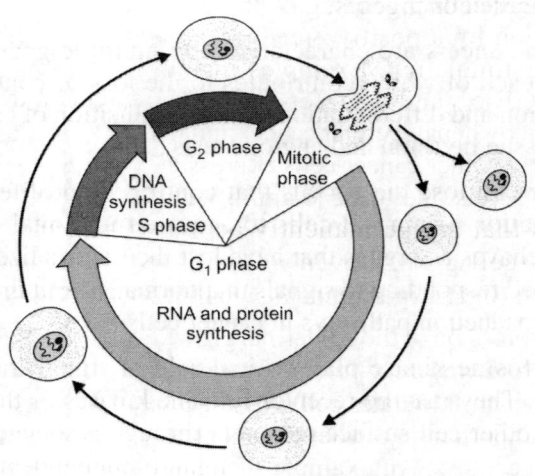

Fig. 18.1: Phases of the cell cycle.

An understanding of the cell cycle has been used to develop chemotherapeutic agents. Actively replicating cells are targeted in cancer therapy, as the DNA during cell division is susceptible to damage or radiation.

Example of chemotherapeutic agents include antimetabolites such as azathioprine and methotrexate, which prevents purines and pyrimidines from becoming incorporated into DNA during the S phase of the cell cycle, thereby arresting cell division.

The miotic spindle poisons vinblastine and vincristine inhibits assembly of tubulin to microtubules, hence disrupting the M phase of the cell cycle.

Other anticancer drugs, such as antibiotics and alkylating agents, affect cell division by a variety of mechanisms.

The cell cycle is also regulated by genes. Abnormal regulation of cell growth in cancer can occur as the result of several mechanisms.

Activation of cell growth

Many cancer cells produce growth factors which drive their own proliferation by a positive feedback loop, a process known as autocrine stimulation. Examples include tumor growth factor-alpha (TGF-α) and platelet-derived growth factor (PDGF) production by hepatocellular cancer and non-small cell lung cancer respectively. Other cancer cells express growth factor receptors at increased levels due to gene amplification or express abnormal receptors that are permanently activated and are capable of abnormal cell growth even in the absence of growth factor stimulation (ligand independent signaling).

Overexpression of the epidermal growth factor receptor (EGFR) and the Her2/neu receptor activate the Ras-Raf-MAP kinase pathway which stimulates cell growth. Understanding these effects has been important in the development of novel therapies targeted to these receptors. An example of ligand independent signaling occurs in the case of Ras mutations, which are present in about 30% of all cancers and cause constitutive activation of MAP kinase signalling, leading to abnormal cell growth.

Advances in the knowledge about the molecular basis of cancer have resulted in the development of a new generation of treatment to block the signalling pathways responsible for the growth of specific tumors. This has created potential to target cancer cells more selectively. Such targeted therapies reduce toxicity to normal tissues.

Inhibitors of tumor suppressor genes

In the normal cells, several proteins inhibit cell growth, these may be inactivated by loss of function mutations or their levels reduced by diverse mechanisms.

For example, retinoblastoma protein (Rb) sequesters transcription factors essential for the cell proliferation and inhibits cell growth. Cancer causes disruption of the Rb signalling circuit (by mutation and loss of transforming growth factor-β (TGF-β) and renders cancer cells insensitive to growth inhibition.

Avoidance of apoptosis

Evasion of apoptosis is a common finding in cancer. Apoptic process requires the role of various molecules, but the BcL-2 family plays a critical role. Some members of the Bcl-2 family (Bcl-2, Bcl-Xi) are antiapoptotic, while others (Bax, Bak) are proapoptotic. In some cancer cells, reduced levels of apoptosis are associated with increased levels of Bcl-2/Bcl-X_L or decreased levels of Bax/Bak.

Another molecule that plays a key role in apoptosis is PTEN. The PTEN molecule is a phosphatase which dephosphorylates Akt (pAkt), a molecule which stimulates cell growth. PTEN also affects the function of the tumor suppressor gene p53, by sequestrating an inhibitory molecule called Mdm-2, allowing p53 to promote apoptosis of cells with damaged DNA. Inactivating mutations of PTEN have been found in a number of different tumors. They cause activation of pAkt and inhibition of the p53 pathway, which stimulates cell growth and inhibits apoptosis.

Maintenance of telomeres

When normal cells replicate, there is progressive shortening of the telomeres; eventually, this prevents the cell from dividing further. Cancer cells can replicate an infinite number of times and this is associated with maintenance of telomere length. There are several mechanisms by which this occurs, the best established being upregulation of the telomerase enzyme, which adds nucleotides to the telomeres and allows cell division to continue.

Angiogenesis

Malignant tumors need to acquire a network of blood vessels for continued growth. This process is known as angiogenesis and is dependent on the production of angiogenic growth factors by the tumor. There are more than 15 angiogenic molecules, the best characterized being vascular endothelial growth factor (VEGF) and PDGF. Both play a central role in producing neovascularisation for the tumor cells and metastasis.

The requirement for tumors to promote angiogenesis has been exploited therapeutically in the development of agents that target angiogenic molecules or their receptors. Examples include bevacizumab (an antibody against VEGF) and sunitinib (a small molecule inhibitor of the PDGF and VEGF receptors). Bevacizumab has been shown to improve survival in metastatic colon, breast and lung cancer, while sunitinib has been shown to be useful in the treatment of renal cell cancer and second-line treatment of gastrointestinal stromal tumor (GIST).

Immune surveillance

The immune system is thought to protect against cancer via a continuous surveillance programme which eliminates cells that have undergone malignant transformation. One of the hallmarks of cancer development is escape from immune surveillance. Tumor cells constantly shed surface antigens into the circulation. Although this would normally evoke a response from the immune system, including the recruitment of cytotoxic T cells, natural killer cells and macrophages, it is thought that tumors escape from immune control for one of three reasons:

- Failure of antigen recognition by immune cells
- Tumor escape from the activity of cytotoxic lymphocytes
- Tumor-induced immune dysfunction.

It has been speculated that the increased risk of some cancers in patients receiving anti-TNF therapy for inflammatory diseases may be due to impairment of immune surveillance.

Invasion and metastasis

The ability of cancer cells to transgress normal tissue boundaries and to spread to other sites is an important process in cancer progression. Cells are attached to one another and to the extracellular matrix (ECM) by cell adhesion molecules (CAM) such as cadherins and integrins. Cell-cell and cell-matrix interactions are critical for the survival of normal cells. In cancer cells, CAMs are absent or dysfunctional, allowing the cell to detach from the primary site and to replicate, despite not being anchored to another cell or to the ECM (anchorage independent growth).

Cancer cells are also able to penetrate the basement membrane by producing enzymes called matrix metalloproteinases (MMP). The MMP degrade the basement membrane, allowing cancer cells to penetrate blood vessels at the primary site and to develop in new sites.

Cancer drugs

Cancer drugs treatments are of four broad types:

Conventional chemotherapy: These agents mainly target DNA structure or segregation of DNA as chromosomes in mitosis.

Targeted agents: These are biological (generally macromolecules such as antibodies or cytokines) designed and developed to interact with a defined molecular target important in either maintaining the malignant state or selectivity expressed by the tumor cells. Targeted therapies attack the activated biochemical pathways that lead to uncontrolled proliferation of tumors through the action of, e.g. oncogene products, loss of cell cycle inhibitors or loss of cell death regulators, thus acquiring the capacity to replicate chromosome indefinitely, invade, metastasize, and evade the immune system.

Hormonal therapies (the first form of targeted therapy) capitalize on the biochemical pathways underlying estrogen and androgen function and action as a therapeutic basis for approaching patients with tumors of breast, prostate, uterus, and ovarian origin.

Anticancer Drugs

Biologic therapies are often macromolecules that have a particular target (e.g. antigrowth factor or cytokine antibodies) or may have the capacity to regulate the growth of tumor cells or induce a host immune response to kill tumor cells. Thus, biologic therapies include not only antibodies but cytokines and gene therapies.

Resistance

Development of resistance to chemotherapeutic drugs may be to pharmacokinetic or pharmacodynamic factors. Pharmacokinetic factors include decreased uptake, decreased transport, increased efflux and metabolism of the drug. Pharmacodynamic factors include the inability of drug lethality because of the lack of the appropriate phase of cell cycle, altered target pathophysiology unconducive to drug action amongst others.

Combination therapy

In order to overcome drug resistance and to limit the side-effects of different drugs, chemotherapy is most commonly given as a combination of agents. Further, combination therapy achieves additive and hopefully supra-additive effect. Combination usually includes drugs from different classes, with the aim of targeting several pathways and getting maximum therapeutic effect.

CHEMOTHERAPEUTIC AGENTS USED FOR CANCER TREATMENT

Use of chemotherapy to treat cancer is generally guided by results of clinical trials in individual tumor types. The complexity of treating cancer has increased over the last decade as more drugs, including those with novel mechanism of action has been developed. Cancer treatment has become a highly specialized field involving particular protocol, planning, and therapy is exclusively administered by a medical oncologist.

The drugs that are listed in Table 18.2 belong to three general categories: those affecting DNA, those affecting microtubules, and molecularly targeted agents. Homone and biologic (other than targeted) therapies have not been included in the table.

Table 18.2: Commonly used cancer chemotherapy drugs

Drug	Clinical use	Delayed toxicity
DIRECT DNA-INTERACTING DRUGS		
ALKINATORS		
Cyclophosphamide	Breast cancer, ovarian cancer, non-Hodgkin's lymphoma, chronic lymphocytic leukemia, soft tissue sarcoma, neuroblastoma, Wilms' tumor, rhabdomyosarcoma	Myelosuppression, hemorrhagic cystitis pulmonary fibrosis, and adrenal insufficiency
Mechlorethamine	Hodgkin's and non-Hodgkin's lymphoma	Moderate depression of peripheral blood count; excessive doses produce severe bone marrow depression with leucopenia
Chlorambucil	Chronic lymphocytic leukemia and non-Hodgkin's lymphoma	
Melphalan	Multiple myeloma, breast cancer, ovarian cancer	Thrombocytopenia, and bleeding; alopecia and hemorrhagic cystitis occasionally occur with
Carmustine (BCNU)	Brain cancer, Hodgkin's and non-Hodgkin's lymphoma	
Lomustine (CCNU)	Brain cancer	Myelosuppression; rarely: interstitial lung disease and interstitial nephritis
Altretamine	Ovarian cancer	Myelosuppression, peripheral neuropathy, flu-like syndrome
Ifosfamide	Same as for cyclophosphamide	CNS effects, somnolence, confusion, and psychosis, myelosuppression, hemorrhagic cystitis

(Contd.)

Table 18.2: Commonly used cancer chemotherapy drugs (Contd.)

Drug	Clinical use	Delayed toxicity
Procarbazine	Hodgkin's and non-Hodgkin's lymphoma, brain tumors	Myelosuppression, hypersensitivity reactions, teratogenicity
Dacarbazine (DTIC)	Hodgkin's lymphoma, melanoma, soft tissue sarcoma	Myelosuppression, alopecia, hepatotoxicity, dermatotoxicity
Temozolomide	Brain cancer, melanoma	Myelosuppression, mild elevation in liver function tests, photosensitivity
Cisplatin	Non-small cell and small cell lung cancer, breast cancer, bladder cancer, gastroesophageal cancer, head and neck cancer, ovarian cancer, germ cell cancer	Nephrotoxicity, peripheral neuropathy, ototoxicity, myelosuppression
Carboplatin	Non-small cell and small cell lung cancer, breast cancer, bladder cancer, head and neck cancer, ovarian cancer	Myelosuppression; rarely: peripheral neuropathy, renal toxicity, hepatic dysfunction.
Oxaliplatin	Colorectal cancer, gastroesophageal cancer, pancreatic	Myelosuppression, peripheral neuropathy, diarrhea
ANTITUMOR ANTIBIOTICS AND TOPOISOMERASE POISONS		
Bleomycin	Hodgkin's and non-Hodgkin's lymphoma, germ cell cancer, head and neck cancer	Skin toxicity, pulmonary fibrosis, mucositis, alopecia

(Contd.)

Table 18.2: Commonly used cancer chemotherapy drugs (Contd.)

Drug	Clinical use	Delayed toxicity
Actinomycin D	Wilms' tumour	Myelosuppression, mucositis, tissue necrosis
Etoposide	Non-small cell and small cell lung cancer; non-Hodgkin's lymphoma, gastric cancer	Alopecia, myelosuppression hypersensitivity reactions
Topotecan	Small cell lung cancer, ovarian cancer	Myelosuppression mucositis, alopecia
Irinotecan	Colorectal cancer, gastroesophageal cancer, non-small cell and small cell lung cancer	Myelosuppression nausea vomiting alopecia, flu-like symptoms
Doxorubicin	Breast cancer, Hodgkin's and non-Hodgkin's lymphoma, soft tissue sarcoma, ovarian cancer, non-small and small cell lung cancer, thyroid cancer, Wilms' tumor, neuroblastoma	Cardiotoxicity, alopecia, myelosuppression, stomatitis
Daunorubicin	Acute lymphoblastic leukemia, Acute myelogenous leukemia	Cardiotoxicity, alopecia, myelosuppression mucositis
Idarubicin	Acute lymphoblastic leukemia, Acute myelogenous leukemia, Chronic myelogenous leukemia in blast crisis	Myelosuppression, mucositis, cardiotoxicity
Mitoxantrone	Breast cancer, Hodgkin's and non-Hodgkin's lymphoma, soft tissue sarcoma, ovarian cancer, non-small and small cell lung cancer, thyroid cancer, Wilms' tumor, neuroblastoma	Cardiotoxicity, alopecia, myelosuppression, stomatitis

(Contd.)

Table 18.2: Commonly used cancer chemotherapy drugs (Contd.)

Drug	Clinical use	Delayed toxicity
INDIRECT DNA-INTERACTING DRUGS		
ANTIMETABOLITES		
Deoxycoformycin	Hairy cell leukemia	Immunosuppression, CNS and renal disorders
6-Mercaptopruine	Acute myelogenous leukemia	Myelosuppresion, immunosuppression, and hepatotoxicity
6-Thioguanine	Acute lymphoblastic leukemia, Acute myelogenous leukemia	Myelosuppresion, immunosuppression, and hepatotoxicity
Azathioprine	Acute myelogenous leukemia myelogenous leukemia	Myelosuppresion, imunosuppression, and hepatotoxicity
2-Chlorodeoxyadenosine	Hairy cell leukemia	Renal failure, CNS dysfunction, immunosuppression
Hydroxyurea	Chronic myeloid leukemia	Myelosuppression, mucositis, skin changes, rare renal, liver, lung, CNS disorders
Methotrexate	Breast cancer, head and neck cancer, osteogenic sarcoma, primary central nervous system lymphoma, non-Hodgkin's lymphoma, bladder cancer, choriocarcinoma	Mucositis, diarrhea, myelosuppression, nephrotoxicity, neurotoxicity, hepatotoxicity, alopecia
5-Fluorouracil (5FU)	Colorectal cancer, anal cancer, breast cancer, gastroesophageal cancer, head and neck cancer, hepatocelular cancer	Nausea, mucositis, diarrhea, bone marrow depression, neurotoxicity

Anticancer Drugs 503

(Contd.)

Table 18.2: Commonly used cancer chemotherapy drugs (*Contd.*)

Drug	Clinical use	Delayed toxicity
ANTIMETABOLITES		
Capecitabine	Breast cancer, colorectal cancer, gastroesophageal cancer, hepatocellular cancer, pancreatic cancer	Diarrhea, hand-foot syndrome, myelosuppression, nausea and vomiting
Cytosine arabinoside	Acute lymphoblastic leukemia, Acute myelogenous leukemia	Gastrointestinal disturbance, myelosuppression
Azacytidine	Leukemia	Myelosuppression, myalgia, CNS and liver disorders
Gemcitabine	Pancreatic cancer, bladder cancer, breast cancer, non-small cell lung cancer, ovarian cancer, non-Hodgkin's lymphoma, soft tissue sarcoma	Nausea, vomiting diarrhea, limited myelosuppression
Fludarabine phosphate	Non-Hodgkin's lymphoma, chronic lymphocytic leukemia	Myelosuppression, immunosuppression, fever, myalgias, arthralgias
Asparaginase	Acute lymphoblastic leukemia	Hepatotoxicity, increased risk of bleeding and clotting, mental depression, pancreatitis, renal toxicity, hyperglycemia
Pemetrexed	Mesothelioma, non-small cell lung cancer	Myelosuppression, skin rash, mucositis, diarrhea, fatigue

(*Contd.*)

Table 18.2: Commonly used cancer chemotherapy drugs (*Contd.*)

Drug	Clinical use	Delayed toxicity
ANTIMITOTIC DRUGS		
Vincristine	ALL, Hodgkin's and non-hodgkins's lymphoma, rhabdomyosarcoma, neuroblastoma, vilms' tumor	Neurotoxicity with peripheral neuropathy, paralytic ileus, alopecia, SIADH
Vinblastine	Hodgkin's and non-Hodgkin's lymphoma, germ cell, cancer, breast cancer, kaposl's sarcoma	Myelosuppression, mucositis, alopecia, SIADH, vascular events
Vinorelbine	Non-small cell lung cancer, breast cancer, ovarian cancer	Myelosuppresion, constipation, SIADH
Paclitaxel	Breast cancer, non-small cell and small cell lung cancer, ovarian cancer, gastroesophageal cancer, prostate cancer, bladder cancer, head and neck cancer	Myelosuppression, peripheral sensory neuropathy
Docetaxel	Breast cancer, non-small cell lung cancer, prostate cancer, gastric cancer, head and neck cancer, ovarian cancer, bladder cancer	Neurotoxicity, fluid retention, myelosuppression with neutropenia
Estramustine phosphate	Advanced prostate cancer	GIT, CVS adverse effects, gynecomastia
Nab-paclitaxel	Breast cancer	Myelosuppression, reversible neurotoxicity
Ixabepilone	Breast cancer	Myelosuppression hypersensitivity reactions, peripheral sensory neuropathy

(*Contd.*)

Table 18.2: Commonly used cancer chemotherapy drugs (Contd.)

Drug	Clinical use	Delayed toxicity
MOLECULARLY TARGETED DRUGS		
RETINOIDS		
Tretinoin	Acute promyelocytic leukemia	Teratogenic, cutaneous disorders
Bexarotene	Cutaneous T cell lymphoma	Teratogenic, cutaneous disorders, hypercholesterolemia, hypertriglyceridemia
TARGETED TOXINS		
Denileukin diffitox	Cutaneous T cell lymphoma	Chills/fever, asthenia, hepatic disorder
TYROSINE KINASE INHIBITORS		
Imatinib	CML, gastrointestinal stromal tumor (GIST), philadelphia chromosome + ALL	Fluid retention with ankle and periorbital edema, diarrhea, myalgias, congestive heart failure, hepatic dysfunction
Gefitinib	Non-small cell lung cancer	Skin rash, diarrhea, anorexia, interstitial lung disease
Erlotinib	Non-small cell lung cancer, pancreatic cancer	Skin rash, diarrhea, anorexia, interstitial lung disease
Dasatinib		
Sorafenib	Renal cell cancer, hepatocellular cancer	Skin rash, fatigue and asthenia, bleeding complication, hypophosphatemia

(Contd.)

Table 18.2: Commonly used cancer chemotherapy drugs (Contd.)

Drug	Clinical use	Delayed toxicity
TYROSINE KINASE INHIBITORS		
Sunitinib	Renal cell cancer, GIST	Skin rash, fatigue and asthenia, bleeding complications, cardiac toxicity leading to congestive heart failure in rare cases
PROTEOSOME INHIBITORS		
Bortezomib	Multiple myelomas and certain lymphomas	Neuropathy, orthostatic hypotension hyponatremia and reversible thrombocytopenia
HISTONE DEACETYLASE INHIBITORS		
Vorinostat	T cell lymphoma	Fatigue, diarrhea, thrombocytopenia embolism
Romidepsin	T cell lymphoma	Nausea, vomiting, cytopenias, cardiac conduction
mTOR INHIBITORS		
Temsirolimus	Renal cancer	Stomatitis, thrombocytopenia, metabolic (glucose, lipid), myelosuppression
Everolimus	Renal cancer	Stomatitis, fatigue, myelosuppression, lung toxicity
MISCELLANEOUS		
Arsenic trioxide	Acute promyelocytic leukemia (APL)	Fatigue, cardiac dysrhythmias, fever, dyspnea, fluid retention and weight gain

SIADH, syndrome of inappropriate antidiuretic hormone

DNA-INTERACTING AGENTS

These are divided into direct and indirect DNA-interacting agents.

Alkylating agents exert their cytotoxic effects via transfer of their alkyl groups to various cellular constituents. Alkylations of DNA within the nucleus lead to DNA strand breakage. Broken or cross-linked DNA is intrinsically unable to complete normal replication or cell division. In addition, alkylating agents are potent activator of cell cycle check-points and further activate cell-signaling pathways that can precipitate apoptosis.

Thus, although alkylating agents are not cell cycle specific, cells are most susceptible to alkylation in G_1 and S phases of the cell cycle and express blockage in G_2.

Resistance

The mechanism of acquired resistance to alkylating agents may involve increased capability to repair DNA lesions, decreased transport of the alkylating agent into the cell and increased production of glutathione and glutathione associated proteins, which are needed to conjugate the alkylating agent or increased glutathione S-transferase activity, which catalyzes the conjugation.

Pharmacologic effects

The adverse effects usually associated with alkylating agents are generally dose-related and occur primarily in rapidly growing tissues such as bone narrow, gastrointestinal tract, and the reproductive system. They differ greatly in a spectrum of normal organ toxicities. As a class they share the capacity to cause "second" neoplasms, particularly leukemia, many years after use, particularly when used in low doses for protected periods.

Cyclophosphamide

Cyclophosphamide is a widely used alkylating agent, and one of the advantages of this compound is that it has high oral bioavailability. It is inactive in its present form, and must be activated to cytotoxic form by liver microsomal enzymes to 4-hydroxycyclophosphamide, which decomposes into an alkylating species, as well as chloroacetaldehyde and acrolein. The latter causes chemical cystitis, therefore excellent hydration must be maintained while using cyclophosphamide. It severe, the cystitis may be effectively treated by mesna (2-mercaptoethanesulfonate). Liver disease impairs drug activation. Sporadic interstitial pneumonotis leading to pulmonary fibrosis can accompany the use of cyclophosphamide, and high doses in conditioning regimens for bone marrow transplantation can cause cardiac dysfunction.

Ifosfamide is a cyclophosphamide analogue also activitated in the liver, but more slowly, and it requires coadministeration of mesna to prevent bladder injury. Central nervous system effects, including somnolence, confusion, and psychosis can follow ifosfamide use.

Several other alkylating agents are less commonly used.

Nitrogen mustard is the prototypic agent of this class. It can be used in cutaneous lymphomas with a notable incidence of hypersensitivity reactions. It causes moderate nausea. Bendamustine is a nitrogen mustard derivative with evidence of activity in chronic lymphocytic leukemia and certain lymphomas.

Chlorambucil causes predictable myelosuppression, azoospermia, nausea and pulmonary side effects. Busulfan can cause myelosuppression, alopecia, and pulmonary toxicity, but is relatively "lymphocytic sparing". Its routine use in treatment of CML has been curtailed in favour of imatinib or dasatinib, but it is still employed in transplant preparation regimens. Melphalan shows variable oral bioavailability and undergoes extensive binding to albumin. Mucositis appears more prominently, however it has prominent activity in multiple myeloma.

Nitrosoureas break down to carbamylating species that not only cause a distinct pattern of DNA base pair-directed toxicity, but also can covalently modify proteins. They share the feature of causing relatively delayed bone marrow toxicity which can be cumulative and long lasting. Lomustine causes direct renal damage. Procarbazine is metabolized in the liver and possibly in tumor cells to yield a variety of free radical and alkylating species. In addition to myelosuppression, it causes hypnotic and other CNS effects.

Altretamine and thiotepa can chemically give rise to alkylating species. Dacarbazine is activated in the liver to yield the highly reactive methyl diazonium cation. It causes only modest myelosuppression but causes prominent nausea. Temozolomide is structurally related to dacarbazine but is activated directly in tumor and is bioavailable orally.

Cisplatin requires administration with adequate hydration, including forced diuresis with mannitol to prevent kidney damage. Gradual decrease in kidney function is common along with noteworthy anemia. Hypocalemia and tetany can occur. Other common toxicities include neurotoxicity, hearing loss and intense emetogenicity. Myelosuppression is less evident than with other alkylating agents. Carboplatin displays less nephro-, oto-, and neurotoxicity. However, myelosuppression is more frequent. Oxaliplatin is a platinum analogue with noteworthy activity in colon cancers refractory to other treatments. It is prominently neurotoxic.

Antitumor antibiotics and topoisomerase poisons

Antitumor antibiotics bind to DNA directly and can frequently undergo electron transfer reactions to generate free radicals in close proximity to DNA, leading to DNA damage in the form of single – strand breaks or cross-links.

Topoisomerase poisons include natural products or semisythetic species derived from plants, and they modify enzymes that regulate the capacity of DNA to unwind to allow normal replication or transcription. These include topoisomerase I, which creates single-strand breaks that then rejoin following the passage of the other DNA strand through the break. Topoisomerase II creates double-strand breaks, through which another segment of DNA duplex passes before rejoining. DNA damage from these agents can occur at any cell cycle phase, but cells tend to arrest in S-phase or G_2 of the cell cycle in cells with p53 and Rb pathway lesions as the result of defective checkpoint mechanisms in cancer cells. Owing to role of topoisomerase 1 in the procession of the replication fork, topoisomerse I poisons cause lethality if the topoisomerase I-induced lesions are made in S-phase.

Doxorubicin can intercalate into DNA, therapy altering DNA structure, replication, and topoisomerase II function. It causes predictable myelosuppression, alopecia, nausea, and mucositis. Cardiotoxicity is rarely of clinical significance.

Daunorubicin is closely related to doxorubicin and is preferable because it causes less muscositis and colonic damage. Idarubicin is also used in myeloid leukemia and may be preferable to daunorubicin in activity.

Bleomycin refers to a mixture of glycopeptides that have the unique feature of forming complexes with Fe^{2+} while also bound of DNA. It remains an important component of curative regimens for Hodgkin's disease and germ cell neoplasms. The drug causes little if any, myelosuppression. Common side effects include fever and chills, facial flush, and Raynand's phenomenon. The most important toxicity is pulmonary fibrosis which is minimally responsive to treatment (e.g. glucocorticoids).

Mitoxantrone, a synthetic compound was developed to have the therapeutic effects doxorubicin, but with less cardiotoxicity. It use is still associated with cardiotoxicity and also alopecia. Cases of acute promyelocytic leukemia (APL) have arisen shortly after exposure of patients to mitoxantrone particularly in the adjuvant treatment of breast cancer.

Etoposide was synthetically derived from the plant product podophyllotoxin: it binds directly to topoisomerase II and DNA. It causes a prominent G_2 arrest, reflecting the action of a DNA damage checkpoint. Adverse effects include myelosuppression, nausea and transient hypotension.

Camptothecin was isolated from a Chinese tree. It shows evidence of toxicity with little antitumor activity. Topotecan is a camptothecin derivative approved for use in gynecologic tumors and small lung cancer. Toxicity is limited to myelosuppression and mucositis. Irinotecan is a camptothecin with evidence of activity in colon carcinoma.

Indirect effectors of DNA function; Antimetabolites

Antimetabolites include compounds with structural similarity to precursors of purine or pyrimidines, or compounds that interfere with folic acid, purine or pyrimidine synthesis. Antimetabolites can cause DNA damage indirectly through misincorporation into DNA, abnormal timing or progression through DNA synthesis, or altered function of pyrimidine and purine biosynthetic enzymes. They tend to convey greatest damage to cells in S-phase, and the degree of toxicity increases with duration of exposure. Common toxic manifestations include stomatitis, diarrhea and myelosuppression. Second malignancies are not associated with their use.

Methotrexate inhibits dihydrofolate reductase, which regenerates reduced folates form the oxidized folates produced when thymidine monophosphate is formed from deoxyuridine monophosphate. Without reduced folates, cells die a "thymine-less" death. Leucovorin can bypass this block and rescue cells from methotrexate. The drug and other reduced folates are transported into cells by folate carrier, and high concentrations of drug can bypass this carrier and allow diffusion of drug directly into cells. These properties have suggested the design of "high-dose" methotrexate regimens with leucovorin rescue of normal marrow and mucosa as part of curative approaches to osteosarcoma in the adjuvant setting and hematopoietic neoplasm in children and adults. To prevent renal toxicity, alkalinization of urine with increased flow by hydration is required for high-dose regimen methotrexate.

Methotrexate, apart from myelosuppression, can cause hypersensitivity like pulmonary syndrome and hepatic fibrosis. Intrathecal methotrexate can cause chemical arachnoiditis and CNS dysfunctions.

Premetrexed is a novel folate-directed antimetabolite. It is "multitargeted" in that it inhibits the activity of several enzymes, including thymidylate synthetase, dihydrofolate reductase, and glycinamide ribonucleotide formyltransferase, thereby affecting the synthesis of both purine and pyrimidine nucleic acid precursors. To avoid significant toxicity to the normal tissues, patients should receive low-dose folate and vitamin B_{12} supplementation. It has notable activity against certain lung cancers and in combination with cisplatin against mesotheliomas. Patatrexate is an antifolate approved for use in T cell lymphoma that is very efficiently transported into cancer cells.

5-Fluorouracil (5FU) is metabolized in cells to 5'FdUMP, which inhibits thymidylate synthesis (TS). In addition misincorporation can lead to single-strand breaks, and RNA can aberrantly incorporate FUMP.

5 FU causes myelosuppression and stomatitis. Leucovorin augments the activity of 5 FU by promoting formation of the tertiary covalent complex of 5 FU, the reduced folate, and TS.

Cytosine arabinoside is incorporated into DNA, resulting in S-phase-related toxicity.

Gemcitabine is a cytosine derivative that is incorporated into DNA after metabolism to the triphosphate, rendering DNA susceptible to breakage and repair synthesis that differs from cytosine in that gemcitabine-induced lesions are inefficiently removed. In contrast to cytosine, it appears to have useful activity in a variety of solid tumors, with limited myelosuppressive toxicity.

Fludarabin phosphate, a prodrug of F-adenine arabinoside (F-ara-A) is incorporated into DNA and can cause delayed cytotoxicity even in cells with low growth fraction, including chronic lymphocytic and follicular B cell lymphoma.

Asparaginase causes breakdown of extracellular asparagine required for protein synthesis in certain leukemic cells. This effectively stops tumor cell DNA synthesis, as DNA synthesis requires concurrent protein synthesis. The outcome of asparaginase action is similar to multiple molecule antimetabolites. Adverse effects include hyperglycemia, clotting function abnormalities, and thromboses particularly affecting the CNS.

Mitotic spindle inhibitors

Microtubules are cellular structures that form the mitotic spindle and in interphase cells. They are responsible for the cellular 'scaffolding' along which various motile and secretary processor occur. Microtubules are composed of repeating non-covalent multimers of a heterodimer of α and β isoform of the protein tubulin. Vincristine binds to the tubulin dimer with the result that microtubules are disaggregated. These results in the block of growing cells in M-phase, however, toxic effects in G1 and

S-phase are also evident, reflecting effects on normal cellular activities of microtubules.

Vinca alkaloids

Vincristine: Neurotoxicity is frequent. Acute neuropathic effects include jaw pain, paralytic ileus, urinary retention, and the syndrome of inappropriate antidiuretic hormone secretion. Myelosuppression is not seen.

Vinblastine: Myelotoxic with more frequent thrombocytopenia and stomatitis and mucositis.

The taxanes include paclitaxal and docetexal. These agents differ from vinca alkaloids in that the taxanes stabilize macrotubules against depolymerization. The 'stabilized' microtubules function abnormally and are not able to undergo the normal dynamic changes of microtubule structure and function necessary for cell cycle completion. Taxanes are among the most broadly active antineoplastic agents for use in solid tumors, with evidence of activity in ovarian cancer, breast cancer, Kaposi's sarcoma and lung tumors.

Resistance to taxanes has been related to emergence of efficient efflux of taxanes from tumor cells through P170 P-glycoprotein or the presence of variant or mutant forms of tubulin.

Epothilones represent a class of novel microtubule-stabilizing agents that have been conscientiously optimized for activity in taxane-resistant tumors. Ixabepilone has clear evidence of activity in breast cancer resistant to taxanes and anthracyclines such as durorubicin. It retains expected side effects, including myelosuppression, and also can cause peripheral sensory neuropathy.

Extramustine, though a mustard derivative, has no interaction with DNA. It causes metaphase arrest by binding to microtubule associated proteins, resulting in abnormal microtubule function. It binds to extramustine-binding proteins (EMBPs) which are notably present in prostate tumor tissue. The drug is used in patients with prostate cancer. GIT and CVS adverse effects related to estrogen moiety occur in up to 10% of patients including worsened heart failure and thrombocytopenia. Gynecomestia and nipple tenderness can also occur.

Targeted therapies

The knowledge of cancer cell biology has led to the development of group of drugs which can target the different stages of the cancer cell proliferation. These include the products of oncogenes and tumor suppressor genes, regulators of cell death pathways, mediators of cellular immortality such as telomerase, and molecules responsible for microenviornmental molding such as proteases or angiogenic factors.

Hematopoietic neoplasms

The tyrosine kinases often play crucial roles in signal transduction pathways in cancer cells. Imatinib is an inhibitor of the tyrosine kinase. It is indicated for the treatment of chronic myelogenous leukemia (CML). This agent also inhibits other receptor tyrosine kinase for platelet-derived growth factor receptor (PDGFR), stem cell factor, and C-Kit.

Imatinib is well absorbed orally, metabolized in the liver, with elimination of metabolites occurring in feces via biliary excretion. It is used as first-line therapy in chronic phase CML, It is fairly well tolerated and side-effects include hepatic dysfunction, diarrhea, and fluid retention. Rarely, it may cause decreased cardiac function.

Nilotinib is a tyrosine protein kinase inhibitor with a similar spectrum of activity to imatinib, but with increased potency and better tolerance by certain patients.

Dasatinib is another inhibitor of several kinases. It differs from imatinib in that binds to active and inactive conformations of the Abl kinase domain and overcomes imatinib resistance. However, some mutant kinases are resistant to Dasatinib for which a new class of inhibitors called aurora kinase inhibitors is in development to address this problem.

Tretinoin (all-trans retinoic acid) is active in patients with acute promyelocytic leukemia (APL) through the induction of terminal differentiation, in which the leukemic promyelocytes lose their ability to proliferate and attenuate the rate of hemorrhagic compilations. Adverse effects include headache with or without pseudotumor cerebri and gastrointestinal and cutaneous toxicities. Another active retinoid is the synthetic retinoid X receptor ligand bexarotene, which has activity in cutaneous T cell lymphoma.

Bortezomib is an inhibitor of the proteasome, the multisubunit assembly of protease activities responsible for the selective degradation of proteins important in regulating activation of transcription factor, including NF-kB and proteins regulating cell cycle progression. It has activity in multiple myeloma and certain lymphomas. Adverse effects include neuropathy, orthostatic hypotension and reversible thrombocytopenia.

Vorinostat is an inhibitor of histone deacetylases, responsible for maintaining the proper orientation of histones on DNA, with resulting capacity for transcriptional readiness. Acetylated histones allow entry of transcription factors and therefore increased expression of genes that are selectively repressed in tumors. The result can be differentiation with the emergence of a more normal cellular phenotype, or cell cycle arrest with expression of endogenous regulators of cell cycle progression. Vorinostat is indicated in cutaneous T cell lymphoma, with dramatic skin clearing and very few side effects. Romidepsin is a distinct molecular class of histone deacetylase inhibitor and also active in T cell lymphoma.

DNA methyltransferase inhibitors including 5-aza-cytidine and 2'-deoxy-5-azacytidine (decitabine) can also increase transcription of genes "silenced" during the pathogenesis of a tumor by causing demethylation of the methylated cytosines that are acquired as an 'epigenetic' (i.e. after the DNA is replicated) modification of DNA. Decitabine is useful in myelodysplastic syndromes and certain leukemias.

Solid tumors

Gefitinib and Erlotinib are small molecule inhibitors of the tyrosine kinase domain associated with EGFR, and both are used in the treatment of non-small cell lung cancer that is refractory to at least one prior chemotherapeutic regimen.

Erlotinib has been approval for use in combination with gemcitabine for the treatment of advanced pancreatic cancer. An acneform skin rash, diarrhea, and anorexia and fatigue are the common adverse effects.

Sorafenib is a small molecule that inhibits multiple receptors tyrosine kinases (RTKs), especially VEGF-R2 and VEGF-R3, platelet-derived growth factor-β (PDGF-β), and raf kinase. It is used in advanced renal cell cancer, and advanced hepatocellular cancer.

Sunitinib is similar to sorafenib in that it inhibits multiple RTKs, although the specific types are somewhat different. They include PDGER-α and PDGER-β VEGER-RI, VEGF-R2, VEGF-R3 and C-kit. It is used for the treatment of advanced renal cancer and gastrointestinal stromal tumors (GIST) after disease progression on or with intolerance to imatinib.

Both sorafenib and sunitinib are metabolized in the liver and eliminated via hepatic with excretion in feces. Each of these agents has potential interaction with drugs that are also metabolized by CY P3A4 system, especially warfarin. Hypertension, bleeding complications, and fatigue are the most common adverse effects. For sunitinib, there is also increased risk of cardiac dysfunction, which may even lead to congestive heart failure.

Temsirolimus and everolimus are mammalian target of rapamycin (mTOR) inhibitors with activity in renal cancers. They produce stomatitis, fatigue, and some hyperlipidemia, myelosuppression, and rare lung toxicity.

Hormonal therapies

Steroid hormone receptors related molecules target small molecules in cancer treatment. When bound to their cognate ligands, these receptors can alter gene transcription and, in certain tissues, induce apoptosis.

Glucocorticoids are generally useful in leukemias and lymphomas where they induce apoptosis in tumor cells. Cushing's syndrome or inadvertent adrenal suppression on withdrawal from high doses glucocorticoids can be significant complications, along with infections common in immunosuppressed patients, in particular pneumocystitis pneumonia, a late complication.

Sex hormones are useful in providing remissions in selected patients with the metastatic breast, prostate, and endometrial cancer and renal cell carcinoma.

Estrogens are now rarely used, although diethylstilbestrol (synthetic estrogen) and its prodrug (fostetrol) are occasionally used in prostate cancer and ethinylestradiol for breast cancer.

Progestogens: Medoxyprogesterone and megestrol actate are the most popular progestogens, which are used orally for endometrial cancer, renal cell carcinoma and as second or third-line treatment for breast cancer. They have also been used for the treatment of cachexia (a profound and marked state of constitutional disorder; general ill health and malnutrition) associated with AIDS. Side effects are minor and include occasional nausea, weight gain and fluid retention.

Androgens are occasionally still used as second or third-line treatments for breast cancer. However, their use is associated with many problems and contraindications.

Sex hormones, now more or less, are seldom indicated in the treatment of breast and prostate cancer, because the safer approach is to block the actions of sex hormones (estrogens and testosterone) at their receptors, which has been made possible with the availability of hormone antagonists.

Hormone antagonists are estrogen receptor antagonists and androgen receptor antagonists as well as the drugs which prevent the production of estrogens and testosterone and have virtually replaced the sex hormones in the treatment of hormone-responsive breast cancer and prostate cancer. In general, hormone antagonists have few serious adverse effects.

Breast cancer

Tamoxifen is a nonsteroidal estrogen receptor antagonist. It is the adjuvant hormonal treatment of choice, particularly in estrogen dependant breast cancer.

Tamoxifen has been reported to reduce the incidence of breast cancer in normal women at high risk. An additional advantage of its long term use may be to prevent osteoporosis and decrease in the incidence of heart disease.

Tamoxifen is prescribed for anovulatory sterility, when the drug is taken on days 2, 3, 4 and 5 of the menstrual cycle.

Side effects are mild and include occasional nausea, hot flushes, fluid retention and a hormone flare (bone pain and hyercalcemia) which subsides within 7 to 10 days. Tamoxifen is contraindicated in breast-feeding and before planned pregnancy.

Long-term use of tamoxifen carries the risk of endometrial cancer and deep vein thrombosis, because of its estrogen receptor agonist action on tissues other than the breast.

Toremifen, an estrogen receptor antagonist, is used to treat hormone-dependent metastatic breast cancer in post-menopausal women.

Aromatase inhibitors inhibit the conversion of androgens to estrogens in the peripheral tissues. The first and second-generation aromatose inhibitors inhibit the steroid synthesis in adrenals and require corticosteroid replacement therapy. Third generation aromatose inhibitors are better tolerated and are more specific since they do not suppress adrenal cortisol production and are used in the treatment of advanced hormone-responsive breast cancer in postmenopausal women.

Two nonsteroidal agents, anastrazole and letrozole and one steroidal agent, exemestane are the third generation aromatase inhibitors that have been found to be active in hormone-sensitive breast cancer. Side effects are usually minimal and include hot flashes and night sweats, but thrombotic episodes may occur.

Prostate cancer

Prostatic carcinoma with metastases, usually, responds to hormonal treatment which deprives the cancer of androgen. With the availability of androgen receptor antagonists and better understanding of gonadotrophin-releasing hormone (GnRH), the treatment is generally carried out by drugs instead of bilateral subcapsular orchidectomy.

GnRH (gonadorelin) causes the release of LH and FSH from the anterior lobe of the pituitary gland. If, however, GnRH is given as a continuous treatment, it shuts down the production of luteinising hormone (LH) and therefore of testosterone.

GnRH agonists: Leuprolide and goserelin are the commonly used GnRH synthetic analogues as monthly SC depot injection for the treatment of metastatic prostate cancer. They cause initial stimulation of LH release by the pituitary, which in turn causes testosterone secretion from the testes; this is followed by inhibition of LH release, thus effectively shutting down testosterone production. During the first 1 to 2 weeks of therapy a number of patients develop a tumor "flare" which may cause spinal cord compression or increased bone pain. To avoid initial flare in tumor symptoms, anti-androgen treatment is started 3 days before GnRH agonists and continued for 3 weeks. Other side effects of GnRH analogues are similar to those of orchidectomy.

Antiandrogens: Flutamide and bicalutamide are anti-androgens which are used in advanced prostate cancer. They are also used to cover the tumor "flare" which may occur after commencing GnRH analogues.

Biologic therapies

Biologic therapies may be distinguished from molecularly targeted agents in that many biologic therapies require an active response (e.g., reexpression of silenced genes, or antigen expression) on the part of the tumor cell or on the part of the host (e.g., immunologic effects) to allow therapeutic effect.

Tumors have a variety of means of avoiding the immune system. Tumor cells are capable of producing a range of soluble molecules, including potential immune targets that can distract the immune system from recognizing the tumor cell or can kill the immune effecter cells. Some of the cell products initially polarize the immune response away from cellular immunity and ultimately lead to defects in T cells that prevent their activation and cytotoxic activity.

Cell mediated immunity

The strongest evidence that the immune system can exert clinically meaningful antitumor effects come from allogenic bone marrow transplantation. Adoptively transferred T cells from the donor expand in the tumor-bearing host, recognize the tumor as being foreign, and can mediate impressive antitumor effects.

Three types of experimental interventions are being developed to take advantage of the ability of T cells to kill tumor cell – bone marrow transplantation of allogenic T cells, manipulated autologous T cell of the tumor-bearing host and development of tumor vaccines aimed at boosting T cell immunity.

Antibodies

Antibodies, normally, are not very effective at killing cancer cells. Cancer patients may have serum antibodies directed at their tumors, but are not present in adequate quantities to influence disease progression. However, the ability to grow very large quantities of high-affinity antibody directed at a tumor by the hybridoma technique has led to the application of antibodies to the treatment of cancer.

Clinical antitumor efficacy has been obtained using antibodies where the antigen-combining regions are grafted into human immunoglobulin gene products. Such humanized antibodies against the CD20 molecule expressed on B cell lymphomas (rituximab) and against human epidermal growth factor receptor 2 (HER-2/nen) is overexpressed in many cancers, especially breast cancer (trastuzumab).

These monoclonal antibodies potentiate the effects of combination chemotherapy given just after their administration.

Antibodies to CD52 are active in chronic lymphoid leukemia and T cell malignancies. EGF-R-directed antibodies (such as cetuximab and paintumumab) have activity in colorectal cancer refractory to chemotherapy and head and neck cancers in combination with chemotherapy and radiotherapy. The mechanism of action is not clear but may involve direct antiproliferative actions, stimulation of host immune mechanism, complement-mediated response to tumor cell bound antibody, and alteration of the release of paracrine factors promoting tumor cell survival.

Side effects include fusion-related hypersensitivity reactions and systemic reactions particularly gastrointestinal and cardiovascular.

Conjugation of antibodies to drugs, toxins, isotopes, photodynamic agents and other killing moieties may also be effective.

Cytokines

Interferons induce the expression of many genes, inihibit protein synthesis, and exerts a number of different effects on diverse cellular processes. The two recombinant forms that are commercially available are IFN-α2a and α2b. Interferon is not curative for any tumor but can induce partial responses in follicular lymphoma, hairy cell leukemia, CHL, myeloma, and Kaposi's sarcoma. It has been used in the adjuvant setting in stage II melanoma, multiple myeloma, and follicular lymphoma, with uncertain effects on survival. It produces fever, fatigue, a flulike syndrome malaise, myelosuppression, depression and clinically significant autoimmune disease.

The antitumor effects of IL-2 are indirectly through augmentation of immune function. Its biologic activity is to promote growth and the activity of T cells and natural killer (NK) cells. High doses of IL-2 can produce tumor regression in certain patients with metastatic melanoma and renal cell cancer. The complete remissions can be durable unlike any other treatment. Major adverse effects include capillary leak syndrome, respiratory distress syndrome and impaired renal and liver function.

Drugs for cytotoxic induced side effects

Myelosuppression

Primary prophylaxis shortly after completing chemotherapy with G-CSF (granulocyte colony stimulation factor) reduces the incidence of febrile neutropenia. However, many patients receive regimens that do not have a high risk of expected febrile neutropenia and do not require primary prophylaxis.

Administration of G-CSF and GM-CSF (granulocyte- macrophage colony stimulating factor) is indicated in patients with documental history of febrile neutropenia, patients older than age 65 years with aggressive lymphoma treated with curative chemotherapy regimens: extensive compromise of marrow by prior radiation or chemotherapy: and patients with active, open wounds or deep-seated infection.

Secondary prophylaxis. CSFs are administered to patients who have experienced a neutropenic complication from a prior cycle of chemotherapy, patients with myeloid leukemia, elderly patients. G-CSF is preferred because of a better safety profile.

Platelet transfusion may be considered in patients with myeloproliferative states.

Certain cytokines have shown an ability to increase platelets (e.g. IL-6, IL-1, thrombopoietin). IL-11 (oprelvekin) is approved for use in the setting of expected thrombocytopenia, but its effects on platelet counts are small and is associated with side effects particularly syncope and cardiac arrhythmias.

Anemia associated with chemotherapy can be treated by transfusion of packed RBCs. The indications of transfusion are: hemoglobin <80 g /L (8 g/dl): end organ function deterioration: coronary artery disease.

Nausea and vomiting

Chemotherapy induced nausea and vomiting requires combination of different classes of agent. Of great importance is psychological approach which augments the action of antiemetic.

Serotonin antagonists (5-HT$_3$), neurokine (NK$_1$) receptor antagonists and dexamethasone are useful in 'high-risk' chemotherapy regimens. The combination acts at both peripheral GIT as well as CNS sites.

Antidopaminergic phenothiazines, and antihistamines can be used routinely on need basis.

Lorazepam, a short-acting benzodiazepine may be useful as an anxiolytic agent.

Metoclopramide acts on peripheral dopamine receptors to augment gastric emptying and is used in high doses for highly emetogenic regimens.

Diarrhea

Hydration, electrolyte repletion and antimotility treatment such as 'high dose' loperamide often is adequate for diarrhea. Patients not responding to loperamide may require octreotide (a somatostatin analogue) or opiate-based preparation.

Mucositis

Topical therapies, including anesthetics and barrier-creating preparations, may provide symptomatic relief in mild cases. Palifermin or keratinocyte growth factor, a membrane of the fibroblast growth factor family is effective in preventing severe mucositis in patients having high dose chemotherapy with stem cell transplantation for hematologic malignancies.

Alopecia

Chemotherapeutic agents vary widely in causing alopecia. Anthracyclines, alkylating agents, and topoisomenase inhibitors cause near-total alopecia when given in therapeutic doses. Antimetabolites are more variably associated with alopecia psychological support and the use of cosmetic appliances need help the patients.

Reproductive functions

Most cytotoxics may cause permanent sterility in man and reversible amenorrhoea in women. They are teratogenic and should not be administered during the first trimester.

19

Vitamins

Vitamins are used for the prevention and treatment of deficiency states which are specific for each particular vitamin. The use of extra vitamins for prevention of epithelial cancers and heart diseases or to increase IQ in children is of unproven value. In fact, the habit of regular use of large doses of multivitamin preparations containing vitamin A or D may be harmful.

Vitamin A (retinol)

Vitamin A is a fat soluble oily liquid which is concerned with the maintenance of healthy epithelium. Its deficiency leads to keratinization of the epithelium of the respiratory tract, changes in the conjunctiva and in the cornea, which may lead to night blindness (xerophthalmia) and increased susceptibility to infections.

Vitamin A in doses of 50,000 IU is given in deficiency states causing night blindness or epithelial changes. Massive overdoses can cause rough skin, dry hair, liver damage, headache and vomiting. Excessive doses may be teratogenic and are best avoided in pregnancy and breast-feeding.

Vitamin B group

These are water-soluble vitamins.

Vitamin B_1 (thiamine)

Thiamine is essential for certain stages in carbohydrate metabolism. Its deficiency leads to a nervous system disorder known as beri-beri, which is characterized, by heart failure and polyneuritis.

Thiamine deficiency may result not only from inadequate intake, but also from disturbances of metabolism such as seen in chronic alcoholism.

Thiamine in high doses (50–100 mg daily) is used in polyneuritis, Wernicke's encephalopathy and Korsakov's psychosis caused by chronic alcoholism. Anaphylactic shock may occasionally occur after parenteral administration.

Vitamin B_2 (riboflavin)

Riboflavin is concerned with the intracellular metabolism and is necessary for antibody production, red blood cell formation, cell respiration and growth.

Deficiency of riboflavin causes several symptoms, including angular stomatitis, glossitis, skin lesions, anemia, neuropathy. The syndrome is called ariboflavinosis. Its deficiency may also result in increased incidence of cataract formation and vascularization of cornea.

Riboflavin is recommended in arteriosclerosis, hypertension, diabetes, obesity, with oral contraceptives and during periods of strenuous exercise.

Vitamin B_3 (niacin)

Niacin (nicotinic acid) is converted to coenzyme, nicotinamide adenine dinucleotide (NAD), which is vital for the proper functioning of a large number of enzymes in the body. It has important roles in the normal secretions of gastric and bile fluids, in the synthesis of sex hormones, in proper functioning of the nervous and circulatory systems. It can lower triglycerides, raise HDL, and lower LDL.

Niacin deficiency leads to a disorder known as pellagra, which may occur in alcoholism and renal failure. Pellagra is characterized by the "3Ds", namely diarrhea, dermatitis and dementia. Its deficiency gives rise to pellagra which is characterized by diarrhea, dermatitis and dementia. Chronic alcoholism, renal failure and deficient diets are the usual cause for its deficiency.

Niacin is particularly useful in combined hyperlipidaemia and in patients with low levels of HDL, treatment of pellagra. Niacin cream is used topically in the treatment of acne vulgaris.

Niacin is a potent vasodilator and requires extensive patient education in hyperlipidaemia, where it causes flushing and tingling of the face, because of the use of large doses (maximum dose up to 2000 mg/day). For the treatment of niacin deficiency, it is available as 50 mg tablets

Niacin should be used with caution in pregnancy, diabetes, liver disease, gout, glaucoma and peptic ulcer.

Vitamin B_6 (pyridoxine)

Pyridoxine is involved in many metabolic processes. It is required for normal functioning of the nervous system, including the brain. It is involved in red blood cell formation and for that of DNA and RNA. It is important in immune function and is the body's mechanisms to prevent atherosclerosis. It blocks the formation of homocysteine, which promotes the deposition of cholesterol around heart muscle.

Deficiency of pyridoxine causes dry and flaking skin, nausea and vomiting, stomatitis, peripheral neuritis, seizures, mental confusion, anemia, seborrhoea like lesions, growth retardation and impaired wound healing. Drugs such as antidepressants, oral contraceptives, isoniazid, and estrogens may lead to deficiency of pyridoxine.

Pyridoxine is commonly used to prevent and treat vomiting of pregnancy or following irradiation, premenstrual syndrome, convulsions in infants and children, polyneuritis associated with drugs like isoniazid, hydralazine, penicillamine and cycloserine and for the wound healing. High doses can damage peripheral nerves and should only be used when indicated for a specific clinical condition.

Vitamin B_{12} (cyanocobalamin)

Cyanocobalamin is the extrinsic factor required for the maturation of RBC. Its deficiency causes megaloblastic anaemia, glossitis, and degenerative changes in the nervous system. It is available as hydroxocobalamin and is given by injection in doses of 1 mg thrice weekly in pernicious anemia.

Vitamin B complex also includes other substances such as amino-benzoic acid, biotin, choline, inositol and pentothinic acid but there is no evidence of their therapeutic value.

Vitamin C (ascorbic acid)

Ascorbic acid is water soluble and is necessary for the formation and maintenance of a cement-like substance between cells. Its deficiency causes a condition known as scurvy, which is characterized by bleeding tendencies due to increased capillary fragility. Bleeding occurs into skin and mucous membranes involving the gums, periosteum of bones and joints producing pain and tenderness. Patient becomes anemic.

Scurvy is treated by giving vitamin C in doses of 500 mg daily. Vitamin C has also been used for promoting wound healing or amelioration of cold.

Vitamin D (calciferol)

Calciferol, a fat soluble vitamin, is essentially concerned with calcium metabolism and bone formation. Its deficiency leads to inadequate calcification of bones, resulting in their becoming soft and easily deformed. Calciferol deficiency causes rickets in children and osteomalacia in adults.

Calciferol requires hydroxylation by the kidney to its active form cacitriol, which is responsible for active calcium absorption in the gut. Calcitriol is effective in promoting calcium absorption and raising the plasma calcium concentrations in patients whose endogenous calcitriol production is impaired. This is the case in renal failure and in hypoparathyroidism (parathyroid hormone is required for renal production of calcitriol from calciferol).

Calcitriol and its analogue alfacalcidol are effective in microgram doses compared with the milligram doses needed with calciferol.

Calcitriol and **alfacalcidol** are indicated in patients with severe renal impairment, in hypoparathyroidism and postmenopausal osteoporosis in doses of 0.25–1 microgram daily.

Calciferol (vitamin D) either by mouth or by a single depot injection of 7.5 or 15 mg is the drug of choice for the treatment of nutritional osteomalacia or rickets.

Overdose with calciferol is dangerous and leads to deposition of calcium in the kidneys and other organs. Symptoms of over dosage include anorexia, lassitude, GIT disorders, weight loss, polyuria, sweating and headache.

Vitamin E (tocopherol)

Deficiency of this fat soluble vitamin rarely occurs in adults and produces no clear clinical syndrome. In children, with congenital cholestasis, vitamin E deficiency is associated with neuromuscular abnormalities, which responds only to parenteral vitamin E.

Vitamin E is an antioxidant and is believed to reduce the incidence of cancer, vascular, neurological and metabolic disorders and increase the life span, but there is little scientific evidence of its value.

Vitamin K (phytomenadione)

Vitamin K is necessary for the production of blood clotting factors (prothrombin and factors VII, IX and X) and proteins necessary for the normal calcification of bone. It is fat soluble and requires bile salts for proper absorption. Vitamin K is also synthesized by the intestinal bacterial flora.

Deficiency of vitamin K may occur in biliary obstruction or hepatic disease. Infants are relatively deficient in vitamin K, because it is not synthesized by the gut bacteria which may lead to haemorrhagic disease of the new born.

Vitamin K is given prophylactically in all new born babies to prevent bleeding. It is used as an antidote to coumarin anticoagulants.

Menadiol sodium phosphae is a synthetic analogue of vitamin K and is water soluble. It is given orally in malabsorption syndromes or states in which bile (necessary for absorption of fat soluble vitamin) is deficient.

Menadiol causes hemolytic anemia in moderate doses especially in G6PD deficiency and vitamin E deficiency. It is contraindicated in neonates and infants and late pregnancy, as neonatal hemolytic anemia may lead to hyperbilirubinemia and kernicterus.

Ginseng

Ginseng is a herbal preparation which is a constituent of many multivitamin tablets. It contains saponins, glycosides and sterols, and is claimed to have a wide variety of actions, including improvement in adrenal, muscular and cerebral functions. Ginseng has been used for its antifatigue and anti-stress action. Its use is not advisable in healthy individuals for long periods as it has estrogen like effects and is liable to cause hypertension.

Antioxidants

Oxidation is a metabolic activity that takes place in all body tissues and is necessary for life.

Oxidation, however, can produce free radicals (oxidants), which are chemically very active and react with a variety of other molecules inactivating proteins, damaging DNA and most importantly inducing lipid peroxidation in the membrane. Oxidants are also known to interact with cycloskeletal elements and interfere with mitochondrial oxidative phosphorylation and cause ATP depletion.

To protect against the free radical damage, a number of defense mechanisms (antioxidants) exist in the body, which are intracellular essential enzymes viz.; superoxide dismutase, catalase, glutathione peroxidase. These endogenous antioxidants trap the free radicals and prevent the chain reaction of destruction of healthy cells. However, excess free radicals may overwhelm endogenous antioxidant defenses and may cause different pathologic diseases.

Experimental studies have shown that oxidants may be involved in the pathogenesis and complications arising from atherosclerosis, cancer, diabetes (IDDM), neurological disorders, age related maculopathy and cataract, pregnancy and eclampsia, aging and some other diseases.

Antioxidants are substances, which are found in green vegetables, carrot and fruits. The well-known antioxidants are Vitamins A, E and C, flavanoids and selenium. At present, there is little evidence that antioxidants have a prophylactic/therapeutic effect, other than a possible reduction of coronary artery disease by vitamin E. The doses of antioxidants are very important, because in higher doses, they act as drugs with different mechanistic actions, side effects and toxicity. Antioxidants should be given in physiologic doses and the available data indicates that the doses of vitamins should not exceed 750 mg of retinol equivalent of vitamin A, 300 mg of vitamin E and 150 mg of vitamin C.

20
Poisons and Management

The management of patients with acute poisoning has become increasingly important in recent years. Acute poisoning is common in suicide cases, in children and due to consumption of illicit liquor and to a lesser extent due to accidental overdose of a drug. Non-specific measures such as maintenance of vital functions and removal and elimination of poisons and specific measures as apply to individual drugs form the treatment of poisoning.

Non-specific measures

Depression of respiration in unconscious patients is a common cause of death in poisoning. Respiratory stimulants do not help and are potentially dangerous. Unobstructed airway, assisted ventilation and oxygen therapy (high concentration, particularly in carbon monoxide and irritant gases poisoning) are the mainstay for maintenance of ventilation.

Many CNS depressants cause circulatory failure. A systolic blood pressure of less than 70 mm Hg may cause irreversible damage to the vital organs such as brain and kidney. Treatment should consist of oxygen therapy and IV fluids. Vasopressor drugs are contraindicated.

Removal and elimination of the poison

Removal of poison from the gut by gastric lavage is not necessary, if the risk of toxicity is small or if the poison has been taken for more than 1 hour. Gastric lavage is contraindicated in corrosive poisoning, poisoning due to petroleum products and in comatose patients, unless a cuffed endotracheal tube protects the danger of inhalation of stomach contents.

Emetics have a very limited role, though ipecacuanha has been used for induction of emesis in conscious patients, when the poison ingested is neither corrosive nor a petroleum distillate, and when gastric lavage is inadvisable or refused or when the poison is not adsorbed by activated charcoal. Salt solutions, copper sulphate, apomorphine and mustard are dangerous and should not be used as emetics.

In general, gastric lavage or emetics do not empty the stomach completely and because of the danger of inhalation of stomach contents, emetics are best avoided in the treatment of poisoning.

Prevention of the absorption by giving **activated charcoal (50 g)** through a nasogastric tube is relatively safe and more effective even though the poison was taken earlier than 1 hour.

Specific drugs

Poisoning can occur with any drug when taken in excessive (toxic) doses. Some of the common drugs, symptoms of poisoning and their antidotes are given in Table 20.1.

Chelating agents

These substances render an ion (generally a metal) biologically inactive by incorporating it into inner ring structure of the molecule. They are used in the treatment of cyanide and heavy metal poisoning.

Dicobalt edetate chelates cyanide ion in the blood. Cyanide causes cellular anoxia by chelating the metallic (Fe^{+++}) part of the intracellular respiratory enzyme, cytochrome P-450 oxidase. Specific therapy consist of dicobalt edetate which is to be used only when patient is tending to loose, or has lost consciousness. Side effects of dicobalt edetate include vomiting, chest pain and anaphylactic shock.

If dicobalt edetate is not available or is ineffective, sodium nitrite followed by sodium thiosulphate is given to convert the cyanide released from methaemoglobin to the inactive thiocyanate.

Oxygen at high pressure (hyperbaric) is given to overcome cellular anoxia.

Table 20.1: Common drugs, poisoning symptoms and their antidotes

Drugs	Symptoms of poisoning	Antidote
Benzodiazepines	Drowsiness, ataxia, dysarthria, short lived coma, cardiorespiratory depression minimal, death rare and more frequent with temazepam	Flunazenil
Barbiturates	Coma, respiratory depression hypotension and hypothermia. Death due to respiratory failure, circulatory collapse or pneumonia at a later stage.	No antidote, charcoal haemoperfusion. Antibiotics for pneumonia
Aspirin	Hyperventilation, tinnitus, vasodilation, sweating. Coma uncommon but indicates very severe poisoning	No antidote, oral activated charcoal, forced alkaline diuresis, haemodialysis.
NSAIDs	Mefenamic acid toxicity leads to convulsions	No antidote, diazepam for convulsions
Paracetamol	Hepatocellular necrosis and less frequently renal tubular necrosis may be fatal	Acetylcystine by IV infusion or methionine orally
Narcotic analgesics (opioids)	Coma, respiratory depression, pin point pupil	Naloxone
Dextropropoxyphene plus paracetamol	Combination one of the commonest causes of fatal poisoning. Symptoms of opioid poisoning, death due to CVS collapse.	Naloxone, acetylcystine
Trycyclic antidepressants (imipramine, amytriptyline)	Coma, hypotension, cardiac arrhythmias, respiratory failure, convulsions, pupils dilated, metabolic acidosis.	No antidote, symptomatic treatment, antiarrhythmic drugs best avoided
Beta-blockers	Bradycardia, hypotension and heart failure	No antidote, IV atropine for bradycardia and hypotension
Phenothiazines (chlorpromazine, etc.)	Hypotension, hypothermia, arrhythmias, distonic reactions, convulsions.	No antidote, symptomatic treatment

(Contd.)

Table 20.1: Common drugs, poisoning symptoms and their antidotes *(Contd.)*

Drugs	Symptoms of poisoning	Antidote
Alcohol (ethanol)	Ataxia, disarthria, nystagmus, drowsiness, coma, hypotension, acidosis, hypoglycemia	No antidote, symptomatic treatment
Methyl alcohol (methanol)	Vomiting, bradycardia, hypotension, delirium, coma, acidosis due to production of formic acid, blindness, respiratory failure	No antidote, haemodialysis, 4-methylpyrazole, calcium leucovorin to retard methanol metabolism and clear toxic formic acid from blood
Carbon monoxide	Confusion or coma usually combined with cyanosis or pallor.	No antidote, 100% oxygen, artificial respiration, I.V. mannitol for cerebral oedema
Pesticides, paraquat (gramoxone)	Progressive renal failure, dyspnoea with pulmonary fibrosis.	No antidote, heavy doses of activated charcoal with a laxative
Organophosphorus insecticides (parathion, malathion, etc.)	Convulsions, coma, pulmonary oedema, hypoxia, arrhythmias, hyperglycemia, with glycosuria	No antidote, atropine to reverse muscarinic actions. Pralidoxime (2-PAM) effective only if given within 24 hours.

Dimercaprol (BAL) contains SH groups which combine with heavy metals and thus spares SH groups of the body. It is used in poisoning by heavy metals antimony, arsenic, bismuth, gold, mercury and possibly thallium. It is also used an adjunct to sodium calcium edetate in lead poisoning. BAL is contraindicated in iron, cadmium or selenium poisoning and hepatic impairment.

Penicillamine chelates toxic metals particularly copper and lead. It is a metabolite of penicillin that contains SH groups so that it is similar to dimercaprol in action. It is used in Wilson's disease, which is due to excessive deposition of copper in the brain and liver. It was also used in rheumatoid arthritis.

Sodium calcium edetate (EDTA) is the chelating agent that combines more avidly with lead than with calcium. Adverse effects with EDTA are fairly common and include lachrymation, nasal stuffiness, chills, myalgia, hypotension and renal damage.

Desferrioxamine is the iron chelating agent used in iron poisoning which may occur as a result of repeated blood transfusion or accidental poisoning in children. Adverse effects are common and include GIT disturbances, arrhythmias, anaphylaxis and convulsions.

21

Drugs for Skin and Eye

Local application of the drugs to the skin and mucus membranes constitutes topical therapy. A topical application generally consists of an active drug in a base or vehicle.

21.1 SKIN

The vehicle affects the degree of hydration of the skin, has a mild anti-inflammatory effect, and aids the penetration of an active drug into the skin. The most commonly used bases or vehicles are soft paraffin, hard paraffin, macrogels, lanolin and oils.

Calamine is native zinc carbonate tinted pink with ferric oxide and is used as a cream or lotion for pruritis.

Barrier creams: These contain water repellent substances such as **dimeticone** or other **silicones**. They are used to protect the skin in areas around stomas, pressure areas in the elderly, bedsores, nappy and urinary rash, minor burns and abrasions, leg ulcers, moist eczema, fissures and a number of related disorders.

Sunscreen preparations

- Solar ultraviolet irradiation can be harmful to the skin. Depending on the wavelengths of ultraviolet radiation, many skin disorders such as eruptions, urticaria, cutaneous porphyria, aggregation of the pre-existing skin disorders, photosensitivity reactions to certain drugs, sunburn and even skin cancer may occur.

Sunscreen preparations are lotions or creams which contain three classes of chemical compounds namely p-aminobenzoic acid

(PABA) and its esters, the benzophenones, and the dibenzol methanes.

Para-aminobenzoic acid and its esters are the most effective available absorbers of ultra-violet B (UVB) wave length, responsible for most of the erythema and tanning associated with skin exposure.

Parosol and **Eusolex**, the dibenzoyl-methanes, absorb wavelengths throughout the longer UVA range and are indicated in patients, with polymorphous light eruption, cutaneous lupus erythematosus and drug induced photosensitivity.

Topical corticosteroids

Topical corticosteroids are widely used in various skin disorders for their anti-inflammatory and antimitotic effects. Corticosteroids come in a variety of strengths and potencies (Table 21.1) and should be prescribed according to the site of application, the age of the patient and the length of time that the corticosteroids are to be used.

Mild topical corticosteroids are used on sensitive sites such as face or genital areas. Superpotent corticosteroids are used under occlusion on chronic persistent lesions much as nodular prurigo. Local side-effects of topical corticosteroids include cutaneous atrophy and telangiectasia.

These are rarely seen and under treatment is a more common problem. As a principle, least potent corticosteroids should be used for the shortest possible time. Corticosteroid-responsive dermatoses should be treated initially with a more potent topical corticosteroid, switching to a less potent one as the condition improves. Long-term treatment is often given intermittently because of tachyphylaxis.

Topical antibacterial agents

Topical antibacterial agents may be useful in:
- Prevention of infection in clean wounds.
- Infected dermatoses and wounds.
- Reduction of colonization of the hares by staphylococci.

Table 21.1: Strengths of some commonly used topical corticosteroids

Corticosteroids	Strength	Common indications
MILD		
Hydrocortisone acetate	0.5%, 1%, 2.5%	Seborrheic dermatitis pruritus ani, intertrigo
Prednisolone	0.5%	As for hydrocortisone. For lesions on face or body folds resistant to hydrocortisone
MODERATE		
Clobetasone butyrate	0.05%	Contact dermatitis, alopic dermatitis
Triamcinolone acetonide	0.1%	Eczema on exterior areas, used for psoriasis with tar seborrheic dermatitis and psoriasis on scalp
POTENT		
Mometasone furoate	0.1%	Nummular dermatitis, allergic contact dermatitis, lichen simplex chronicus
Betamethasone dipropionate	0.1%	
Fluticasone propionate	0.005%, 0.05%	
VERY POTENT		
Clobetasol propionate	0.05%	For lesions resistant to potent corticosteroids, lichen planus, insert bites

- Axillary deodorization.
- Management of acne.

The pathogens isolated from most infected dermatoses are group A β-hemolytic streptococci, *Staphylococcus aureus*, or both.

Most topical antibacterial preparations contain multiple antibiotics, which have the advantage of efficacy in mixed infections, broader coverage of infections due to undetermined pathogens, and delayed microbial resistance to any single component antibiotic.

Bacitracin and Gramicidin

Bacitracin and gramicidin are active against gram-positive cocci, most anaerobic cocci, neisseria, tetanus and diphtheria bacilli.

Bacitracin is generally used in combination with neomycin, polymyxin, or both.

Microbial resistance may develop following prolonged use. Allergic contact dermatitis occurs frequently. Bacitracin is poorly absorbed through the skin so systemic toxicity is rare.

Gramicidin is only available for topical use, in combination with other drugs. The incidence of sensitization following topical use in therapeutic concentration is exceedingly low.

Mupirocin

Most gram-positive aerobic bacteria, including methicillin-resistant *S. aureus* (MRSA) are sensitive to mupirocin. It is effective in impetigo caused by *S. aureus* and group A β-hemolytic streptococci.

Mupirocin is not absorbed after topical application to intact skin.

Polymyxin B sulfate

Polymyxin B is effective against gram-negative organisms including *P. aeruginosa*, *E. coli*, *Enterobacter*, and *Klebsiella*. Most strains of proteus and serratia are resistant, as are all gram-positive organism.

It is generally used in combination with other antibiotic and hypersensitivity to topically applied polymyxin B sulfate is uncommon.

Neomycin and gentamycin

These are aminoglycoside antibiotics active against gram-negative organisms, including *E. coli*, proteus, klebsiella, and enterobacter. Gentamycin is more effective than neomycin against *P. aeruginosa* and also against staphylococci and group A β-hemolytic streptococci.

Neomycin is available in numerous topical formulations, both alone and in combination with polymyxin, bacitracin, and other antibiotics. Neomycin frequently causes sensitization, particularly if applied to eczematous dermatoses. Gentamycin is available as an ointment or cream and absorption is possible if the drug is applied to large areas of denuded skin, as in burn patients.

Tropical antibiotics in acne

Patients with minor degrees of acne vulgaris require antibiotic therapy, either systemic or local. Topical antibiotics (clindamycin or erythromycin) are used more widely than previously and should be considered prior to systemic antibiotics or in relatively minor disease, and in combination with other topical agents.

Clindamycin

Clindamycin is active against acnes which accounts for its beneficial effect in acne therapy. About 10% of an applied dose is absorbed, and rare cases of bloody diarrhea and pseudomembranous colitis have been reported following topical application. The water-based gel and lotion preparations are well tolerated and less likely to cause irritation.

Clindamycin is also available in combination topical gels with benzoyl peroxide, and with tretinoin.

Erythromycin

Topical erythromycin water-based gel alone or in combination with benzoyl peroxide may be used in inflammatory acne vulgaris.

The possible complication of topical therapy is the development of antibiotic-resistant strains of organism, including staphylococci. Allergic hypersensitivity is uncommon.

Metronidazole

Topical metronidazole is effective in the treatment of rosacea. Oral metronidazole has been shown to be a carcinogen and its topical use is not recommended during pregnancy and by nursing mothers and children.

Silver sulphadiazine

Silver sulphadiazine is used in the treatment of burn infections. It is contraindicated in pregnancy and breast feeding, hypersensitivity to sulphonamides and in neonates.

ANTIVIRAL AGENTS

Acyclovir or **penciclovir** cream is the treatment of choice for herpes simplex infection of the skin, treatment should begin as early as possible. Contact with the eyes and mucous membranes should be avoided.

Fungal infections

Dermatophytes are fungi capable of causing superficial infections known as ringworm or dermatophylosis. Topical and systemic antifungal therapy is used for the treatment of ringworm infection.

Topical therapy

Azoles and allylamines are effective, but nystatin is not effective against ringworm infection. Topical therapy is generally effective for uncomplicated tinea corporis (involvement of which body), tinea cruris (groin involvement) and limited tinea pedis (involvement of feet). It is not effective as monotherapy for tinea capitis (scalp involvement) or onychomycosis (nail involvement).

Allylamines (ciclopirox, butenafine and terbinafine) are more effective and have faster and higher cure rates than azoles (clotrimazole, miconazole, econazole, ketoconazole and sulconazole).

Topicals are applied as 1 to 2% lotion or cream twice daily and treatment in continued 1 week beyond clinical resolution of the infection.

Oral therapy

Oral antifungals are required for the infections involving the hair and nails and for other infections unresponsive to topical therapy.

All oral drugs may cause hepatotoxicity and should not be used in women who are pregnant or breastfeeding.

Criseofulvin is the drug of choice for dermatophyte infections involving the skin and hair. It is given daily in doses of 500 mg with a fatty meal for 2 weeks for tinea corporis and 8–12 weeks for tinea capitis.

Griseofulvin, due to high relapse rates, is seldom used for nail infections. Common side effects include gastrointestinal distress headache, and urticaria.

Itraconazole and terbinafine are used for nail infections. Itraconazole (200 mg/day) is given with food for 2 weeks. Itraconazole has the potential for serious interactions with other drugs requiring the P450 enzyme system for metabolism. Terbinafine (250 mg/daily) for 6 to 12 weeks is given for nail infections and has fewer drug-drug interactions.

ANTIPARASITIC AGENTS

Scabies

Permethrin or **malathion** are the drugs of choice. Two applications overnight 1week apart of an aqueous solution of either permethrin (1% cream) or malathion (0.5% lotion) to the whole body excluding the head, are usually successful. Adverse reactions include transient burning, stinging, and pruritis.

It there is poor compliance, immunocompromise or heavy infestations, systemic treatment with **ivermectin** (200 mg/kg) as a single dose on empty stomach may be necessary. A second dose 7–10 days later gives better results.

Gamma benzene hexachloride (lindane) is no longer preferred because of its toxicity, particularly neurotoxicity and hematotoxicity.

Sulfur is an effective scabicide which is nonirritating, but has unpleasant odor, cause staining and thus disagreeable to use.

It has been replaced by more aesthetic and effective scabicides, but still remains an alternative drug for use in infants and pregnant women. The usual formulation is 5% precipitated sulfur in petrolatum.

Pediculosis (lice)

Head lice

Malathion, permethrin and **carbaryl** in a lotion or aqueous formulation, applied on two separate occasions at 7–10 days interval, constitute the standard treatment. A contact time or overnight treatment is required to kill lice emerging form surviving eggs.

Body lice

These live on clothing, particularly in seem, and feed on the skin. Itch is the principal symptoms. The skin is excoriated and secondary infection is common.

The management of body lice lies in the insecticide treatment of clothes and management of skin disorders by antihistamine and antibacterial agents.

Pubic lice

The treatment of choice is aqueous-based malathion or carbaryl applied on two occasion to the whole body, as body hair also liable to be infested.

TOPICAL CIRCULATORY PREPARATIONS

Heparinoid cream (**Hirudoid**) or ointment (**Lasonil**) are used to improve local circulation in conditions such as bruising, superficial thrombophlebitis, chilbains and varicose veins. Their therapeutic value is questionable.

TOPICAL DISINFECTANTS

There are a large number of agents used to destroy the vegetative bacteria on skin and mucous membranes. They are used during surgical procedures for skin and hand disinfection, mouth wash, bladder irrigation, wound cleansing and many other conditions which require antisepsis. These are:

Iodine is an effective disinfectant and is largely used for skin disinfection. It rarely causes skin sensitization. Its regular use is contraindicated in patients with thyroid disorders or under lithium therapy. The only preparation of iodine used is providone-iodine in alcoholic or aqueous solution, as it is non-staining and less irritant. It is used as a 10% solution for pre and postoperative skin disinfection and as a 7.5% solution for surgical scrub and scalp and skin cleanser.

Chlorhexidine is a useful skin disinfectant. It may cause occasional sensitivity. It is used in varying dilutions ranging from 0.02 to 4% solution for disinfection of skin, surgical scrub, cleansing and disinfecting wounds and burns, mouth wash, bladder irrigation and as an obstetric antiseptic and lubricant cream.

Hexachlorophene is used as 3% cream for preoperative scrub of hands. It should not be used on badly burned or excoriated skin, in pregnancy and children under 2 years.

Cationic surface acting disinfectants emulsify fats and posses bactericidal action. **Cetrimide** is the most widely used skin disinfectant. Combined with chlorhexidine (**Savlon**), it is one of the most popular hospital disinfectants for surgical procedures, instruments and utensils. It may cause skin irritation and sensitization.

Oxidizing agents. **Hydrogen peroxide** and **potassium permanganate** liberate oxygen which oxidizes bacterial protoplasm. They are mainly used for cleansing and deodorizing wounds and ulcers.

There are a large number of other disinfectants like alcohol, saline, chlorinated solutions, weak acids, metallic salts and dyes which are of limited value.

ACNE

Acne vulgaris occurs in at least 90% of adolescents. Acne depends on the action of androgens on sebaceous glands. Excess production of sebum, its retention and hyperkeratosis may result in the formation of comedones. The choice of treatment depends on whether the acne is predominantly inflammatory or comedonal and its severity. Mild to moderate acne is treated by topical preparations. Oral therapy is required for moderate to severe acne, or when topical preparations are not tolerated or ineffective.

Topical preparations

Benzoyl peroxide is effective in both inflammatory lesions and comedones. It possesses antimicrobial and anticomedonal properties. Adverse effects include local skin irritation which tends to subside with continued treatment.

Retinoids: These are synthetic vitamin A derivatives and include **tretinoin** and **adapalene**. Retinoids have a dramatic effect on the production of sebum, reducing the size of sebaceous glands by 90% in the first month of treatment. Inhibition of sebaceous gland activity is the main reason for their efficacy in acne. Retinoids also cause desquamation of the skin which accounts for their use in hyperkeratotic hyperproliferative skin disorders such as psoriasis. Adapalene and tretinoin are applied locally in mild to moderate acne. Tazarotane gel is another topical retinoid preparation used for the treatment of psoriasis and acne and may be used in patients intolerant of the other retinoids.

Topical retinoids give rise to local reactions including erythema with resultant sore, pain or marked dermatitis or desquamation.

Azelaic acid is as effective as benzoyl peroxide and retinoids without causing their irritant side effects.

Antibiotics: Topical antibiotics are generally less effective than their oral counterparts and do not appear to be more effective than topical azelaic acid or retinoids. **Erythromycin** and **clindamycin** lotion or gel may produce mild irritation, rarely sensitization and antibiotic resistance and are not the drugs of choice for local application. Topical corticosteroids should not be used.

Topical **metronidazole** is effective in the treatment of rosacca. Oral metronidazole has been shown to be a carcinogen and its topical use is not recommended during pregnancy and by nursing mothers and children.

Oral preparations

Antibiotics: Patients with moderate to severe acne with a prominent inflammatory component, in addition to topical therapy, shall require oral antibidics such as doxycycline 100 mg twice daily. The antibiotic has anti-inflammatory effect independent of its antibacterial effect.

Hormonal treatment is no more effective than oral antibiotics. Hormonal manipulation is often successful in women who fail to respond to antibiotics and require oral contraceptives. **Cyproterone acetate**, an antiandrogen combined with **ethinylestradiol** is indicated in women refractory to oral antibiotics.

Patients with severe nodulocystic acne unresponsive to antibiotic and hormonal therapies may benefit with retinoid isotretinoin. The dose is based on the patient's weight and it is given once daily for 5 months. Isotretinoin is highly effective, but may cause serious adverse effects such as severe depression. Isotretinoin is teratogenic and is contraindicated is pregnancy.

Acne rosacea is not comedonal. The pustules and papules respond effectively to topical metronidazole. Oral broad-spectrum antibiotics for prolonged periods are also effective, but their use is associated with usual antibiotic disadvantages.

PSORIASIS

Psoriasis is one of the most common dermatologic disease, affecting up to 2% of the world's population. It is a non-infectious, chronic inflammatory disease of the skin, characterized by well-defined erythematous plaques with silvery scale, with a predilection for the extensor surfaces and scalp, and a chronic fluctuating course.

Certain drugs, such as beta-blockers, antimalarials, statins and lithium may flare or worsen psoriasis. In the vast majority of cases, psoriasis is not life-threatening and therefore if the treatment is worse than the disease, it should be stopped.

Treatment can be classified into following four categories:

Topical agents

Emollients, corticosteroids, vitamin D agonists, 'weak' tar or dithranol preparations.

UV therapies

UNB or PUVA

Systemic agents

- Methotrexate, retinoids
- Immunosuppressives, e.g. ciclosporin, mycophenolate
- Newer 'biological' agents, e.g. infiximab, etanercept

Intensive inpatient or day-patient care

Topical agents and UVR under medical supervision

Topical agents

A large number of topical agents are used to treat psoriasis. Emollients have a modest effect in reducing scale and diminishing itch, and many patients feel more comfortable using them.

Standard topical treatment for psoriasis includes coal tar and dithranol alone or in combination with salicylic acid.

Coal tar is more potent keratolytic than salicylic acid and has anti-inflammatory and antiscaling properties. It is used as an ointment or paste in combination with an emollient (calamine) or salicylic acid. It should not be used in sore, acute or pustular psoriasis or in presence of infection.

Dithranol is highly effective in psoriasis. The most useful advancement in the topical treatment has been "short contact dithranol treatment". High concentration dithranol (2–4%) is applied to lesion and then washed off between 15 and 30 minutes. Its use is contraindicated in hypersensitivity and in acute and pustular psoriasis.

The main clinical limitation of dithranol is its proinflammatory action on normal skin, which causes 'burning' with pain and erythema that peaks 72 hours after application. Use of dithranol or coal tar has drastically diminished due to low patient acceptability, the increasing use of outpatient phototherapy and therapeutic options available with newer immunomodulatory drugs.

Calcipotriene is a synthetic Vitamin D_3 derivative that is effective in the treatment of plaque-type psoriasis. It seldom clears plaques but reduces plaques thickness and diminishes scaling. It is applied twice or once daily and, providing no more than 100 g of ointment each week. It does not cause hypercalcemia or hypercalciuria. Irritation, usually transient, is the main side effect. It is a mainstay of primary care of management of psoriasis and may be combined with betamethasone.

Corticosteroids may cause local skin atrophy, and when they are stopped the psoriasis tends to return. Nevertheless, they are invaluable for many sites, particularly the flexures, and short bursts of moderately potent corticosteroids can be invaluable. Use of potent topical corticosterioids on the face or hair margins requires close medical supervision.

Systemic corticosteroids should never be used for the treatment of psoriasis due to potential for developing life-threatening pustular psoriasis when theropy is discontinued.

Ultraviolet and PUVA therapy

Ultraviolet radiation (UVR) is the mainstay of outpatient management of those with moderate to severe psoriasis. The main risks are burning in the short term, and increased skin cancers in the long term therapy.

Photochemotherapy (PUVA). It consists of administration of psoralen (usually **methoxsalen**) either by mouth or topically combined with ultraviolet A irradiation (UVA) for the treatment of plaque psoriasis. Adverse effects include short-term hazard of severe burning and long-term hazards of development of skin cancer and cataract formation, unless protected.

Systemic treatment

There are now a large number of systemic agents that can be used for psoriasis. These range from the classical agents, such as methotrexate and hydroxyurea, through standard immunosuppressive such as cyclosporin and mycophenolate to the newer 'biological' therapies.

Methotrexate

Methotrexate is highly effective and is given once weekly. The main hazards are immunosuppression and bone marrow suppression. Long-term use is associated with hepatic fibrosis and cirrhosis. An alternative is hydroxyurea, but this is less effective and carries an increased risk of bone marrow suppression.

Oral retinoids

Acitretin, a third generation retinoid, is a metabolite of etretinate (tigason). It has a marked effect on keratinizing epithelium. Its mode of action is unknown. In psoriatic skin mitosis is reduced and acanthosis is diminished.

Acitretin is effective in generalized pustular psoriasis, and in chronic disabling form of pustular psoriasis, palmoplanter psoriasis, severe chronic plaque psoriasis and erythrodermic psoriasis. Rates of relapses are high on stopping the treatment.

Acitretin is teratogenic and is contraindicated in pregnancy. Hyperlipidemia and hepatotoxicity may occur and acitretin is not used in hepatic and renal impairment.

Cyclosporin

Cyclosporin is an immunosuppressive drug used in proriasis and other inflammatory skin disease. Side-effects include hypertension, nephrotoxicity and immunosuppression, leading to opportunistic infections and an increased risk of skin and other cancers in the long-term. Cyclosporin is highly effective but continuous use is difficult to justify its use. It may be used over a 3–4 month period to induce clearance or prior to treatment with other systemic agents.

Biologic drugs

A range of new agents, including monoclonal antibodies, fusion proteins and cytokine, have been found to have striking activity against psoriasis and are as effective as classical drugs. However, their long term toxicity has still to be established.

The drugs in use include T-cell modulators **alefacept** and the TNF-α inhibitors-**etanercept**, **infliximab** and **adalimumab**, They are all given parenterally.

Etanercept is a human recombinant TNF receptor fusion protein, infliximab a human-murine anti-TNF-α monoclonal antibody and adalimumab a human anti-TNF-α monoclonal antibody. All bind TNF, preventing its actions, and are highly effective in clearing prosiasis. They have to be given either by infusion or by subcutaneous injection, which may cause adverse reactions. Potential side effects include reactivation of latent tuberculosis and the development of other opportunistic infections.

Treatment of psoriasis requires the use of potentially toxic drugs, since psoriasis is not a life threatening disease; treatment should be individualized so that the treatment is not worse than the disease.

MISCELLANEOUS SKIN PREPARATIONS

A large number of drugs are available for application to the skin. Some of the common skin disorders and drugs used are:

- Topical antihistamines and local anesthetics are not very effective in pruritus and may occasionally cause sensitization. Topical corticosteroids are useful in treating insect stings. Calamine lotion is not useful.
- Irritants and counterirritants were used for relief of local muscle and joint pain, but have been largely replaced by topical NSAIDs. The ingredients of counterirritants include volatile oils, menthol, camphor, methylsalicylates, capsicum and canthridin.

IMMUNOMODULATORS

Imiquimod, an immunomodulator, stimulates peripheral mononuclear cells to release interferon and to stimulate macrophages to produce interleukins and tumor necrosis factor-α (TNF-α).

It is applied to wart tissue three times per week and left on the skin for 6–10 hours prior to washing. Actinic keratosis is treated with twice-weekly applications on the contagcous area of involvement.

Imiquimod is applied five-times per week to the tumor for treatment of superficial basal cell carcinoma.

Adverse side effects consist of local inflammatory reactions.

KERATOLYTIC AND DESTRUCTIVE AGENTS

Salicylic acid is an effective keratolytic agent in concentration of 3–6%. It solubilizes cell surface proteins resulting in desquamation of keratotic debris. The total amount of salicylic acid applied and the frequency of application should be limited, particularly in children, to prevent intoxication. Topical use may be associated with local irritation acute inflammation, and even ulceration with the use of high concentration of salicylic acid.

Propylene glycol alone in concentration of 40–70% or in gel with 6% salicylic acid is keratolytic.

Propylene glycol is an effective keratolytic agent for the removal of hyperkeratotic debris. It is also effective humectants and increases the water content of the stratum corneum. It is used with 6% salicylic acid for the treatment of ichthycosis, palmar and plantar keratoderma, psosiasis, pityriasis, keratosis pilaris, and hypertrophic lichen planus.

Urea is a lubricant and also keratolytic. As a kerotolytic agent, it is used in 20% concentrations in diseases such as ichthyosis vulgaris, hyperkeratosis of palms and soles, xerosis, and keratosis pilaris.

Podophyllum resin and Podofilox

Podophyllum resin is cytotoxic and in concentration of 25% in compound tincture of benzonin is used for the treatment of condyloma acuminatum. Application should be confined to wart tissue only, as being lipid soluble is rapidly absorbed and widely distributed throughout the body including central nervous system.

Toxic symptoms associated with excessively large application may result in neurological symptoms, coma, and even death.

Podofilox is pure podophyllotoxin and is used in 0.5% concentration for application by the patient in the treatment of genital condylomas.

Fluorouracil is pyrimidine antimetabolite and is used topically for the treatment of multiple actinic keratoses. It is available in multiple formulations containing 0.5%, 1%, 2% and 5% concentration. Topical application results in inflammatory reaction, ulceration, necrosis, and finally reepithelization.

Other drugs useful in actinic keratoses include topical 3% **diclofenac** (NSAID) and **aminolevulinic acid** 20% solution and blue light photodynamic illumination therapy.

MELANIZING AGENTS

They increase sensitivity to solar radiation and promote repigmentation of vitiliginous areas of skin. Psoralens (methoxsalen) or photo activation (sunlight or UV radiation) stimulates melanocytes and their proliferation.

MINOXIDIL

Minoxidil is a potent vasodilator antihypertensive drug. Topically, it may stimulate limited hair growth in male pattern baldness (men and women) but only as long as it is used. It may cause irritant dermatitis and allergic contact dermatitis.

Eczema

The terms 'eczema' and 'dermatitis' are synonymous.

Regular use of bland *emollients* (e.g. emulsifying ointment) is the mainstay of treatment in all forms of eczema. They prevent excessive loss of water from an already dry skin and help to reduce the amount of local corticosteroids used.

Low to midpotency *topical corticosteroid* lotions or cream in acute eczema and ointments in chronic, are usually applied once or twice daily. The side effects of strong or extensive local corticosteroid therapy are important when used as a long-time measure and include skin atrophy, enhanced or disguised infections and systemic absorption causing suppression of the hypothalamic-pituitary-adrenal axis and cushingoid features.

Two nonsteroidal anti-inflammatory drugs are available: *Tacrolimus* ointment and *pimecrolimus* cream. These drugs are macrolide immunosuppressants that do not cause skin atrophy or corticosteroid advance effects, if absorbed. However, concerns have emerged regarding the potential for lymphos in patients treated with these drugs. These drugs should only be used when other topical treatments are ineffective. Treatment should be limited to affected area and duration to be as brief as possible. They should not be used in patients with known immunosuppression, HIV infection, bone marrow and organ transplantation and those with a prior history of lymphoma.

Secondary infection of eczematous skin is generally with *S. aureus*, which requires treatment with systemic antibiotics.

Control of pruritus is essential and require systemic sedative antihistamines. Systemic corticosteroids should only be limited to severe exacerbations not responding to topical therapy.

21.2 EYE

A large number of topical drugs are available for use in various ophthalmic diagnosis and treatment.

CONJUNCTIVITIS

Conjunctivitis is the most common eye disease. Most cases are due to viral or bacterial infections. Other causes include keratoconjunctivitis, allergic and chemical irritant.

Viral conjunctivitis

Adenovirus is the most common cause of viral conjunctivitis. It may also be due to herpes simplex virus (HSV).

Herpes simplex virus keratitis responds to topical anti-viral eye drops. There is no specific treatment for adenoviral infection.

Topical ocular antiviral drugs include acyclovir ointment, ganciclovir gel and trifluridine solution.

Bacterial conjunctivitis

The most commonly organisms involved include staphylococci, streptococci (especially *S. pneumonia*), *Hemophilus* species, pseudomonas and moraxella.

Mild cases of bacterial conjunctivitis usually are treated empiricaly with broad-spectrum topical antibiotics such as sulfacetamide 10%, molifloxacin 0.5%, polymyxin-bacitracin, or trimethoprim-polymyxin combination. Smears and cultures usually are reserved for severe, resistant or recurrent cases of conjunctivitis.

Other topical ocular antibiotics include cetazolin, chloramphenicol, erythromycin, ciprofloxacin, levofloxacin, olfloxacin, gatifloxacin, fusidic acid, gentamycin, neomycin and tobramycin.

Gonococcal conjunctivitis

Gonococcal conjunctivitis is an ophthalmic emergency because corneal involvement may rapidly lead to perforation.

A single 1 g dose of intramuscular ceftriaxone is usually adequate (fluoroquinolone resistance is common). Topical antibodies such as **erythromycin** and **bacitracin** may help in clearing the infections.

Chlamydial keratoconjunctivitis

Trachoma is the most common infectious cause of blindness. Single-dose therapy with oral **azithromycin**, 20 mg/kg, is the preferred treatment. Local treatment is not necessary.

Inclusion conjunctivitis

The agent of inclusion conjunctivitis is a common cause of genital tract disease in adults. Treatment is with a single dose of **azithromycin** given orally.

DRY EYES

This is a common disorder, particularly in older women. Hypofunction of the lacrimal glands, causing loss of the aqueous component of tears, may be due to aging, hereditary disorders, systemic disease (e.g. Sjögren syndrome) or systemic drugs. Other causes include abnormalities of the lipid component of the tear film as in blepharitis, mucin deficiency due to vitamin A deficiency.

Aqueous deficiency can be treated with various types of artificial tears. The simplest preparations are physiologic (0.9%)

or hypo-osmotic (0.45%) solutions of **sodium chloride** instilled frequently.

More prolonged duration of action can be achieved with drops containing **methylcellulose, polyvinyl alcohol** or **polyacrylic** acid (carbomers) or by using petroleum ointment or a **hydroxypropyl cellulose** insert.

Artificial tear preparations are generally very safe and without side effects.

Preservatives to maintain sterility are potentially toxic and allergenic and may cause keratitis and conjunctivitis.

Allergic eye diseases

Allergic eye diseases are common and include allergic conjunctivitis, viral keratoconjunctivitis and atopic conjunctivitis.

Symptoms caused by allergic conjunctivitis can be alleviated with topical antihistamones, mast cell stabilizers and immunomodulator.

Topical glucocorticoids provide dramatic relief of immune-mediated forms of conjunctivitis, but their long-term use is ill advised because of the complications of glaucoma, cataract and secondary infection. Tropical nonsteroidal anti-inflammatory drugs (NSAIDs) are better and safer alternatives.

The available topical ocular anti-allergic preparations are:

- *Antihistamines:* Azelastine HCl, bepotastine besilate, emedastine diflumarate, epinastine HCl and levocabastine HCl.
- *Mast cell stabilizers:* Cromolyn sodium, ketotifen fumarate, lodoxamide tromethamine, nedocromil sodium and olopatadine HCl.
- *Immunomodulators:* Cyclosporin and tacrolimus
- *Glucocorticoids:* Dexamethasone sodium phosphate, fluorometholone, loteprednol etabopate, prednisolone acetate and rimexolone
- *NSAIDs:* Bromfenac, diclofenac sodium, flubiprofen sodium, ketorolac tromethamine and nepafenac.

Systemic corticosteroid or other immunosuppressant therapy and even plasmapheresis may be required in severe atopic keratoconjunctivitis.

CORNEAL ULCER

Corneal ulcer is most commonly due to infection by bacteria, virus, fungi, or amebas.

Bacterial keratitis

It is generally due to prolonged use of contact lens wear or corneal trauma.

The pathogens most commonly isolated are *P. aeruginosa*, pneumococcus, moraxella species, and staphylococci. Fluoroquinolones eye drops are commonly used as first-line agents. The fourth generation fluoroquinolines moxifloxacin and gatifloxacin are also active against myocobacteria but may not be preferable.

Gram-positive cocci can be treated with a cephalosporin and gram-negative bacilli with an aminoglycoside.

Herpes simplex keratitis

Herpes simplex keratitis is an important cause of ocular morbidity. Treatment consists of topical antivirals with long-term oral antivirals.

Topical corticosteroids may be required in combination with antiviral therapy to control stromal disease.

Herpes zoster ophthalmicus

High doses oral antiviral therapy is required. Anterior uveitis requires treatment with topical corticosteroids and cycloplegics.

Fungal keratitis

Natamycin, amphotericin B and voriconazole are the most commonly used topical agents.

Acanthamoeba keratitis

Acanthamoeba infection is an important cause of keratitis in contact lens wearers. Topical biguanides are probably the only effective primary treatment. Topical corticosteroids may be beneficial.

Acute angle closure glaucoma

Primary acute angle-closure glaucoma occurs only with closure of a pre-existing narrow anterior chamber angle, for which the predisposing factors are age, owing to enlargement of crystalline lens, farsightedness and inheritance. It is precipitated by factors which cause papillary dilation such as darkened condition, stress, drugs.

Secondary acute-angle closure glaucoma may occur in anterior uveitis, dislocation of lens or topiramate therapy.

Initial treatment of primary angle-closure glaucoma is reduction of intraocular pressure by intravenous 500 mg **acetazolamide** followed by 250 mg orally four times a day. Osmotic diuretics such as oral **glycerin** and intravenous urea or mannitol may be necessary, if there is no response to acetazolemide. Once the intraocular pressure has started to fall, topical **pilocarpine** is used to reverse the underlying dosure.

In secondary acute angle-closure glaucoma, systemic acctazolamide is used, with or without osmotic agents.

Chronic glaucoma

Chromic glaucoma is characterized by gradually progressive excavation ("cupping") and pallor of the optic disk with loss of vision to complete blindness.

In chronic open-angle glaucoma, the intraocular pressure is increased due to reduced drainage of aqueous fluid through the trabecular meshwork. (In chronic angle-closure glaucoma, flow of aqueous fluid into the anterior chamber angle is obstructed.)

Five general groups of drugs – pararympathomimetics, α agonists, β blockers and prostaglandin F_{2a} analogs have been found useful in reducing intraocular pressure.

Topical prostaglandin analogs (page 189) once daily at night are commonly used as first-line therapy because of their efficacy, lack of systemic side-effects as well as the convenience of once-daily dosing. Prostaglandin analogs may produce conjunctival hyperemia, permanent darkening of the iris and eye-brow color, and increased eyelash growth. **Latanoprost** has been associated with reactivation of uveitis and macular edema

Topical β adrenergic blocking drops may be used in combination with a prostaglandin analog. They are contraindicated in patients with reactive airway disease or heart failure.

Topical selective α_1 agonist and topical carbonic anhydrase inhibitors (*see* page 208) can be used as initial therapy, when prostaglandin analog and β blockers are contraindicated.

α_1 agonists are associated with allergic reactions.

Combination drops of prostaglandins and β blockers once daily and α_1 agonists and β blockers twice daily improve compliance.

Apraclonidine (alpha$_2$ agonist) is commonly used to control acute rises in intraocular pressure such as after laser therapy.

Pilocarpine, adrenalin and the prodrug dipivefrin are rarely used because of adverse effects.

Oral carbonic anhydrase inhibitor may be used on long-term basis if topical therapy is inadequate and surgical or laser therapy is inappropriate.

UVEITIS

Anterior uveitis responds to topical corticosteroids. Occasionally, periocular corticosteroid injections or even systemic corticosteroid may be required.

Posterior uveitis more commonly requires systemic or intravitreal corticosteroid therapy and occasionally systemic immunosuppression with drugs such as **azathioprine**, **tacrolimus**, **cyclosporine**, or **mycophenolate**. The role of biologic therapies is under investigation.

Age-related macular degeneration

Antioxidants (vitamin A [beta-carotene], vitamin C and vitamin E), and zinc and copper reduces the risk of disease progression in patients with moderate age-related maculopathy. High dietary consumption of other carotenoids, lutein and zeaxanthine, and omega-$_3$ long-chain polyunsaturated fatty acid, folic acid, vitamin B$_6$ and vitamin B$_{12}$ also helps to check disease progression in women.

Inhibitors of vascular endothelial growth factors (VEGF) reverse the chorodial neovascularization, resulting in stabilization and less frequently improvement in vision in neovascular degeneration. They are administered monthly by intravitreal injection.

Intravitreal injection of VEGF inhibitors is also beneficial in chromic macular edema.

AIDS

CMV retinitis is treated with oral vaganciclovir or intravitreal injection of ganciclovir or sustained-release intravitreal implant of ganciclovir.

Precautions in management of ocular disorders

Use of local anesthetics

Unsupervised self-administration of local anesthetics may lead to injury and may also interfere with normal healing process.

Pupillary dilation

Dilation of pupil may precipitate acute glaucoma in patients with narrow anterior chamber angle closure. If required a short-acting mydriatic such as tropicamide should be used. Acute closure glaucoma is more likely to occur if pilocarpine is used to overcome papillary dilation than if the pupil is allowed to constrict naturally.

Corticosteroid therapy

Repeated use of local corticosteroids presents several hazards: herpes simplex (dendritic) keratitis, fungal infection, open-angle glaucoma, and cataract formation. Futhermore, perforation of the cornea may occur when the corticosteroids are used for herpes simplex keratitis. The potential for causing or exacerbating systemic hypertension, diabetes mellitus, gastritis, osteoporosis, or glaucoma must always be borne in mind when systemic corticosteroids are prescribed such as for uveitis or giant cell arteritis.

Contaminated eye medications

There is always a risk of contamination, particularly with solution of tetracaine, proparacaine, fluorescein, and any preservative-free preparation. The most dangerous is fluorecein, as this solution is frequently contaminated with *P. aeruginosa*, which can rapidly destroy the eye. Sterile fluorescein filter paper strips are recommended for use in place of fluorescein solution.

Eye solution should not remain in use for long periods after opening of the bottle. Four weeks after the opening should be the maximal time to use a solution containing preservatives before discarding. Preservative-free preparations should be kept refrigerated and should be used within one week after opening.

Toxic and hypersensitivity reactions to topical therapy

Patients having inadequate tear secretion may be amenable to toxic or hypersensitivity reactions.

An antibiotic instilled into the eye can sensitize the patient to the drug and cause an allergic reactions upon systemic administration.

Systemic effects of ocular drugs

Opthalmic solution of the non-selective β blockers, e.g. timolol may worsen bradycardia, heart failure or asthma. Phenylephrine eye drops may precipitate hypertensive crisis and angina.

Index

Aacmprosate 179
Abacavir 442
Abatacept 101
Abciximab 245
Acarbose 330
Acebutolol 43, 223
Acetazolamide 111, 209
Acetaminophen 85
Acetohexamide 325
Acetylcholine 50
Acetylcystine 534
Acipimox 250
Acitretin 550
Actinomycin D 502
Acyclovir 279,436,542
Adalimumab 100, 292, 463, 550
Adapalene 546
Adenosine 269
Adrenalin 27
Albendazole 485
Albuterol 304
Alcohol 178
Aldosterone 338
Alefacept 550
Alemtuzumab 463
Alendronate 95, 374
Alesleukin 460
Alfacalcidol 528
Alfentanil 89,166
Alginates 280
Aliskiren 200, 213
Allopurinol 105
Almotriptan 109
Aloes 297
Aloserton 295
Alprazolam 65
Alprostadil 190,360
Alteplase 258,262
Altretamine 510
Aluminium hydroxide 279
Alvimopan 299
Amakinra 100, 103, 463
Amantadine 124, 439
Amebonium 54

Amethocaine 156
Amidulafungin 434
Amikacin 401, 421
Amiloride 207
Aminolerulinic acid 553
Aminophylline 308
Aminosalicylate 289
Amiodarone 210, 267
Amitriptyline 108,143
Amitryptiline 94,110,143
Amlodipine 216,223,256
Amodiaquine 474
Amoxapine 143
Amoxicillin 286, 392
Amphetamine 33,173
Amphotericin 279,429,482, 557
Ampicillin 392
Amprenavir 442
Amylin 330
Anakinra 100, 463
Anastrazole 519
Anidulafungin 435
Anit-D immunoglobin 459
Antabuse 178
Anthracenes 297
Antioxidants 530, 559
Antisera 457
Apixaban 241
Apomorphine 123, 150
Apraclomidine 559
Apriso 289
Ardeparin 238
Arecgikube 53
Argatroban 239
Aripiprazole 129,136
Arsenic trioxide 507
Artemether 472
Artemisinins 471
Artesunate 472
Articaine 154,157
Asacol 289
Ascorbic acid 528
Asenapine 129
Asparaginase 504, 513

Aspart 317
Aspirin 84, 243, 253, 260, 262
Atazanavir 442
Atenolol 43, 223, 261, 267
Atomoxetine 34
Atopaxar 246
Atovaquone 475
Atracurium 156
Atropine 58, 62, 269
Atrovastatin 247
Augmentin 393
Azacytidine 504
Azapropazone 91
Azathioprine 98,291, 559
Azelaic acid 546
Azelastine 556
Azithromycin 407, 477, 555
Azlocillin 393
Aztreonam 398

Bacitracin 413, 540, 555
Baclofen 171
Balsalazide 289
Barbiturates 178
Barrier creams 537
Basiliximab 463
BCG vaccine 456
Beclomethasone 211
Bendamustine 509
Bendrofluazide 201
Bendroflumethiazide 200, 223
Benidipine 216
Benserazide 120
Benzamide 150
Benzathine penicillin 390
Benzbromarone 105
Benzhexol 127
Benzocaine 157
Benzodiazepines 63
Benzoyl peroxide 546
Benzqiunamide 129
Benzthiazide 201

Index

Benztropine Mesylate 127
Benzydamine 278
Benzylpenicillin 388
Bepotastine 556
Beraprost 187
Betahistine 153
Betamethasone 344, 539
Betaxolol 43
Bethanechol 52
Bexarotene 506, 516
Bhang 176
Bicalutamide 520
Bimatoprost 189
Biophosphonates 373
Biperiden 127
Bisacodyl 298
Bismuth subsalicylate 285, 300
Bisoprolol 43, 210, 223
Bivalirudin 239
Bleomycin 511
Bortezomib 516
Botulinum toxin A 109, 173
Bran 296
Brinzolamide 209
Bromfenac 556
Bromhexine 301
Bromocriptine 123, 184, 186, 363
Brompheniramine 302
Budesomide 290, 311
Bumetamide 205
Bupivacaine 156
Buprenorphine 78
Bupropion 143
Buspirone 68,185
Busulfan 509
Buterafine 542
Butyrophenones 129

Cabergoline 364
Caffeine 174,307
Calamine 537
Calchew D3 376
Calciferol 528
Calcipotriene 547
Calcitonin 371
Calcitriol 528

Camptothecin 511
Candesartan 109, 199, 210
Cangrelor 245
Cannabis 176
Capecitabine 504
Capreomycin 421
Capsaicin 92
Capsofungin acetate 431
Captopril 198
Carbachol 52
Carbamazepine 94, 114, 140
Carbapenems 389
Carbaryl 544
Carbergoline 123
Carbidopa 120
Carbimazole 337
Carbocisteine 301
Carboplatin 510
Carboprost 361
Carisoprodol 172
Carmustine 500
Carprofen 91
Carvedilol 43, 210
Caspofungin 432
Castoroil 298
Cefaclor 395
Cefadroxil 394
Cefalexin 394
Cefamandole 395
Cefazolin 394
Cefdinir 396
Cefditoren pivoxil 396
Cefepime 397
Cefmetazole 395
Cefoperazone 396
Cefotaxime 396
Cefotetan 395
Cefoxitin 395
Cefpodoxine proxetil 396
Cefprozil 395
Cefradine 394
Cefriaxone 396
Ceftaroline 397
Ceftazidime 396
Ceftibuten 396
Ceftizoxime 396
Ceftobiprole 397

Ceftriaxone 396
Cefuroxime 395
Cefuroximeaxeril 395
Celecoxib 87
Celiprolol 43
Centchroman 357
Centrimide 545
Cephalosporins 394
Certolizumab 292
Certoparin 238
Cetrizine 182
Cetuximab 521
Charas 176
Charcoal 533
Chloral hydrate 70
Chlorambucil 509
Chloramphenicol 405
Chlordiazeboxide 65
Chlorhexidine 278, 545
Chlorodeoxyadencsine 503
Chloroquine 473, 479
Chlorothiazide 201
Chlorotrianisene 352
Chlorpheniramine 182
Chlorphenamine 258
Chlorphenesin 172
Chlorpromazine 129
Chlorpropamide 325
Chlortetracycline 402
Chlorthalidone 201
Chlorzoxazone 172
Cholecalciferol 370
Cholestyramine 249, 300
Choline salicylate 85
Cholinsalicylate 278
Chromolyn 311
Ciclopirox 542
Cidofovir 438
Cilazopril 198
Cilostazol 245
Cimetidine 281
Ciprofloxacin 290, 386
Cisapride 185, 281, 299
Cisatracarium 168
Cisplatin 510
Citalopram 143
Clarithromycin 286, 407
Clavulanic acid 391, 393

Clevidipine 216, 230
Clindamycin 408, 476, 541, 546
Clobazan 111
Clobetasone 539
Clofazimine 426
Clomiphene 351
Clomipramine 143
Clonazepam 65, 116
Clonidine 31, 41, 227
Clopidogrel 243, 253, 200
Clotrimazole 436
Cloxacillin 391
Clozapine 129, 135
Coaltar 548
Co-artemether 472
Cocaine 150, 175
Co-danthramer 298
Codeine 76, 302
Colchicine 102
Colesevelam 249, 331
Colestipol 249
Colistin 411
Colloidal bismuth subcitrate 285
Colocynth 298
Co-proxamol 76
Corticosteroid 57, 151, 309
Cortisol 338
Cortisone 342
Co-trimaxozole 382
Cromolyn 311, 556
Cyanocobalamin 273, 527
Cyclizine 182
Cyclobenzaprine 172
Cyclopentolate 62
Cyclophosphamide 98, 508
Cycloserine 422, 560
Cyclosporin 292, 550, 559
Cyproheptadine 182, 185
Cyproterone acetate 359, 547
Cytokines 460, 522
Cytomegelovirus immunoglobulin 459
Cytosine arabinoside 504, 513

Dabigatran 241
Dacarbazine 510
Daclizumab 463
Dalbavancin 410
Dalfopristin 411
Dalteparin 238
Danazol 358
Dantrolene 172
Dapsone 425
Daptomycin 412
Darbepoetin alfa 273
Darifenacin 51
Darunavir 442
Dasatinib 515
Daunorubicin 511
Debrisoquine 40
Decitabine 516
Deferasirox 272
Dehydroemetine 478
Delavirdine 442
Demecarium 54
Demeclocycline 402
Denosumab 376
Deoxycoformycin 503
Desfemoxamine 272, 536
Desflurane 164
Desipramine 143
Desloratidine 182
Desogestrel 354
Desvenlafaxine 143
Dexamethasone 94, 343, 556
Dexfenfluramine 185
Dexlausoprazole 283
Dexmedetomidine 31
Dextromethorphan 302
Dextropoxyphene 76
Diamox 209
Diazemuls 118
Diazepam 65, 171
Diclofenac 88, 556
Dicloxacillin 391
Dicobalt edetate 533
Dicyclomine 61, 294
Didanosine 442
Diethylcarbamazine 489

Diethylstilbestrol 352, 518
Diflumisal 88
Digibind 195
Digitoxin 191
Digoxin 191, 211, 269
Dihydroartemisinin 472
Dihydrocodeine 76
Dihydroergotamine 169, 186
Diloxanide fluroate 479
Diltiazem 216, 223, 268
Dimercaprol 535
Dimeticone 537
Dinoprostone 361
Diphenhydramine 182, 302
Diphtheria vaccine 457
Dipyridamole 245
Dirithromycin 407
Disopyramide 264
Distigmine 54
Disulfiram 178
Dithranol 548
D-lysergic acid diethylamide, 176
Dobutamine 32
Docetexel 514
Docosanol 437
Docusate 296
Dolasetron 151
Domperidone 281
Donepezil 55
Dopamine 31
Dorzolamide 209
Dosvenlafaxine 140
Doxacurium 168
Doxapram 174
Doxazosin 89, 226
Doxepin 143
Doxorubicin 511
Doxycycline 402, 476, 490, 546
Doxylamine 182
Dramamine 182
Dronedarone 268
Dulcolax 298
Duloxetine 58, 143
Dutasteride 40
Dyflos 50

Index

Echinocandins 432
Echothiophate 49
Ecstasy 177
Efavirenz 442
Eicosapentaenoic acid 252
Elamercept 100
Eletriptan 107
Emedastine 556
Emetine 478
Emtricitabine 442
Enalapril 198, 223
Endrophonium 54
Enflurane 164
Enfuvirtide 442
Enoxaparin 238
Entacapone 125
Ephedrine 32
Epinastine 556
Eplerenone 206, 211
Epoetin alfa 273
Epoprostenol 189
Epothilones 514
Eptifibatide 245
Ergometrine 186, 363
Ergonovine 187, 362
Ergotamine 108, 186
Ergotoxine 362
Erlotinib 516
Ertapenem 399
Erythromycin 406, 541, 546
Erythropoietin 271
Escitalopram 143
Eserine 53
Esmolol 43, 229, 267
Esomeprazole 283
Estradiol 352
Estriol 352
Estrogens 372
Estrone 352
Etanercept 550
Ethacrynic acid 206
Ethambutol 417
Ether 165
Ethinylestradiol 352, 547
Ethionamide 421
Ethosuximide 115
Etidocame 157

Etodolac 90
Etomidate 161
Etoposide 511
Etoricoxib 87
Etravirine 442
Everolimus 517
Exemestane 519
Exenatide 327
Extramustine 514
Ezetimibe 249

Famciclovir 437
Famotidine 281
Fansidar 476
Febuxostat 106
Felodipine 216
Fenofibrate 250
Fenoldopam 27, 33
Fentanyl 77, 166
Ferrous fumarate 270
Ferrous gluconate 270
Ferrous glycine sulphate 270
Ferrous sulphate 270
Fesoterodine 61
Fexofenadine 182
Fibroblast growth factor 371
Filgrastim 274
Finasteride 359
Fish oil 252
5-Fluorouracil 513, 552
Flecainide 265
Flubiprofen 88, 556
Flucloxacillin 391
Fluconazole 279, 431
Flucytosine 430
Fludarabine phosphate 513
Flumazenil 67
Flunisolide 311
Fluorescein 560
Fluorometholone 556
Fluoroquinolones 385, 420
Fluoxetine 143
Fluphenazine 129
Flurazepam 65, 69
Flutamide 359, 520

Fluticasone 311, 539
Fluvastatin 247
Fluvoxamine 143
Folic acid 273
Folinic acid 274
Follitropin 350
Fondaparinu 239
Fonmoterol 305
Fosamprenavir 442
Fosaprepitant 152
Foscarnet 438
Fosinopril 198
Fosphenytoin 118
Fostetrol 518
Fostomycin 412
Frovatriptan 107
Furosemide 205, 223

Gabapentin 94, 110, 111
Galantamine 55
Gamma benzene hexachloride 541
Gamma hydroxybutyrate 177
Ganciclovir 438
Gantacurium 168
Gatifloxacin 387
G-CSF 522
Gefitinib 516
Gemcitabine 513
Gemfibrozil 250
Gentamycin 401, 540
Gestodene 354
Ginseng 530
Glandosane 277
Glargine 318
Glicalzide 326
Glimepiride 326
Glipizide 325
Glucocorticoid 95, 103, 372, 517
Glyburide 325
Glycine 172
Glycopyrronium 158
Glycylcyclines 404
GM-CSF 522
Gonadorelin 350, 519
Goserelin 350, 520

Gramicidin 540
Granisetron 151
Griseofulvin 435, 543
Guanethidine 40

Halofantrine 471
Haloperidol 129
Halothane 163
Hashish 176
Heparin 236
Hepatitis b vaccine 455
Heroin 76
Hexachlorophene 545
Hexamethonium 40
Hirudoid 544
Histamine 180
Histrelin 350
Homatropine 62
Hydralazine 227, 229
Hydrochlorothiazide 201
Hydrocortisone 278, 342, 539
Hydroflumethiazide 201
Hydrogen peroxide 278, 545
Hydroxocobalamin 273
Hydroxychloroquine 97
Hydroxyprogesterone 354
Hydroxypropyl cellulose 556
Hydroxyurea 503
Hydroxyzine 182
Hyoscine 152
Hyoscyamine 61

Ibandronate 374
Ibuprofen 89
Idarubiucin 511
Idrocilamide 169
IFN-α2a 462, 522
IFN-α2b 462, 522
Ifosfamide 509
Iloprost 189
Imatinib 515
Imidapril 198
Imipenem 399
Imipramine 143
Imiquimod 551

Immunoglobin 458
Incretins 327
Indapamide 201, 223
Indinavir 442
Indomethacin 89
Infelximab 100, 292, 462, 550
Insulin 315
Interferons 450, 462, 522
Iodine 544
Iodoquinol 480
Ipecacuanha 150
Ipratropium 51, 307
Irbesartan 199, 223
Irinotecan 511
Iron dextran 271
Iron sucrose 271
Isocarboxazid 143
Isoflurane 164
Isoniazid 414
Isoprenaline 31
Isoproterenol 31
Isosorbide dinitrate 233
Isosorbide mononitrate 233
Ispaghula 296
Isradipine 216
Itraconazole 279, 431, 543
Ivermectin 490, 543
Ixabepilone 514

Kanamycin 401, 421
Kaolin 300
Ketamine 94, 162
Ketolides 409
Ketoprofen 90
Ketorolac 90, 556

Labetalol 43, 229
Lacidipine 216
Lactulose 298
Lamivudine 442
Lamotrigine 116, 140
Lansoprazole 283
Lasix 205
Lasonil 544
Latanoprost 189
Leflunomide 99
Lepirudin 239

Lercanidipine 216
Letrozole 519
Leucovorin 512
Leukotrience 312
Leuprolide 350, 520
Levetiracetam 117
Levocabastine 556
Levocetrizine 182
Levodopa 119
Levofloxacin 387, 420
Levonorgestrel 354
Levothyroxine 335
Lialda 289
Lidocaine 155, 265
Lindane 543
Linezolid 412, 423
Lingocaine 155, 265
Liothyronine 335
Liquid paraffin 297
Liraglutide 327
Lisinopril 198, 210, 223
Lispro 317
Lisuride 123
Lithium 137
Lodoxamide 556
Lofexidine 178
Lomefloxacin 386
Lomotil 300
Lomustine 509
Loperamide 294
Lopinavir 442
Loracarbef 396
Loratidine 182
Lorazepam 64, 117
Losartan 199, 210
Loteprednol 556
Lovastatin 247
Loxapine 129
Lubiprostone 296, 299
Luborant 277
Lugol's solution 336
Lumefantrine 471
Lysergic acid diethylamide 186

Macrolides 406
Madopar 120
Magnesium carbonate 279

Magnesium choline
   salicylate 85
Magnesium sulphate 118
Magnesium trisilicate 279,
   298
Malarone 475
Malathion 543, 544
Mannitol 210
Maraviroc 442
Marijuana 176
MDMA 177
Mebendazole 486
Mecamylamine 39
Mechlorethamine 500
Meclizine 182
Meclofenamate 91
Mecysteine 301
Medroxyprogesterone
   354, 518
Mefloquine 470
Megestrol 354, 518
Meloxicam 87
Melphalan 509
Menadiol sodium
   phosphate 529
Meperidine 77
Mepivacaine 157
Mepivacame 289
Meptazinol 79
Mercaptopurine 291
Meropenem 399
Meropenem 399
Mesalamine 289
Mescaline 176
Mesna 509
Mestranol 352
Metaproterenol 304
Metformin 328
Methacholine 52
Methadone 77
Methallenestril 352
Methamphetamine 34
Methenamine 383
Methimazole 337
Methionine 534
Methocarbamol 172
Methotrexate 97, 291,
   512, 549

Methoxamine 30
Methoxsalen 549
Methyclothiazide 201
Methylcellulose 296, 556
Methyldopa 31, 41, 226
Methylergometrine 363
Methylnaltrexone 73, 299
Methylphenidate 34, 174
Methylprednisolone 96,
   103, 343
Methysergide 110, 186
Metoclopramide 108, 158,
   281
Metolazone 201, 210
Metopranolol 43
Metoprolol 43, 210, 267
Metronidazole 286, 290,
   383, 478, 541, 546
Mexiletine 265
Micafungin 435
Miconazole 279, 435
Midazolam 64
Midodrine 30
Miglitol 330
Miltefosine 357, 483
Minocycline 402
Minoxidal 227, 553
Mirtazepine 143
Misoprostol 286, 361
Mitoxantrone 511
Mivacurium 156, 166
MMR vaccine 454
Moclobemide 146
Modafinil 34
Moexipril 198
Molindone 129
Mometasone 311, 539
Monte lukast 190, 313
Morphine 72, 259
Moxifloxacin 387, 420
Mupirocin 413, 540
Muromonab 463
Muscarine 52
Mycophenolate mofetil
   98, 559

Nabilone 153
Nabumetone 90
Nadolol 43

Nadroparin 238
Nafarelin 350
Nafcillin 391
Naftifine 435
Nalbuphine 78
Nalidixic acid 385
Naloxone 79
Naltrexone 80, 178
Naphazoline 30
Naproxen 90, 107
Naratriptan 107
Natalizumab 292
Natamycin 557
Nateglinide 326
Nedocromil 311, 556
Nefazodone 143
Nelfinavir 442
Neomycin 295, 402, 540
Neostigmine 53
Nepafenac 556
Nesiritide 227
Netimicin 401
Neuroleptanesthesia 166
Nevirapine 442
Niacin 250, 526
Nicardipine 216, 229
Nicroandil 257
Nidosamide 488
Nifedipine 216, 223
Nikethamide 174
Nilotinib 515
Nisoldipine 216
Nitazoxamide 479
Nitrazepam 65, 69
Nitreridipine 216
Nitrofurantoin 383
Nitrogen mustard 509
Nitroglycerine 229, 233,
   254, 260
Nitroprusside 229
Nitrosoureas 509
Nitrous oxide 163
Nizatidine 281
Noradrenalin 29
Norethisterone 354
Norfloxacin 386
Norgestimate 354
Norgestrel 354

Nortryptyline 143
Nystatin 279, 435
Octreotide 300
Ofloxacin 386
Olanzapine 129, 135
Olmesartan 199
Olopatadine 556
Olsalazine 289
Omalizumab 313
Omega-3 fatty acids 252
Omeprazole 283
Omnopon 77
Ondansetron 151, 186
Opioids 178
Opium 72
Opreleukin 276, 462, 524
Organophosphates 50
Orlistat 333
Ornidazole 479
Orphenadrine 127, 172
Oxacillin 391
Oxaliplantin 510
Oxaprozin 90
Oxazepam 64
Oxcarbamazepine 115
Oxcarbazepine 14
Oxetacain 280
Oxitocin 362
Oxprenolol 47
Oxymetazoline 30
Oxytetracycline 402
Oxytocin 362

Paclitaxal 514
Paintumumab 521
Palifermin 524
Paliperidone 129
Palonosetron 151
Pamidronate 374
Pamoate 488
Pancuronium 169
Pantoprazole 283
Papaveretum 77
Papaverine 360
Para-amino salicylic acid 422
Paracetamol 85

Paraldehyde 70
Parathyroid hormone 367
Paromomycin 480, 483
Parosol 538
Paroxetine 143
PAS 422
Patatrexate 512
Pectin 300
Pegfilgrastim 275
Pegloticase 106
Pemetrexed 512
Penciclovir 437, 542
Penicillamine 535
Penicillin 388
Pentazocine 78
Pentsa 289
Pergolide 123
Perindopril 198
Permethoin 543
Permethrin 544
Perphenazine 129
Pethidine 77
Phenelzine 110, 143
Phenobarbital 111
Phenolphthalin 298
Phenothiazines 132
Phenoxybenzamine 38
Phenoxymethyl penicillin 390
Phentolamine 38
Phenylephrine 30, 561
Phenylpropanolamine 33
Phenytoin 111
Pholocodeine 302
Physostigmine 53
Phytomenadione 529
Pilocarpine 52, 277
Pimecrolimus 553
Pimozide 129
Pindolol 43
Pioglitazone 330
Pipecuronium 168
Piperacillin 393
Piperaquine 474
Piracetam 111
Pirbuterol 304
Pirenzepine 486
Piroxicam 90

Plasmapheresis 56
Podofilox 552
Podophyllum 552
Poliomyclitis vaccine 454
Polyacrylic acid 556
Polyethylene glycol 298
Polymyxin 411, 540
Polysaccharide iron complex 270
Polythiazide 201
Polyvinyl alcohol 556
Posaconazole 432
Povidone-iodine 278
Pralidoxime 56
Pramipexole 124
Pramlintide 330
Pranlukast 190
Prasugrel 243
Pravastatin 247
Praziquantel 486
Prazosin 38, 226
Prednisolone 343, 539
Prednisone 95, 291, 342, 427, 556
Pregabalin 111
Preglylated interferon 452
Premetrexed 512
Premetrexed 512
Prilocaine 156
Primidone 111
Probenecid 104
Probiotics 295
Procaine 157
Procaine benzylpenicillin 390
Procarbazine 509
Prochlorperazine 109, 134
Procyclidine 127
Progabide 169
Progesterone 354
Proguanil 475
Promethazine 70, 134, 153, 182
Propafenone 266
Propofol 109, 161
Propranolol 43, 110, 266
Propylene glycol 552
Propylthiouracil 337

Prosligmine 53
Protamine sulphate 239
Prucalopride 299
Pseudoephedrine 313
Psilocybin 176
Psoralen 549
Psyllium 293, 296
Pyrazinamide 416
Pyridostigmine 54
Pyridoxine 525, 527
Pyrilamine 182
Pyrimethamine 476

Quetiapine 129, 136
Quinagolide 364
Quinestrol 352
Quinethazone 201
Quinidine 264, 467
Quinine 467
Quinolones 385
Quinupristin 411
Qunapril 198

Rabeprazole 283
Rabies Immunoglobulin 459
Rabies vaccine 455
Radioactive iodine 336
Raloxifene 357, 375
Raltegravir 442
Ramipril 198, 223
Ranitidine 281
Ranolazine 256
Rasagiline 125
Remifentanil 77, 166
Repaglinide 326
Reserpine 40
Reteplase 258
Retinoids 548
Retinol 525
Reviparin 238
Rhubarb 297
Riboflavin 526
Rifabutin 417
Rifampin 415, 427
Rifapentine 418
Riluzole 140
Rimexolone 556

Rimonabant 333
Risedronate 374
Risperidone 129, 136
Ritalin 34, 174
Ritodrine 32, 364
Ritonavir 442
Rituximab 101, 521
Rivaroxaban 239
Rivastigmine 55
Rizatriptan 107
Rocuronium 160, 168
Rofecoxib 87
Romidepsin 516
Romiplostin 276
Ropinirole 124
Ropivacaine 156
Rosiglitazone 330
Rosuvastatin 247
Rotigotine 121
Rubella vaccine 455

Sabin vaccine 454
Saheli 357
Salbutamol 304
Salbutamol 364
Salicylic acid 552
Salicylsalicylate 85
Salk vaccine 454
Salmeterol 305
Saquinavir 442
Sargamostim 274
Savlon 545
Saxagliptin 328
Saxagliptin 328
Scopolamine 59
Selegiline 125, 143
Selegiline 143
Senna 297
Sertindole 127
Sertraline 143
Sevoflurane 164
Sibutramine 34, 333
Sildenafil 360
Silver sulfadiazine 381, 542
Simethicone 280
Simvastatin 249, 253
Sinemet 120
Sitagliptin 328

Sodium bicarbonate 280
Sodium calcium edentate 536
Sodium choloride 556
Sodium ferric gluconate 271
Sodium fusidate 409
Sodium iron edentate 270
Sodium nitrate 533
Sodium nitroprusside 131
Sodium perborate 278
Sodium salicylate 85
Sodium stibogluconate 482
Sodium thiosulphate 533
Sodium valproate 112
Solifenacin 61
Sorafenib 517
Sorbitrate 234
Sotalol 43, 267
Sparfloxacin 387
Spectinomycin 401
Spironolactone 206, 211
Stalevo 124
Stavudine 442
Sterculia 296
Streptokinase 257
Streptomycin 402, 418
Strontium ranelate 374
Succinylcholine 168
Sucralfate 285
Sugammadex 167
Sulbactum 391
Sulfacetamide 381, 556
Sulfadiazine 382
Sulfadoxine 382
Sulfamethoxazole 382
Sulfametopyrazine 381
Sulfasalazine 97, 289, 381
Sulfinpyrazone 104
Sulfisoxazole 381
Sulfonamides 380
Sulfonylureas 323
Sulindac 91
Sulphur 543
Sulpride 129
Sumatriptan 107
Sunitinib 517
Syntocinon 362

570 Pharmacology for Undergraduates

Tacrine 146
Tacrolimus 293, 553, 556, 559
Tamoxifen 357, 518
Tamsulosin 39
Tazobactum 391
Teclopidine 243
Tegaserod 185, 295, 299
Teicoplanin 411
Telavancin 410
Telithromycin 409
Telmisartan 199
Temazepam 64, 158
Temozolomide 510
Temsirolimus 517
Tenecteplse 258, 261
Tenoxicam 91
Terazosin 39, 226
Terbinafine 435, 542
Terbutaline 304, 364
Testosterone 358
Tetanus immunoglobulin 467
Tetanus toxoid 457
Tetracaine 152
Tetracycline 278, 286, 402
Thalidomide 427
Thebain 71
Theobromine 307
Theophylline 307
Thiabendazole 488
Thiamine 525
Thioguanine 503
Thiopental sodium 161
Thioridazine 129
Thiotepa 510
Thiothixene 129
Thrombopoietin 523
Thymol 277
Thyroxine 335
Tiagabine 117
Tibolone 353
Ticagrelor 245
Ticarcillin 393
Ticlopidine 243
Tigecycline 404
Timolol 43, 109, 561

Tinidazole 479
Tinzaparin 238
Tirofiban 245
Tizanidine 31, 171
Tobramycin 401
Tocainide 153
Tocopherol 529
Tolazamide 325
Tolbutamide 325
Tolcapone 125
Tolerogens 464
Tolterodine 61
Topiramate 110, 116
Topotecan 511
Torcilizumab 101
Toremifen 519
Torsemide 206
Tramadol 79
Trandolapril 198
Tranylcypromine 143
Trastuzumab 521
Travaprost 189
Trazodone 143
Treprostinil 189
Tretinoin 515, 546
Triachlormethiazide 201
Triamcinolone 103, 278, 311, 343, 539
Triamterene 207
Triazolam 64
Tribavirin 439
Trifluoperazine 124
Trifluridine 438
Trihexyphenidyl 127
Trimethaphan 40, 230
Trimethobenzamide 150
Trimethoprim 382
Triodothyronine 335
Triptorelin 350
Tropicamide 62
Tubocurarine 168
Tumor necrosis factor 462

Uniphyllin 308
Unofollitropin 350
Unoprostone 189
Urea 552

Vaccines 453
Vaglibose 330
Valaciclovir 437
Valethamate 61
Valganciclovir 438
Valproic acid 110, 139
Valsartan 199, 210, 223
Vancomycin 410
Varicella zoster immunoglobulin 459
Vecuronium 168
Velafaxine 68
Venlafaxine 143
Verapamil 216, 223, 268
Viagra 360
Vigabatrin 117
Vildagliptin 328
Vinblastine 514
Vincristine 514
Vinonelbine 505
Vitamin A 525
Vitamin B complex 528
Vitamin D 370
Vorapaxar 246
Voriconazole 431, 557
Vorinostat 516

Warfarin 240, 253
Whooping cough vaccine 456

Xenon 165
Xipamide 204
Xylocaine 155

Zafirlucast 190
Zalcitabine 442
Zaleplon 69
Zanamivir 439
Zidovudine 442
Zileuton 312
Ziprasidone 129, 136
Zoledronic acid 374
Zolmitriptan 107
Zolpidem 69
Zopiclone 70
Zosyn 393